Practical Guide to

INTERVENTIONAL PULMONOLOGY

Practical Guide to
INTERVENTIONAL PULMONOLOGY

Momen M. Wahidi, MD, MBA
Professor of Medicine
Division of Pulmonary and Critical Care Medicine
Duke University School of Medicine;
Director, Interventional Pulmonology and Bronchoscopy
Duke University Medical Center
Durham, North Carolina

David E. Ost, MD
Professor of Pulmonary Medicine
MD Anderson Cancer Center
Houston, Texas

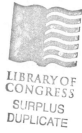

ELSEVIER

Elsevier
1600 John F. Kennedy Blvd.
Ste 1800
Philadelphia, PA 19103-2899

PRACTICAL GUIDE TO INTERVENTIONAL PULMONOLOGY   ISBN: 978-0-323-70954-5

Content Strategist: Robin Carter
Content Development Specialist: Shilpa
Publishing Services Manager: Shereen Jameel
Project Manager: Beula Christopher
Design Direction: Patrick C. Ferguson
Cover Artist: Eric Hirsh

Printed in India

Last digit is the print number: 9   8   7   6   5   4   3   2   1

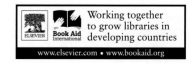

CONTRIBUTORS

Matthew Aboudara, MD
Interventional Pulmonology
Division of Pulmonary and Critical Care Medicine
St. Luke's Health System;
Assistant Professor of Medicine
University of Missouri at Kansas City
Kansas City, Missouri

Megan Acho, MD
Assistant Professor
Division of Pulmonary Allergy and Critical Care
    Medicine
University of Pittsburgh School of Medicine
Pittsburgh, Pennsylvania

Jason Akulian, MD, MPH, MBA
Assistant Professor of Medicine
Division of Pulmonary and Critical Care Medicine
Department of Medicine
University of North Carolina at Chapel Hill
Chapel Hill, North Carolina

A. Christine Argento, MD
Associate Professor
Johns Hopkins University
Baltimore, Maryland

Waqas Aslam, MD
Interventional Pulmonology
Department of Interventional Pulmonology
Lahey Hospital and Medical Center
Burlington, Massachusetts

Jason Beattie, MD
Assistant Attending Physician
Interventional Pulmonology
Memorial Sloan Kettering Cancer Center
New York, New York

Allen Cole Burks, MD
Assistant Professor of Medicine
Division of Pulmonary and Critical Care Medicine
Department of Medicine
University of North Carolina at Chapel Hill
Chapel Hill, North Carolina

Alexander Chen, MD
Associate Professor of Medicine
Division of Pulmonary and Critical Care,
Division of Cardiothoracic Surgery
Washington University School of Medicine
St. Louis, Missouri

George Z. Cheng, MD, PhD
Associate Professor of Medicine
Department of Pulmonary, Critical Care, and Sleep
University of California–San Diego
La Jolla, California

Kevin Ross Davidson, MD
Attending Physician
Department of Pulmonary and Critical Care
WakeMed Health Hospitals
Raleigh, North Carolina

Neeraj R. Desai, MD, MBA, FCCP
Interventional Pulmonology
Chicago Chest Center of Suburban Lung Associates/
    AMITA Health
Elk Grove Village, Illinois;
Clinical Associate Professor of Medicine
Division of Pulmonary, Critical Care, Sleep
    and Allergy
University of Illinois at Chicago
Chicago, Illinois

Michael Dorry, MD
Instructor in Medicine
Interventional Pulmonology
Division of Pulmonary, Allergy and
    Critical Care Medicine
Duke University School of Medicine
Durham, North Carolina

Crystal Ann Duran, MD
Physician
The Oregon Clinic
Portland, Oregon

Kim D. French, MHSA, CAPPM, FCCP
Executive Director
Chicago Chest Center of Suburban Lung Associates/
    AMITA Health
Elk Grove Village, Illinois

Coral X. Giovacchini, MD
Assistant Professor
Division of Pulmonary, Allergy and Critical Care
Department of Medicine
Duke University Medical Center
Durham, North Carolina

Alexander Gregor, MD
Division of Thoracic Surgery
Toronto General Hospital;
University Health Network
Toronto, Ontario, Canada

Kevin Haas, MD
Assistant Professor of Medicine
Division of Pulmonary and Critical Care
University of Illinois at Chicago
Chicago , Illinois

Terunaga Inage, MD, PhD
Division of Thoracic Surgery
Toronto General Hospital;
University Health Network
Toronto, Ontario, Canada

Tsukasa Ishiwata, MD, PhD
Division of Thoracic Surgery
Toronto General Hospital;
University Health Network
Toronto, Ontario, Canada

Shaheen Islam, MD, MPH
Professor and Chief
Division of Pulmonary, Critical Care and Sleep
    Medicine
Medical College of Georgia, Augusta University
Augusta, Georgia

Edward Kessler, MD
Interventional Pulmonology
Chicago Chest Center of Suburban Lung Associates/
    AMITA Health
Elk Grove Village, Illinois;
Division of Pulmonary, Critical Care, Sleep and Allergy
University of Illinois at Chicago
Chicago, Illinois

Kevin L. Kovitz, MD, MBA, FCCP, FACP, ASTF
Professor of Medicine and Surgery
Division of Pulmonary, Critical Care, Sleep and Allergy
University of Illinois at Chicago College of Medicine
Chicago, Illinois;
Founder, Chicago Chest Center of Suburban Lung
    Associates/AMITA Health
Elk Grove Village, Illinois

Carla R. Lamb, MD, FACP, FCCP
Director of Interventional Pulmonology
Pulmonary and Critical Care
Lahey Hospital and Medical Center
Burlington, Massachusetts

Donald R. Lazarus, MD
Assistant Professor of Medicine
Baylor College of Medicine;
Director of Interventional Pulmonology
Michael E. DeBakey VA Medical Center
Houston, Texas

Pyng Lee, MD, PhD, FRCP (UK), FCCP
Associate Professor
Yong Loo Lin School of Medicine, National University
    of Singapore;
Division of Respiratory and Critical Care Medicine
Department of Medicine
National University Hospital
Singapore

Kamran Mahmood, MD, MPH
Assistant Professor of Medicine
Division of Pulmonary, Allergy and Critical Care
Department of Medicine
Duke University Medical Center
Durham, North Carolina

Adnan Majid, MD
Chief, Section of Interventional Pulmonology
Beth Israel Deaconess Medical Center
Boston, Massachusetts

Fabien Maldonado, MD
Professor of Medicine, Thoracic Surgery and
    Mechanical Engineering
Division of Allergy, Pulmonary and Critical Care
    Medicine
Vanderbilt University Medical Center
Nashville, Tennessee

Russell Jason Miller, MD
Interventional Pulmonologist
Naval Medical Center San Diego;
University of California San Diego
San Diego, California

Lakshmi Mudambi, MBBS
Director
Interventional Pulmonology
VA Portland Health Care System;
Assistant Professor
Department of Medicine
Oregon Health and Science University
Portland, Oregon

David E. Ost, MD
Professor of Pulmonary Medicine
MD Anderson Cancer Center
Houston, Texas

Jasleen Pannu, MBBS
Assistant Professor of Medicine
Interventional Pulmonology;
Pulmonary Critical Care and Sleep Medicine
Ohio State University
Columbus, Ohio

Tenzing Phanthok, MD, MS
Physician
Athens Pulmonary and Sleep
Athens, Georgia

Otis B. Rickman, DO
Associate Professor
Department of Allergy, Pulmonary, and Critical Care
Vanderbilt University Medical Center
Nashville, Tennessee

Roy Semaan, MD
Director of Interventional Pulmonology
Division of Pulmonary, Allergy, and Critical Care
    Medicine
University of Pittsburgh School of Medicine
Pittsburgh, Pennsylvania

Ajay Sheshadri, MD, MSCI
Associate Professor
Department of Pulmonary Medicine
The University of Texas MD Anderson Cancer Center
Houston, Texas

Samira Shojaee, MD, MPH
Assiociate Professor of Medicine
Internal Medicine – Pulmonary and Critical Care
    Medicine
Virginia Commonwealth University
Richmond, Virginia

Sean B. Smith, MD
Assistant Professor
Northwestern University, Feinberg School of Medicine
Chicago, Illinois

Momen M. Wahidi, MD, MBA
Professor of Medicine
Division of Pulmonary and Critical Care Medicine
Duke University School of Medicine;
Director, Interventional Pulmonology and
    Bronchoscopy
Duke University Medical Center
Durham, North Carolina

Lonny Yarmus, DO
Associate Professor of Medicine
Division of Pulmonary and Critical Care Medicine
Johns Hopkins University School of Medicine
Baltimore, Maryland

Kazuhiro Yasufuku, MD, PhD, FRCSC
Division Head
Division of Thoracic Surgery
Toronto General Hospital;
University Health Network
Toronto, Ontario, Canada

Video Contributor

Abdul Hamid Alraiyes, MD, FCCP
Medical Director for Interventional Pulmonology
Interventional Pulmonology/Critical Care,
Associate Professor of Medicine
Rosalind Franklin University
North Chicago, Illinois

CONTENTS

VIDEO TABLE OF CONTENTS

Introduction

Momen M. Wahidi and David E. Ost

INTERVENTIONAL PULMONOLOGY

Interventional pulmonology (IP) has evolved over the past decade to become a recognized discipline offering advanced consultative and procedural services to patients with thoracic malignancy, anatomic airway disease, and pleural disease. As with many procedurally oriented medical disciplines, there are not always data to inform every aspect of how to perform a given IP procedure. Consequently, there exists significant variation between physicians in how procedures are performed. Many publications focus on the evidence of efficacy of IP interventions but fail to provide practical advice on how to perform the procedures. Procedural details are often relegated to a single paragraph in the methods section of original research. This leaves trainees and practicing physicians who are learning a new procedure with a paucity of practical information on how to actually do them.

In this book, we aim to present a practical approach to IP procedures with a focus on patient selection, preprocedural preparation (including equipment, staff, and setting), procedural techniques, complications, and a brief summary of the evidence. The book is organized in chapters covering diagnostic and therapeutic IP procedures, as well as multimodality approaches to malignant and benign airway obstruction, and finishes with some practical advice on how to build and lead an IP program. We designed the procedural chapters to flow in a similar fashion and consistently cover the aforementioned practical steps of IP procedures. We further supplemented the book with colored images and original illustrations.

The goal of this book is to capture the procedure "craft" of IP practice as well as the science. Procedure craft in this context really refers to how to do a procedure. It includes tips and tricks from experienced physicians that may not reach the level of evidence necessary for a guideline but are nonetheless helpful and often essential for everyday practice. To achieve this goal, each chapter is written by experts in the field who use these techniques in their everyday practice. After all, when learning to fly a plane, who would you rather learn from: a PhD aerospace engineer or an experienced pilot who flies the same type of plane you are going to fly?

This book covers the most frequently performed IP procedures, but some rare IP procedures are not included. Although the content may be viewed as ideal for beginners in IP procedures, such as trainees in pulmonary medicine, interventional pulmonology, and thoracic surgery, it is truly a fantastic review for clinicians already performing these procedures. It is an opportunity to evaluate whether there are different styles of performing certain procedures or just a refresher on the entire spectrum of IP procedures: old and new. Grab that cup of coffee or tea this Sunday morning and immerse yourself in easy-to-read rich content with tips and tricks from experts in the field.

Advanced Diagnostic
Bronchoscopy Procedures

Linear Endobronchial Ultrasound

Kazuhiro Yasufuku, Terunaga Inage,
Alexander Gregor, and Tsukasa Ishiwata

INTRODUCTION

In 2002, a new bronchoscope was developed by integrating a convex-type ultrasound probe on its tip and introduced into clinical practice.[1] The convex probe endobronchial ultrasound (CP-EBUS), also known as linear EBUS, can be combined with a dedicated biopsy needle for real-time endobronchial ultrasound-guided transbronchial needle aspiration (EBUS-TBNA) of centrally located peribronchial lung lesions, mediastinal lymph nodes, and hilar lymph nodes. EBUS-TBNA using a linear transducer is a well-established minimally invasive modality for diagnosis and staging of lung cancer. Lung cancer guidelines recommend combined EBUS-TBNA with endoscopic ultrasound-fine-needle aspiration (EUS-FNA, also called EUS-B-FNA if an EBUS bronchoscope is used in the combined procedure) as the best first test for mediastinal nodal staging in lung cancer. Over the past 20 years, the role of this minimally invasive modality has been expanding to include restaging after neoadjuvant therapy and additional sample acquisition for biomarker testing. Advances in ultrasonography image analysis have expanded the capabilities of linear EBUS. As such, EBUS-TBNA has now also become a minimally invasive diagnostic tool for lymphoma, sarcoidosis, tuberculosis, mediastinal cysts, and other intrathoracic malignancies. New biopsy needles will further expand the potential capabilities of EBUS-TBNA in pulmonary medicine. Use of linear EBUS as a therapeutic modality, via transbronchial injection, has likewise seen growing interest and evidence. Linear EBUS continues to play an essential role in disease diagnosis but is taking on novel indications with potentially significant clinical implications.

PREPROCEDURE PREPARATION

Indications for Linear Endobronchial Ultrasound

The initial indication for linear EBUS is diagnosis and nodal staging of lung cancer.[2] Suspicion for other intrathoracic malignancies, such as lymphoma,[3] sarcoma,[4] mesothelioma,[5] and other mediastinal metastases,[6,7] as well as benign conditions, such as sarcoidosis,[8] tuberculosis,[9] and mediastinal cysts,[10] can also be considered as indications for biopsy by EBUS-TBNA. EBUS-guided therapeutic interventions[11] are under investigation. Several EBUS bronchoscopes exist. However, in general, the size and flexibility of currently available EBUS bronchoscopes most reliably provide access to central lesions and in many circumstances the mid-lung of the lower lobes. The accessibility of current EBUS bronchoscopes to specific bronchi is more limited than that of regular bronchoscopes, especially when a biopsy needle is inserted into the working channel. Acce ss to the upper lobes, particularly the peripheral upper lobe, can be more challenging. More flexible EBUS bronchoscopes and needles with improved access to the periphery are under development.

Equipment

- Linear endobronchial ultrasound bronchoscope
- Universal ultrasound processor
- EBUS-TBNA needle (19-gauge [G], 21-G, 22-G, and/or 25-G)

Staff

- Bronchoscopist
- Endoscopy/respiratory technician
- Sedation nurse or anesthesia team
- Cytopathologist (optional)
- Cytopathology technician (optional)

Setting

The procedure can be performed in an endoscopy suite or operating room, with either moderate/conscious sedation or general anesthesia. The linear endobronchial ultrasound bronchoscope may be inserted into the airway via the oral route. An endotracheal tube or laryngeal mask airway can be selected optionally.

PROCEDURAL TECHNIQUES

General Linear EBUS/EBUS-TBNA Preparation

A dedicated latex balloon is attached to the probe tip of the EBUS bronchoscope using the balloon applicator and inflated with normal saline during EBUS-TBNA. A 20-mL syringe and extension tube filled with saline is connected to the balloon channel. Approximately 0.3 to 0.5 mL of saline is needed to achieve appropriate balloon inflation. Because the balloon is made of latex, it cannot be used in patients with allergy to latex.

EBUS-TBNA can be performed under either local anesthesia with mild conscious sedation or general anesthesia. With local anesthesia, the EBUS scope is inserted orally and 1% lidocaine (a 2-mL bolus dose) is gently administered into the airway through the instrument channel. With general anesthesia, an endotracheal tube (at least 8.0 mm in internal diameter) or a laryngeal mask airway (#4) is generally used. General anesthesia with these airway devices provides some advantages such as easier EBUS scope insertion and reduced coughing. This must be balanced against the logistic and safety considerations of general anesthesia.

After sedation or induction of anesthesia, a regular flexible bronchoscope is first inserted into the airway. The initial diagnostic bronchoscopy facilitates safe EBUS through clearance of secretions, identification of airway lesions, verification of bronchial tree anatomy, and administration of additional local anesthetic, if required. Once complete, the flexible bronchoscope is removed, and EBUS-guided biopsy can begin. Insertion

and manipulation of the EBUS bronchoscope can be more challenging than a conventional flexible bronchoscope. The EBUS bronchoscope optical system is limited by the forward oblique angle relative to the scope neutral position and ultrasound probe. Flexing the bronchoscope downward to provide a traditional "end-on" view during EBUS scope advancement can result in inadvertent injury from forceful dragging of the ultrasound probe. Rather, the EBUS bronchoscope should be advanced in a neutral position, with intermittent pausing and downward flexion to confirm position, if needed.

EBUS/EBUS-TBNA of Specific Lesions

If EBUS is being performed to acquire tissue from a specific lung or mediastinal lesion, the EBUS bronchoscope is navigated to the planned area identified on preprocedural imaging review. The ultrasound balloon should be gently inflated and the bronchoscope upward flexed to maximize contact with the bronchial wall. Once the lesion is centered on the ultrasound image, the EBUS needle sheath is advanced beyond the working channel, followed by the biopsy needle. Care should be made to monitor both the white-light and ultrasound image during advancement, as the bronchoscope may move as the needle is pushed forward. Ideally, for mediastinal lesions, the needle should be deployed in the gaps between cartilage rings.

EBUS/EBUS-TBNA of Lymph Nodes for Lung Cancer Staging

Lymph node staging should be performed in a consistent, systematic fashion to promote accurate staging. Lymph nodes are examined by EBUS for documentation of their station, size, and other ultrasound features (see later), in accordance with the American Joint Committee on Cancer (AJCC)/Union for International Cancer Control (UICC) staging systems. EBUS-TBNA has limited access to lymph nodes far from the central airways such as the prevascular nodes (station 3a), subaortic/paraaortic nodes (stations 5 and 6), and paraesophageal/pulmonary ligament nodes (stations 8 and 9). However, both transbronchial and transesophageal endosonographic procedures can be performed with a single EBUS scope, often referred to as EUS-B-FNA, which can facilitate access to stations 8 and 9 as well as alternative access routes for other stations.[12,13] EUS-B-FNA offers potential logistic advantages. However, if EUS-B-FNA is being considered, we recommend performing the esophageal portion *after* the bronchoscopic portion of the procedure to avoid contamination of the respiratory system.

A dedicated TBNA needle is inserted through the working channel of the EBUS bronchoscope, and the designated lymph node is punctured under real-time EBUS guidance. The aspirated material can then be submitted for cytologic/pathologic diagnosis. There is a theoretical risk for contamination of the biopsy needle or channel as the bronchoscope is moved from one lymph node to the next, risking over-staging. It is therefore generally recommended that N3 nodes be biopsied first, then N2, then N1. Although not necessary, an on-site cytopathologist may be able to provide immediate feedback on the quality of the biopsy specimen and potentially a preliminary diagnosis. This information may be used to inform decisions on repeating a biopsy during the same procedure.

COMPLICATIONS

EBUS-TBNA with linear EBUS is a safe and well-established minimally invasive modality for sampling centrally located peribronchial lesions. Complication rates are very low, but major complications including bleeding, infection, recurrent nerve paralysis, and mortality have been reported.[14,15]

EVIDENCE

Lung Cancer
Nodal Staging in Lung Cancer

The prognosis and operability of a lung cancer patient is influenced by the presence of mediastinal lymph node metastases. One meta-analysis calculated a pooled sensitivity of 0.93 (95% confidence interval [CI], 0.91–0.94) and a pooled specificity of 1.00 (95% CI, 0.99–1.00) for detection of mediastinal nodal disease across 11 studies.[2] The sensitivity, specificity, and accuracy of EBUS-TBNA were superior to positron emission tomography (PET) or PET-computed tomography (PET-CT) in two prospective trials.[16,17] The combination of EBUS-TBNA and EUS-FNA has a higher staging accuracy than either procedure alone for patients with lung cancer, with a sensitivity of 0.86 (95% CI, 0.82–0.90) and a specificity of 1.00 (95% CI, 0.99–1.00) in a meta-analysis covering

eight studies.[18] In the ASTER trial, combined staging with upfront EBUS-TBNA plus EUS-FNA followed by surgical staging showed higher diagnostic yield and fewer unnecessary thoracotomies than surgical staging alone.[19] Recently published guidelines for primary mediastinal staging in lung cancer recommend that ultrasonography-guided needle biopsy (EBUS-TBNA and/or EUS-FNA) be the first-choice modality over surgical staging.[20–22] However, if EBUS/EUS biopsy results are negative, surgical staging via mediastinoscopy or video-assisted mediastinoscopy is recommended.

Ultrasound Image Analysis of Lymph Nodes

During EBUS-TBNA, ultrasonographic features are helpful to differentiate malignant and benign lymph nodes. Several features on B-mode imaging, such as size (short axis), shape (oval vs. round), margin (indistinct vs. distinct), echogenicity (homogeneous vs. heterogeneous), central hilar structure (CHS) (present vs. absent), and coagulation necrosis sign (present vs. absent), have been shown to be good predictive markers for lymph node metastasis in non–small cell lung cancer (NSCLC). Fujiwara et al. reported round shape, distinct margin, heterogeneous echogenicity, and presence of coagulation necrosis sign as independent risk factors for metastasis.[23] Alici et al. integrated grayscale texture (anechoic, hypoechoic, isoechoic, or hyperechoic) with the previous six features to create a modified algorithm.[24] This algorithm's sensitivity, specificity, positive predictive value (PPV), negative predictive value (NPV), and diagnostic accuracy for detecting metastatic lymph nodes were 100%, 51.2%, 50.6%, 100%, and 67.5%, respectively.[24] Doppler imaging permits assessment of blood flow and nodal vascular patterns. Nakajima et al. classified lymph nodes by Doppler findings: grade 0, no blood flow or small amounts of flow; grade I, a few main vessels running toward the center of the lymph node from the hilum; grade II, a few cuneiforms or rod-shaped flow signals, or a few small vessels found as a long strip of a curve; and grade III, rich flow with more than four vessels of differing diameters and/or twist-/helical-low signal.[25] The sensitivity, specificity, and diagnostic accuracy of this grading system (grade 0/I benign vs. grade II/III malignant) were 87.7%, 69.6%, and 78.0%, respectively. Wang et al. classified Doppler vascular patterns into avascular, hilar, and nonhilar (central, capsular, or mixed); the authors combined these vascular features with the previous six sonographic features to predict benign lymph node status.[26] The sensitivity, specificity, PPV, and NPV for predicting benign lymph nodes were 81.3%, 90.9%, 85.3%, and 88.2%, respectively.

Elastography is a strain imaging technique to assess tissue stiffness, which is displayed as a color overlay on the B-mode ultrasound image. Most systems identify hard, intermediate, and soft tissues as blue, green, and yellow/red, respectively.[27] Izumo et al. categorized elastography image patterns into type 1 (predominantly nonblue), type 2 (part blue, part nonblue), and type 3 (predominantly blue). The sensitivity, specificity, PPV, NPV, and diagnostic accuracy of this classification system (type 1 benign vs. type 3 malignant) were 100.0%, 92.3%, 94.6%, 100.0%, and 96.7%, respectively. Nakajima et al. compared nodes by stiff area ratio (stiff blue area divided by total lymph node area) and found the mean stiffness ratios were significantly greater for metastatic lymph nodes (0.48) than benign lymph nodes (0.22, $P = 0.0002$).[28] When a cut-off ratio of 0.31 was used, sensitivity and specificity were 81% and 85%, respectively.

A growing area of focus is the application of artificial intelligence technologies to risk-stratify EBUS images by malignant potential. A 2008 study by Tagoya et al. developed an artificial neural network to predict the presence of nodal metastases using linear EBUS B-mode images, which ultimately developed a 91% diagnostic accuracy.[29] The sensitivity, specificity, and accuracy of this system were 87.0%, 82.1%, and 85.4%, respectively. The application of artificial intelligence may enable significant future advances in EBUS image analysis.

Restaging After Neoadjuvant Therapy

At present, the recommended treatment for stage IIIA-cN2 NSCLC is chemoradiotherapy.[30] However, surgical resection after neoadjuvant chemotherapy or chemoradiotherapy may improve the survival of patients with stage IIIA-cN2 disease.[31,32] Accurate restaging of the mediastinal lymph nodes in these cases is critical to confirm mediastinal down-staging prior to consideration for surgery. Repeat mediastinoscopy may also be considered; however, mediastinoscopy following neoadjuvant therapy can be challenging and the diagnostic yield is reduced due to development of fibrosis and adhesions.[33–35] A systematic review of five studies calculated the pooled sensitivity, specificity, and false-negative rate of remediastinoscopy after neoadjuvant therapy as 63%, 100%, and 22%, respectively.[36] Transcervical extended mediastinal lymphadenectomy has shown a

sensitivity of 96.6% for mediastinal restaging in patients with NSCLC after neoadjuvant therapy.[37] Mortality and morbidity were 0.3% and 6.4%, respectively. Similarly, restaging with EBUS-TBNA after neoadjuvant therapy has been reported to have lower sensitivity compared with EBUS-TBNA used during initial lung cancer staging.[38,39] A systematic review and meta-analysis including 10 studies found that endosonographic-guided needle biopsy (EBUS-TBNA, EUS-FNA, or combined endoscopic and endobronchial ultrasound [CUS]) for mediastinal restaging has a pooled sensitivity of 67% (95% CI, 56–77) and pooled specificity of 99% (95% CI, 89–100).[40] The discrepancy of diagnostic yields between initial staging and restaging may relate to difficulty obtaining adequate samples from down-staged nodes, which may be smaller, fibrotic, and/or necrotic following neoadjuvant therapy. There is also difficulty differentiating the sonographic appearance of metastases from postinflammatory adhesions and degenerative changes. Combined EBUS-TBNA and EUS-FNA could enable more accurate minimally invasive mediastinal restaging. Current guidelines recommend EBUS-TBNA and/or EUS-FNA for mediastinal restaging after neoadjuvant therapy, avoiding remediastinoscopy.[21,22]

Molecular Testing Using EBUS-TBNA Samples

As the treatment of advanced NSCLC has shifted toward molecular targeted therapy, biomarker testing has become necessary for determining the optimal treatment of patients newly diagnosed with NSCLC. Sensitizing mutations in the *EGFR* gene were first described in 2004, serving as the first class of molecular targeted therapy.[41] Since then, anaplastic lymphoma kinase (*ALK*) gene fusion,[42] *ROS1* gene rearrangements,[43] and *BRAF* mutations[44] were identified as potential treatment targets. Combination therapies, including cytotoxic chemotherapy and targeted gene therapy, have improved overall response rates, increased progression-free survival, and may be associated with improved overall survival in advanced NSCLC when compared with cytotoxic chemotherapy alone.[45] The National Comprehensive Cancer Network (NCCN) 2018 Clinical Practice Guidelines for NSCLC recommend concomitant diagnosis, staging, and acquisition of adequate material for molecular profiling to improve care of patients with NSCLC.[46] The importance of obtaining tissue for molecular profiling is clear. A systematic review and meta-analysis including 33 studies (2698 participants in total) found that use of EBUS-TBNA for molecular profiling of *EGFR* mutation status had a pooled probability of obtaining sufficient tissue of 94.5% (95% CI, 93.2%–96.4%). For identification of *ALK* mutations, the pooled probability was 94.9% (95% CI, 89.4%–98.8%).[47] There are several emerging molecular targets and therapies in NSCLC, such as *PIK3CA* mutation, *AKT1 KRAS* mutation, *RET* rearrangements, *MET* exon 14 skipping mutations, and activating *HER2* mutations. Therefore, the NCCN 2018 guidelines recommend testing using broad-based genomic sequencing, such as next-generation sequencing (NGS). A study including 54 TBNA/FNA samples showed a 50-gene assay panel was successful in 97.5% and 100% of 22-G and 25-G samples, respectively. A larger 1231-gene panel was successful in 91.3% and 100% of 22-G and 25-G samples, respectively.[48] Another study including 115 samples undergoing a large (341–469 gene) NGS-based panel found EBUS-TBNA obtained sufficient tissue in 86.1% of samples.[49] Rebiopsy by EBUS-TBNA for follow-up molecular profiling can be performed safely after initial treatment. In the era of biomarker-driven management of cancer, the ability to analyze EBUS-TBNA specimens for multiple biomarkers is critical in selecting an optimal, personalized treatment plan for each patient.

Lymphoma

Approximately 10% of lymphomas are first diagnosed in the chest, often as a mediastinal tumor. Subclassification, which guides treatment and prognosis, is based on morphologic, phenotypic, genotypic, and molecular features. Early diagnosis and staging are key to improving patient survival in those diagnosed with lymphoma. When available, EBUS-TBNA is a useful alternative approach for the diagnosis and subclassification of intrathoracic lymphoma compared to "gold standard" approaches of mediastinoscopy, thoracoscopy, and/or thoracotomy. In a systematic review and meta-analysis including 14 studies, the overall sensitivity and specificity of EBUS-TBNA for diagnosis of lymphoma were 66.2% (95% CI, 55%–75.8%) and 99.3% (95% CI, 98.2%–99.7%), respectively.[3] In subgroup analysis, sensitivity and specificity of EBUS-TBNA for the *initial* diagnosis of lymphoma were 67.1% (95% CI, 54.2%–77.9%) and 99.6% (95% CI, 99.1%–99.8%), respectively. EBUS-TBNA performed slightly better for diagnosing lymphoma *recurrence*, with a sensitivity of 77.8% (95% CI, 68.1%–85.2%) and specificity of 99.5% (95% CI, 98.9%–99.8%). These

diagnostic metrics are comparable to historical data on using mediastinoscopy for the diagnosis of mediastinal lymphoma.[50] For subtyping lymphoma, EBUS-TBNA obtained sufficient samples for ancillary testing (e.g., flow cytometry, fluorescence in situ hybridization) in 63% of histologically positive samples.[3] This suggests that EBUS-TBNA is an appropriate first-choice modality in patients with suspected lymphoma for the diagnosis of both initial and recurrent disease.

Sarcoidosis

The diagnosis of sarcoidosis requires the following criteria be met: a compatible clinical and radiologic presentation, pathologic evidence of noncaseating granulomas, and exclusion of other diseases with similar findings (e.g., infections, malignancy).[51] Conventional transbronchial biopsy (TBB) and TBNA were historically the most common procedures for obtaining pathologic evidence of noncaseating granulomas. The diagnostic yields of TBNA and TBNA + TBB are reported to be 62% and 83%, respectively.[52] EBUS-TBNA is particularly useful for stage I/II sarcoidosis, for which lymphadenopathy is a common feature. A meta-analysis including 15 studies found that EBUS-TBNA had a pooled diagnostic accuracy of 79% (95% CI, 71%–86%).[53] Performance of EBUS-TBNA was superior to TBNA or TBB alone.[51] However, a separate meta-analysis including 16 studies found the diagnostic yield of combined EBUS-TBNA + TBB + endobronchial biopsy (EBB) was 89.7% and more effective than EBUS-TBNA alone (82.7%) for the diagnosis of sarcoidosis.[54] The pooled diagnostic odds ratio for the two groups was 0.55 (95% CI, 0.39–0.78, $P = 0.0007$). These results suggest EBUS-TBNA, when combined with TBB and/or EBB, can be an effective minimally invasive approach for confirming the diagnosis of sarcoidosis.

Tuberculosis, Mediastinal Cysts, and Other Malignant Diseases

Pulmonary tuberculosis is often associated with mediastinal or hilar lymphadenopathy. The potential utility of EBUS-TBNA for diagnosis of tuberculosis has been previously reported.[55] A recent meta-analysis revealed the pooled sensitivity and specificity of EBUS-TBNA for diagnosis of intrathoracic tuberculosis were 80% (95% CI, 0.74–0.85) and 100% (95% CI, 0.99–1.00), respectively.[9]

A systematic review including 26 studies and 32 cases outlined the utility of diagnostic and therapeutic transbronchial ultrasound approaches for the diagnosis of mediastinal cysts.[10] However, four cases of postprocedural infection were identified after TBNA.

Rice et al. reported a cases series of nodal staging by EBUS-TBNA in malignant pleural mesothelioma, including 38 EBUS-TBNA and 50 mediastinoscopy cases.[5] The sensitivity and NPV were 28% and 49% for mediastinoscopy versus 59% and 57% for EBUS, respectively. Czarnecka-Kujawa et al. likewise published a case series including 48 patients with malignant pleural mesothelioma who underwent EBUS-TBNA for nodal staging.[56] The sensitivity, specificity, PPV, NPV, and diagnostic accuracy were 16.7%, 100%, 100%, 68.8%, and 70.6%, respectively. Although there is no large cohort study investigating the performance of EBUS-TBNA for the diagnosis of sarcoma, several authors have described successful tissue acquisition in small case series.[4,57,58]

EBUS Needles

Several EBUS needles are currently available across a range of sizes (25-, 22-, 21-, or 19-G). The size of the needle may affect the quantity of tissue obtained, degree of tissue trauma, amount of aspirated blood (which can affect the quality of the specimen), diagnostic yield, and maximal angulation range of the EBUS bronchoscope (Fig. 2.1). The increasing number of EBUS-TBNA needles has prompted several investigations

on their comparative diagnostic performance. The most common needles are 22-G and 21-G needles; however, there are little data supporting the use of one over another for its size. A large cohort of 1299 patients showed no differences in the diagnostic yield of 22-G and 21-G needles for the diagnosis and staging of NSCLC.[59] Adequate samples were obtained in 94.9% of the 22-G needle group and in 94.6% of the 21-G needle group ($P = 0.81$). A pathologic diagnosis was obtained in 51.4% of the 22-G group and 51.3% of the 21-G group ($P = 0.98$). These results suggest there is little difference when selecting between 22-G and 21-G needles for cytologic evaluation via TBNA.

19-G EBUS-TBNA Needle

The 19-G EBUS-TBNA needle is considered a histology needle, with the hypothesis that obtaining a core biopsy could improve diagnostic yield. Kinoshita et al. retrospectively evaluated two prototype 19-G EBUS-TBNA needles.[60] In this study, including 82 target lesions (72 lymph nodes and 10 lung tumors) in 45 patients, the authors found the pooled diagnostic yield of the 19-G EBUS-TBNA needles was 100%, with 28% of specimens being sufficient for histopathologic diagnosis. Recently, an EBUS-TBNA-specific 19-G needle (NA-U402SX-4019; Olympus, Tokyo, Japan) has become commercially available. This needle has a flexible tip segment that better preserves scope angulation[61] while maintaining a larger inner diameter (0.69 mm vs.

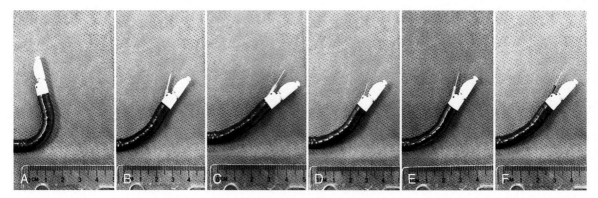

Fig. 2.1 Flexibility of endobronchial ultrasound-guided transbronchial needle aspiration (EBUS-TBNA) needles and maximal up-angulation of an EBUS bronchoscope (BF-UC180F, Olympus, Tokyo, Japan). (A) BF-UC180F without a needle. (B) ViziShot2 FLEX 19-G needle (Olympus Surgical Technologies America, Westborough, MA, USA). (C) ViziShot 22-G needle (Olympus, Tokyo, Japan). (D) ViziShot2 25-G needle (Olympus, Tokyo, Japan). (E) Expect Pulmonary 25-G needle (Boston Scientific, Marlborough, MA, USA). (F) EchoTip ProCore HD 25-G (Cook Medical, Bloomington, IN, USA).

0.41 mm with 22-G needles).[62] Several studies have since reported on the performance of this commercial 19-G needle (Table 2.1). Doom et al. demonstrated excellent diagnostic yield (39/39 100%) that was identical to using a 21-G needle (39/39 100%) in a randomized control trial.[62] In this study, they found that the 19-G tissue specimens were bloodier and had a larger tissue surface area than 21-G specimens. Another prospective randomized trial including 107 patients similarly found that 19-G samples contained significantly more tissue than 21-G samples (20.0 vs. 10.2 mg, $P = 0.0119$).[63] However, the larger needle size was once again associated with significantly bloodier samples ($P = 0.029$). The diagnostic yields were similar with both needles. These results suggest that, given the already excellent performance of cytologic 22- and 21-G needles, the added benefit of 19-G needles is not related to improved diagnostic yield. Rather, the reliable acquisition of greater tissue volumes

may facilitate use of multiple molecular (e.g., NGS) and pathologic tests (e.g., programmed death-ligand 1 [PD-L1] staining). Further investigation is needed to evaluate such use.

25-G EBUS-TBNA Needle

Currently, three types of 25-G EBUS-TBNA needles are commercially available: the EchoTip ProCore HD (Cook Medical, Bloomington, IN, USA), the Expect Pulmonary needle (Boston Scientific, Watertown, MA, USA), and the ViziShot2 (Olympus, Tokyo, Japan) (Fig. 2.2). The underlying justification for the development of these needles was to reduce injury to biopsied nodal and lung tissue, as well as reduce contamination. However, only a limited number of studies have been published (Table 2.2). A retrospective study by Di Felice et al. evaluated 158 lymph nodes, finding that 25-G and 22-G needles achieved comparable specimen adequacy ($P = 1$)

TABLE 2.1 Studies on the Diagnostic Performance of 19-G Needles

Reference	Year	Study Design	Number	Overall Diagnostic Yield	Diagnostic Yield for Malignancy	Diagnostic Yield for Nonmalignancy	Complication
Pickering et al.[64]	2019	Prospective observational	47	16/47 (97%)	N/A[a]	N/A[a]	None
Dooms et al.[62]	2018	Randomized control trial	39	39/39 (100%)	32/32 (100%)	7/7 (100%)	None
Tremblay et al.[65]	2018	Retrospective	154	119/154 (77%)	N/A[a]	N/A[a]	One moderate bleeding
Jones et al.[66]	2018	Retrospective	100	96/100 (96%)	N/A[a]	N/A[a]	None
Balwan et al.[67]	2018	Retrospective	15	14/15 (93%)	N/A[a]	14/15 (93%)	None
Garrison et al.[68]	2018	Retrospective	48	45/48 (94%)	N/A[a]	N/A[a]	None
Minami et al.[69]	2018	Retrospective	11	9/11 (81%)	N/A[a]	N/A[a]	None
Chaddha et al.[70]	2017	Prospective observational	56 lymph nodes	52/56 (93%)	N/A[a]	N/A[a]	None
Tyan et al.[61]	2017	Retrospective	47	42/47 (89%)	24/27 (89%)	18/20 (90%)	One moderate bleeding
Gnass et al.[71]	2017	Retrospective	22	22/22 (100%)	15/15 (100%)	7/7 (100%)	None
Trisolini et al.[53]	2017	Retrospective	13	13/13 (100%)	12/12 (100%)	1/1 (100%)	One mild bleeding
Pooled diagnostic yield			$n = 552$	84.6%			

[a]N/A, not assessed

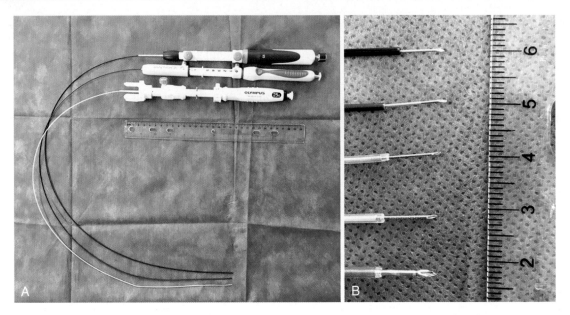

Fig. 2.2 Comparison of endobronchial ultrasound-guided transbronchial needle aspiration (EBUS-TBNA) needles. (A) From top to bottom, the Expect Pulmonary 25-G needle (Boston Scientific, Marlborough, MA, USA), EchoTip ProCore HD 25-G (Cook Medical, Bloomington, IN, USA), and ViziShot2 25-G needle (Olympus, Tokyo, Japan) are shown. (B) From top to bottom, Expect Pulmonary 25-G needle (Boston Scientific, Marlborough, MA, USA), the EchoTip ProCore HD 25-G (Cook Medical, Bloomington, IN, USA), ViziShot2 25-G needle (Olympus, Tokyo Japan), ViziShot 22-G needle (Olympus, Tokyo, Japan), and the ViziShot2 FLEX 19-G needle (Olympus Surgical Technologies America, Westborough, MA, USA).

TABLE 2.2	Studies and Cases of 25-G Needles				
Reference	**Year**	**Study Design**	**Number**	**Diagnostic Yield**	**Complication**
Di Felice et al.[72]	2018	Retrospective	79	73/79 (92%)	None
Matsumoto et al.[73]	2017	Retrospective	29	29/29 (100%)	N/[a]
Okubo et al.[74]	2017	Case report	1	1/1 (100%)	None
Waheed et al.[75]	2017	Case report	1	1/1 (100%)	None

[a]N/A, not assessed

with similar diagnostic accuracy ($P = 0.7$); the sensitivity, specificity, NPV, and diagnostic accuracy of the 25-G needle were 88.9% (95% CI, 51.8%–99.7%), 100% (95% CI, 92.1%–100%), 97.8% (95% CI, 87.6%–99.7%), and 98.2% (95% CI, 90.1%–100%), respectively.[72] By comparison, the sensitivity, specificity, NPV, and diagnostic accuracy in the 22-G group were 77.8% (95% CI, 40%–97.2%), 100% (95% CI, 86.8%–100%), 92.9% (95% CI, 79.3%–97.8%), and 94.3% (95% CI, 80.8%–99.3%), respectively. Another retrospective study also found similar diagnostic accuracy with 25-G (100%, 25/25) and 22-G (90.7%, 68/75) needles.[73] Stoy et al. retrospectively evaluated 104 patients, finding that 25-G needles

provided adequate samples for NGS as frequently as 22-G needle samples.[48] Further study evaluating more detailed features of the 25-G needle and biopsy samples is needed.

Therapeutic Endobronchial Ultrasound-Guided Transbronchial Needle Injection

Transbronchial needle injection (TBNI) via conventional bronchoscope has been previously used to administer various therapeutic agents for the treatment of bronchial malignancies or fistulas.[76] EBUS-TBNI is a relatively new technique that has been described for the treatment of recurrent NSCLC.[77] Mehta et al.

described cisplatin injection into a total of 41 sites in 36 patients by EBUS-TBNI.[78] Complete or partial response was observed in 69% (24/35) and median survival for the group was 8 months (95% CI, 6–11 months). EBUS-TBNI may potentially have utility for benign conditions as well, though data are also limited to case reports. Parikh et al. described a 71-year-old female with an aspergilloma who received intralesional amphotericin B (total dose 175 mg; 2.5 mg/kg) by EBUS-TBNI.[79]

SUMMARY

EBUS-TBNA via linear EBUS brought about a paradigm shift in nodal staging in lung cancer. The use of EBUS-TBNA has since expanded to include tissue acquisition for the diagnosis of a growing number of intrathoracic diseases and biomarker testing for precision medicine. More recently, the potential utility of linear EBUS as a therapeutic modality (via TBNI) has received growing attention. Its broad indications and low complication rate make EBUS a vital technical skill for physicians specializing in interventional pulmonary procedures.

REFERENCES

1. Yasufuku K, Chiyo M, Sekine Y, et al. Real-time endobronchial ultrasound-guided transbronchial needle aspiration of mediastinal and hilar lymph nodes. *Chest.* 2004;126(1):122–128.
2. Gu P, Zhao YZ, Jiang LY, Zhang W, Xin Y, Han BH. Endobronchial ultrasound-guided transbronchial needle aspiration for staging of lung cancer: A systematic review and meta-analysis. *Eur J Cancer.* 2009;45(8):1389–1396.
3. Labarca G, Sierra-Ruiz M, Kheir F, et al. Diagnostic accuracy of endobronchial ultrasound transbronchial needle aspiration in lymphoma. A systematic review and meta-analysis. *Ann Am Thorac Soc.* 2019;16(11):1432–1439.
4. Shingyoji M, Ikebe D, Itakura M, et al. Pulmonary artery sarcoma diagnosed by endobronchial ultrasound-guided transbronchial needle aspiration. *Ann Thorac Surg.* 2013;96(2):e33–e35.
5. Rice DC, Steliga MA, Stewart J, et al. Endoscopic ultrasound-guided fine needle aspiration for staging of malignant pleural mesothelioma. *Ann Thorac Surg.* 2009;88(3):862–868. discussion 868–869.
6. Liberman M, Hanna N, Duranceau A, Thiffault V, Ferraro P. Endobronchial ultrasonography added to endoscopic ultrasonography improves staging in esophageal cancer. *Ann Thorac Surg.* 2013;96(1):232–236. discussion 236–238.
7. Val-Bernal JF, Martino M, Romay F, Yllera E. Endobronchial ultrasound-guided transbronchial needle aspiration in the diagnosis of mediastinal metastases of clear cell renal cell carcinoma. *Pathol Res Pract.* 2018;214(7):949–956.
8. Agarwal R, Srinivasan A, Aggarwal AN, Gupta D. Efficacy and safety of convex probe EBUS-TBNA in sarcoidosis: A systematic review and meta-analysis. *Respir Med.* 2012;106(6):883–892.
9. Ye W, Zhang R, Xu X, Liu Y, Ying K. Diagnostic efficacy and safety of endobronchial ultrasound-guided transbronchial needle aspiration in intrathoracic tuberculosis: A meta-analysis. *J Ultrasound Med.* 2015;34(9):1645–1650.
10. Maturu VN, Dhooria S, Agarwal R. Efficacy and safety of transbronchial needle aspiration in diagnosis and treatment of mediastinal bronchogenic cysts: Systematic review of case reports. *J Bronchology Interv Pulmonol.* 2015;22(3):195–203.
11. Kinsey CM. Endobronchial ultrasound-guided-transbronchial needle injection for direct therapy of lung cancer. *AME Med J.* 2018
12. Hwangbo B, Lee GK, Lee HS, et al. Transbronchial and transesophageal fine-needle aspiration using an ultrasound bronchoscope in mediastinal staging of potentially operable lung cancer. *Chest.* 2010;138(4):795–802.
13. Oki M, Saka H, Ando M, et al. Transbronchial vs transesophageal needle aspiration using an ultrasound bronchoscope for the diagnosis of mediastinal lesions: A randomized study. *Chest.* 2015;147(5):1259–1266.
14. Kuijvenhoven JC, Leoncini F, Crombag LC, et al. Endobronchial ultrasound for the diagnosis of centrally located lung tumors: A systematic review and meta-analysis. *Respiration.* 2020;99(5):441–450.
15. Vaidya PJ, Munavvar M, Leuppi JD, Mehta AC, Chhajed PN. Endobronchial ultrasound-guided transbronchial needle aspiration: Safe as it sounds. *Respirology.* 2017;22(6):1093–1101.
16. Yasufuku K, Nakajima T, Motoori K, et al. Comparison of endobronchial ultrasound, positron emission tomography, and ct for lymph node staging of lung cancer. *Chest.* 2006;130(3):710–718.
17. Hwangbo B, Kim SK, Lee HS, et al. Application of endobronchial ultrasound-guided transbronchial needle aspiration following integrated PET/CT in mediastinal staging of potentially operable non-small cell lung cancer. *Chest.* 2009;135(5):1280–1287.

18. Zhang R, Ying K, Shi L, Zhang L, Zhou L. Combined endobronchial and endoscopic ultrasound-guided fine needle aspiration for mediastinal lymph node staging of lung cancer: A meta-analysis. *Eur J Cancer*. 2013;49(8):1860–1867.

19. Annema JT, van Meerbeeck JP, Rintoul RC, et al. Mediastinoscopy vs endosonography for mediastinal nodal staging of lung cancer: A randomized trial. *JAMA*. 2010;304(20):2245–2252.

20. Vilmann P, Clementsen PF, Colella S, et al. Combined endobronchial and esophageal endosonography for the diagnosis and staging of lung cancer: European Society of Gastrointestinal Endoscopy (ESGE) guideline, in cooperation with the European Respiratory Society (ERS) and the European Society of Thoracic Surgeons (ESTS). *Endoscopy*. 2015;47(6):545–559.

21. De Leyn P, Dooms C, Kuzdzal J, et al. Revised ESTS guidelines for preoperative mediastinal lymph node staging for non-small-cell lung cancer. *Eur J Cardiothorac Surg*. 2014;45(5):787–798.

22. Silvestri GA, Gonzalez AV, Jantz MA, et al. Methods for staging non-small cell lung cancer: Diagnosis and management of lung cancer, 3rd ed: American College of Chest Physicians evidence-based clinical practice guidelines. *Chest*. 2013;143(5 Suppl):e211S–e250S.

23. Fujiwara T, Yasufuku K, Nakajima T, et al. The utility of sonographic features during endobronchial ultrasound-guided transbronchial needle aspiration for lymph node staging in patients with lung cancer: A standard endobronchial ultrasound image classification system. *Chest*. 2010;138(3):641–647.

24. Alici IO, Yilmaz Demirci N, Yilmaz A, Karakaya J, Ozaydin E. The sonographic features of malignant mediastinal lymph nodes and a proposal for an algorithmic approach for sampling during endobronchial ultrasound. *Clin Respir J*. 2016;10(5):606–613.

25. Nakajima T, Anayama T, Shingyoji M, Kimura H, Yoshino I, Yasufuku K. Vascular image patterns of lymph nodes for the prediction of metastatic disease during EBUS-TBNA for mediastinal staging of lung cancer. *J Thorac Oncol*. 2012;7(6):1009–1014.

26. Wang L, Wu W, Teng J, Zhong R, Han B, Sun J. Sonographic features of endobronchial ultrasound in differentiation of benign lymph nodes. *Ultrasound Med Biol*. 2016;42(12):2785–2793.

27. Izumo T, Sasada S, Chavez C, Matsumoto Y, Tsuchida T. Endobronchial ultrasound elastography in the diagnosis of mediastinal and hilar lymph nodes. *Jpn J Clin Oncol*. 2014;44(10):956–962.

28. Nakajima T, Inage T, Sata Y, et al. Elastography for predicting and localizing nodal metastases during endobronchial ultrasound. *Respiration*. 2015;90(6):499–506.

29. Tagaya R, Kurimoto N, Osada H, Kobayashi A. Automatic objective diagnosis of lymph nodal disease by B-mode images from convex-type echobronchoscopy. *Chest*. 2008;133(1):137–142.

30. Ettinger DS, Wood DE, Aisner DL, et al. Non-small cell lung cancer, version 5.2017, NCCN clinical practice guidelines in oncology. *J Natl Compr Canc Netw*. 2017;15(4):504–535.

31. Betticher DC, Hsu Schmitz SF, Totsch M, et al. Mediastinal lymph node clearance after docetaxel-cisplatin neoadjuvant chemotherapy is prognostic of survival in patients with stage IIIA pN2 non-small-cell lung cancer: A multicenter phase II trial. *J Clin Oncol*. 2003;21(9):1752–1759.

32. Lorent N, De Leyn P, Lievens Y, et al. Long-term survival of surgically staged IIIA-N2 non-small-cell lung cancer treated with surgical combined modality approach: Analysis of a 7-year prospective experience. *Ann Oncol*. 2004;15(11):1645–1653.

33. De Leyn P, Stroobants S, De Wever W, et al. Prospective comparative study of integrated positron emission tomography-computed tomography scan compared with remediastinoscopy in the assessment of residual mediastinal lymph node disease after induction chemotherapy for mediastinoscopy-proven stage IIIA-N2 non-small-cell lung cancer: A Leuven Lung Cancer Group study. *J Clin Oncol*. 2006;24(21):3333–3339.

34. Marra A, Hillejan L, Fechner S, Stamatis G. Remediastinoscopy in restaging of lung cancer after induction therapy. *J Thorac Cardiovasc Surg*. 2008;135(4):843–849.

35. De Waele M, Serra-Mitjans M, Hendriks J, et al. Accuracy and survival of repeat mediastinoscopy after induction therapy for non-small cell lung cancer in a combined series of 104 patients. *Eur J Cardiothorac Surg*. 2008;33(5):824–828.

36. de Cabanyes Candela S, Detterbeck FC. A systematic review of restaging after induction therapy for stage IIIA lung cancer: Prediction of pathologic stage. *J Thorac Oncol*. 2010;5(3):389–398.

37. Zielinski M, Szlubowski A, Kolodziej M, et al. Comparison of endobronchial ultrasound and/or endoesophageal ultrasound with transcervical extended mediastinal lymphadenectomy for staging and restaging of non-small-cell lung cancer. *J Thorac Oncol*. 2013;8(5):630–636.

38. Nasir BS, Bryant AS, Minnich DJ, Wei B, Dransfield MT, Cerfolio RJ. The efficacy of restaging endobronchial ultrasound in patients with non-small cell lung cancer after preoperative therapy. *Ann Thorac Surg*. 2014;98(3):1008–1012.

39. Herth FJ, Annema JT, Eberhardt R, et al. Endobronchial ultrasound with transbronchial needle aspiration for restaging the mediastinum in lung cancer. *J Clin Oncol*. 2008;26(20):3346–3350.

40. Muthu V, Sehgal IS, Dhooria S, Aggarwal AN, Agarwal R. Efficacy of endosonographic procedures in mediastinal restaging of lung cancer after neoadjuvant therapy: A systematic review and diagnostic accuracy meta-analysis. *Chest.* 2018;154(1):99–109.

41. Lynch TJ, Bell DW, Sordella R, et al. Activating mutations in the epidermal growth factor receptor underlying responsiveness of non-small-cell lung cancer to gefitinib. *N Engl J Med.* 2004;350(21):2129–2139.

42. Soda M, Choi YL, Enomoto M, et al. Identification of the transforming EML4-ALK fusion gene in non-small-cell lung cancer. *Nature.* 2007;448(7153):561–566.

43. Rimkunas VM, Crosby KE, Li D, et al. Analysis of receptor tyrosine kinase ROS1-positive tumors in non-small cell lung cancer: Identification of a FIG-ROS1 fusion. *Clin Cancer Res.* 2012;18(16):4449–4457.

44. Marchetti A, Felicioni L, Malatesta S, et al. Clinical features and outcome of patients with non-small-cell lung cancer harboring BRAF mutations. *J Clin Oncol.* 2011;29(26):3574–3579.

45. Blumenthal GM, Karuri SW, Zhang H, et al. Overall response rate, progression-free survival, and overall survival with targeted and standard therapies in advanced non-small-cell lung cancer: US Food and Drug Administration trial-level and patient-level analyses. *J Clin Oncol.* 2015;33(9):1008–1014.

46. Ettinger DS, Aisner DL, Wood DE, et al. NCCN guidelines insights: Non-small cell lung cancer, version 5.2018. *J Natl Compr Canc Netw.* 2018;16(7): 807–821.

47. Labarca G, Folch E, Jantz M, Mehta HJ, Majid A, Fernandez-Bussy S. Adequacy of samples obtained by endobronchial ultrasound with transbronchial needle aspiration for molecular analysis in patients with non-small cell lung cancer. Systematic review and meta-analysis. *Ann Am Thorac Soc.* 2018;15(10):1205–1216.

48. Stoy SP, Segal JP, Mueller J, et al. Feasibility of endobronchial ultrasound-guided transbronchial needle aspiration cytology specimens for next generation sequencing in non-small-cell lung cancer. *Clin Lung Cancer.* 2018;19 (3):230–238. e232.

49. Turner SR, Buonocore D, Desmeules P, et al. Feasibility of endobronchial ultrasound transbronchial needle aspiration for massively parallel next-generation sequencing in thoracic cancer patients. *Lung Cancer.* 2018;119:85–90.

50. Elia S, Cecere C, Giampaglia F, Ferrante G. Mediastinoscopy vs. anterior mediastinotomy in the diagnosis of mediastinal lymphoma: A randomized trial. *Eur J Cardiothorac Surg.* 1992;6(7):361–365.

51. Statement on sarcoidosis Joint statement of the American Thoracic Society (ATS), the European Respiratory Society (ERS) and the World Association of Sarcoidosis and Other Granulomatous Disorders (WASOG) adopted by the ATS board of directors and by the ERS executive committee, February 1999. *Am J Respir Crit Care Med.* 1999;160(2):736–755.

52. Agarwal R, Aggarwal AN, Gupta D. Efficacy and safety of conventional transbronchial needle aspiration in sarcoidosis: A systematic review and meta-analysis. *Respir Care.* 2013;58(4):683–693.

53. Trisolini R, Lazzari Agli L, Tinelli C, De Silvestri A, Scotti V, Patelli M. Endobronchial ultrasound-guided transbronchial needle aspiration for diagnosis of sarcoidosis in clinically unselected study populations. *Respirology.* 2015;20(2):226–234.

54. Hu LX, Chen RX, Huang H, et al. Endobronchial ultrasound-guided transbronchial needle aspiration versus standard bronchoscopic modalities for diagnosis of sarcoidosis: A meta-analysis. *Chin Med J (Engl).* 2016;129(13):1607–1615.

55. Navani N, Molyneaux PL, Breen RA, et al. Utility of endobronchial ultrasound-guided transbronchial needle aspiration in patients with tuberculous intrathoracic lymphadenopathy: A multicentre study. *Thorax.* 2011;66(10):889–893.

56. Czarnecka-Kujawa K, de Perrot M, Keshavjee S, Yasufuku K. Endobronchial ultrasound-guided transbronchial needle aspiration mediastinal lymph node staging in malignant pleural mesothelioma. *J Thorac Dis.* 2019;11(2):602–612.

57. Sanchez-Font A, Chalela R, Martin-Ontiyuelo C, et al. Molecular analysis of peripheral lung adenocarcinoma in brush cytology obtained by EBUS plus fluoroscopy-guided bronchoscopy. *Cancer Cytopathol.* 2018;126(10):860–871.

58. Dalal S, Nicholson 3rd CE, Jhala D. Unusual presentation of poorly differentiated primary pulmonary synovial sarcoma (PD-PPSS) diagnosed by EBUS-TBNA with cytogenetic confirmation–a diagnostic challenge. *Diagn Cytopathol.* 2018;46(1):72–78.

59. Yarmus LB, Akulian J, Lechtzin N, et al. Comparison of 21-gauge and 22-gauge aspiration needle in endobronchial ultrasound-guided transbronchial needle aspiration: Results of the American College of Chest Physicians quality improvement registry, education, and evaluation registry. *Chest.* 2013;143(4):1036–1043.

60. Kinoshita T, Ujiie H, Schwock J, et al. Clinical evaluation of the utility of a flexible 19-gauge EBUS-TBNA needle. *J Thorac Dis.* 2018;10(4):2388–2396.

61. Tyan C, Patel P, Czarnecka K, et al. Flexible 19-gauge endobronchial ultrasound-guided transbronchial needle aspiration needle: First experience. *Respiration.* 2017;94(1):52–57.

62. Dooms C, Vander Borght S, Yserbyt J, et al. A randomized clinical trial of Flex 19G needles versus 22G needles for endobronchial ultrasonography in suspected lung cancer. *Respiration*. 2018;96(3):275–282.

63. Wolters C, Darwiche K, Franzen D, et al. A prospective, randomized trial for the comparison of 19-G and 22-G endobronchial ultrasound-guided transbronchial aspiration needles; introducing a novel end point of sample weight corrected for blood content. *Clin Lung Cancer*. 2019;20(3):e265–e273.

64. Pickering EM, Holden VK, Heath JE, Verceles AC, Kalchiem-Dekel O, Sachdeva A. Tissue acquisition during EBUS-TBNA: Comparison of cell blocks obtained from a 19G versus 21G needle. *J Bronchology Interv Pulmonol*. 2019;26(4):237–244.

65. Tremblay A, McFadden S, Bonifazi M, et al. Endobronchial ultrasound-guided transbronchial needle aspiration with a 19-G needle device. *J Bronchology Interv Pulmonol*. 2018;25(3):218–223.

66. Jones RC, Bhatt N, Medford ARL. The effect of 19-gauge endobronchial ultrasound-guided transbronchial needle aspiration biopsies on characterisation of malignant and benign disease. The Bristol experience. *Monaldi Arch Chest Dis*. 2018;88(2):915.

67. Balwan A. Endobronchial ultrasound-guided transbronchial needle aspiration using 19-G needle for sarcoidosis. *J Bronchology Interv Pulmonol*. 2018;25(4):260–263.

68. Garrison G, Leclair T, Balla A, et al. Use of an additional 19-G EBUS-TBNA needle increases the diagnostic yield of EBUS-TBNA. *J Bronchology Interv Pulmonol*. 2018;25(4):269–273.

69. Minami D, Ozeki T, Okawa S, et al. Comparing the clinical performance of the new 19-G ViziShot FLEX and 21- or 22-G ViziShot 2 endobronchial ultrasound-guided transbronchial needle aspiration needles. *Intern Med*. 2018;57(24):3515–3520.

70. Chaddha U, Ronaghi R, Elatre W, Chang CF, Mahdavi R. Comparison of sample adequacy and diagnostic yield of 19- and 22-G EBUS-TBNA needles. *J Bronchology Interv Pulmonol*. 2018;25(4):264–268.

71. Gnass M, Sola J, Filarecka A, et al. Initial polish experience of flexible 19 gauge endobronchial ultrasound-guided transbronchial needle aspiration. *Adv Respir Med*. 2017;85(2):64–68.

72. Di Felice C, Young B, Matta M. Comparison of specimen adequacy and diagnostic accuracy of a 25-gauge and 22-gauge needle in endobronchial ultrasound-guided transbronchial needle aspiration. *J Thorac Dis*. 2019;11(8):3643–3649.

73. Matsumoto Y, Okubo Y, Tanaka M, et al. The utility of new 25 gauge endobronchial ultrasound-guided transbronchial needle in lymph node staging. Respirology. 2017;22(S3):27.

74. Okubo Y, Matsumoto Y, Nakai T, et al. The new transbronchial diagnostic approach for the metastatic lung tumor from renal cell carcinoma-a case report. *J Thorac Dis*. 2017;9(9):E762–E766.

75. Waheed SA, Goyal A. A case of adapting to antiplatelets: Successful diagnosis of nocardia via endobronchial ultrasound using a 25 gauge needle. D31. Interventional pulmonary: Case reports II. *Am J Respir Crit Care Med*. 2018;197:A6430–A6430.

76. Seymour CW, Krimsky WS, Sager J, et al. Transbronchial needle injection: A systematic review of a new diagnostic and therapeutic paradigm. *Respiration*. 2006;73(1):78–89.

77. Khan F, Anker CJ, Garrison G, Kinsey CM. Endobronchial ultrasound-guided transbronchial needle injection for local control of recurrent non-small cell lung cancer. *Ann Am Thorac Soc*. 2015;12(1):101–104.

78. Mehta HJ, Begnaud A, Penley AM, et al. Treatment of isolated mediastinal and hilar recurrence of lung cancer with bronchoscopic endobronchial ultrasound guided intratumoral injection of chemotherapy with cisplatin. *Lung Cancer*. 2015;90(3):542–547.

79. Parikh MS, Seeley E, Nguyen-Tran E, Krishna G. Endobronchial ultrasound-guided transbronchial needle injection of liposomal amphotericin B for the treatment of symptomatic aspergilloma. *J Bronchology Interv Pulmonol*. 2017;24(4):330–333.

3

Radial Endobronchial Ultrasound

Alexander Chen and Kevin Haas

INTRODUCTION

Radial probe endobronchial ultrasound (rEBUS) is a small ultrasound probe placed through the working channel of a bronchoscope used to locate peripheral lung abnormalities, such as pulmonary nodules. The probe provides a circumferential 360-degree view of its surrounding structures (Fig. 3.1).

Normal lung is filled with air, which is highly reflective of ultrasound waves (Fig. 3.2). When the radial probe is placed within or adjacent to a solid lesion in the periphery of the lung, a hyperechoic image with a clear border will be seen. If the radial probe is placed within the lesion, a concentric ultrasound view will be obtained (Fig. 3.3). If the radial probe is placed adjacent to the lesion, an eccentric ultrasound view will be obtained (Fig. 3.4). Radial EBUS allows for real-time localization of the target lesion. The rEBUS probe must be removed from the working channel prior to sampling. It is important to recognize that rEBUS does not provide the bronchoscopist with a road map to the target nodule; rather, the bronchoscopist will have to charter a path based on their own review of the chest computed tomography (CT) or use a guidance system such as navigational bronchoscopy. Radial EBUS is used once the bronchoscopist feels that the tip of the scope or guide sheath is close to the lesion and can confirm in real time whether the nodule has been reached based on an ultrasound image.

The American College of Chest Physicians Lung Cancer Guidelines recommend rEBUS as an adjunct imaging modality for patients suspected of having lung cancer, who have a peripheral lung nodule, and a tissue diagnosis is required due to uncertainty of diagnosis or poor surgical candidacy.[1]

PREPROCEDURE PREPARATION

Patient Selection

Patient selection is dependent on the location and size of the lesion, the experience of the bronchoscopist, and weighing the risk of complications versus the probability of a diagnosis. The presence of a bronchus sign, a visible airway on the CT scan leading to the peripheral lesion, should favor the use of rEBUS because of the higher probability of finding and diagnosing the lesion (Fig. 3.5). Lesions located adjacent to the chest wall should be considered for CT-guided percutaneous needle aspiration, though the decision to proceed with rEBUS is dependent on the comfort level of the bronchoscopist. Operator inexperience and inability to tolerate procedural sedation are contraindications to rEBUS.

Equipment

- Radial endobronchial ultrasound probe
- Probe driving unit
- Universal ultrasound processor
- Bronchoscope
- Fluoroscopy
- Sampling instrument (forceps, brush, needle)
- Guide sheath kit (optional)
- Guiding double-hinged curette (optional).

Staff

- Bronchoscopist
- Endoscopy/respiratory technician
- Sedation nurse or anesthesia team.

Setting

The procedure can be done in an endoscopy suite or operating room. Anesthesia can be with either

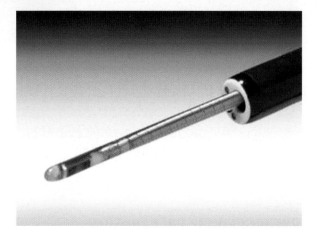

Fig. 3.1 Radial probe endobronchial ultrasound through the working channel of a bronchoscope.

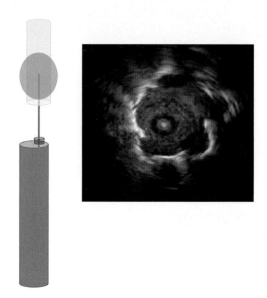

Fig. 3.3 Concentric radial probe endobronchial ultrasound view. The radial probe is placed within the lesion.

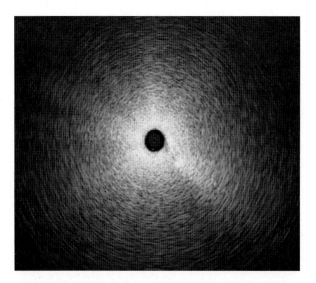

Fig. 3.2 Radial probe endobronchial ultrasound surrounded by normal lung.

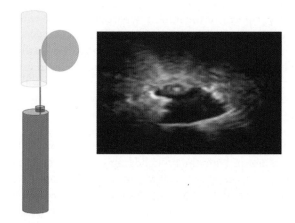

Fig. 3.4 Eccentric radial probe endobronchial ultrasound view. The radial probe is placed adjacent the lesion.

moderate/conscious sedation, monitored anesthesia care, or general anesthesia. The bronchoscope can be inserted into the airway with a nasal or oral approach. The use of an endotracheal tube or laryngeal airway mask is optional. These practices are variable among institutions.

PROCEDURAL TECHNIQUES

Radial EBUS Without Guide Sheath

Prior to starting the bronchoscopy, the operator will need to determine where the lesion is located. Lesion localization can be performed with navigational

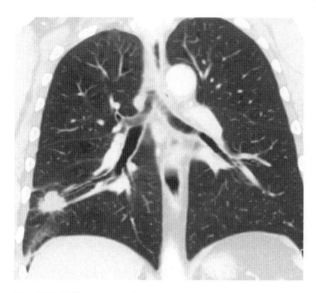

Fig. 3.5 CT bronchus sign.

assistance or by CT-anatomic correlation using coronal, sagittal, and axial planes. If navigation is being used for localization, the rEBUS probe can be used to confirm in real time the lesion location prior to sampling. When using CT imaging as a reference for lesion localization, the majority of nodules can be identified with rEBUS. A retrospective review of 467 peripheral nodule bronchoscopy cases found that when using CT imaging for lesion localization, 96% of nodules were identified with rEBUS; however, this level of expertise requires ample practice.[2]

The bronchoscope is inserted into the target lobe and segment. The proceduralist will need to be in eyesight of their endoscopic, radial ultrasound, and fluoroscopic views (fluoroscopy is optional but recommended). Using the endoscopic and fluoroscopic views, the radial probe is inserted sequentially into the preplanned target airways until a lesion is identified with radial ultrasound. The bronchoscopist should aim to obtain a concentric ultrasound image because of the increased diagnostic yield compared with an eccentric ultrasound image. If an eccentric image is obtained, the bronchoscopist should attempt to reposition the radial probe in nearby airways seeking to obtain a concentric ultrasound view. Unfortunately a concentric ultrasound view is not always achievable, and an eccentric ultrasound image may occur in nearly half of patients.[2] When satisfied

with the rEBUS image, the bronchoscope is positioned a few centimeters proximal to the lesion if possible. The closer the bronchoscope is to the lesion, the more likely the sampling instruments will follow the same path as the radial probe.

Before removing the radial probe to sample the lesion, a static or "still frame" of the fluoroscopic image may be captured and projected adjacent to the "live" fluoroscopy. The still frame of the radial probe localizing the lesion can be used as a template for sampling the lesion. The radial probe is then removed and a sampling instrument is placed into the working channel. Using "live" fluoroscopy, the sampling instrument is advanced to the lesion in a similar manner as the radial probe, aiming to replicate the still frame. When sampling, the goal is to place the sampling tool (with live fluoroscopy) in the same location as the radial probe (still frame).

rEBUS can also be done without fluoroscopy. Once the lesion is located, the radial probe is removed and the length can be measured from the working channel insertion site. A sampling tool is then placed into the working channel and samples are taken at the same length of the radial probe.

rEBUS can be done with any size bronchoscope, though thinner bronchoscopes improve access deeper into the periphery of the lung. Ultrathin bronchoscopes with a 3-mm outer diameter are also an option and have been shown to increase diagnostic yield.[3]

Radial EBUS Plus Guide Sheath

If the bronchoscope cannot be placed in close proximity to the peripheral lesion, a guide sheath can be used. A guide sheath is an optional tool that can be utilized with rEBUS. The guide sheath is a plastic catheter with a distal radio-opaque marker placed through the working channel of the bronchoscope. The radial probe and sampling instruments can then pass independently through the guide sheath. Only one instrument can be placed in the guide sheath at a time. Once the target lesion is identified with rEBUS, the radial probe is withdrawn and the guide sheath is kept in place just proximal to the lesion. Fluoroscopy is optional and can be used to guide sampling. Transbronchial needle aspiration, forceps biopsy, and brushings can be placed through the guide sheath. Two guide sheath sizes are available, with the smaller size being compatible with a working channel of 2 mm.

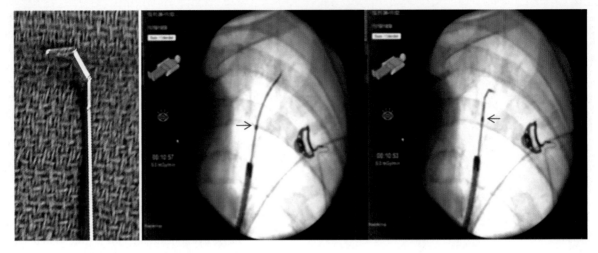

Fig. 3.6 Guiding curette. *Arrows* indicate guide sheath tip.

Radial EBUS Plus Guide Sheath and Guiding Curette

If there is difficulty locating a peripheral lesion, a guiding curette can be used to enter airways not directly accessible with the radial probe or bronchoscope. The guiding curette is placed through the guide sheath and can be flexed, extended, or rotated to access more acutely angled airways. This is most easily performed using fluoroscopic guidance. Once the curette has accessed the airway, the guide sheath is advanced over the curette into the airway. The curette is then withdrawn and the radial probe is inserted into the guide sheath to examine the newly accessed airway (Fig. 3.6).

COMPLICATIONS

Radial EBUS itself is very safe due to the soft and pliable end of the radial probe. Complications can result from transbronchial biopsies, needle aspirations, and brushings. These sampling methods are performed no differently than conventional sampling, and therefore have the same rate of complications. Complications primarily include bleeding that does not require intervention and pneumothorax in 1%–2.8% of cases.[4–6] Many of the pneumothorax cases do not require chest tube placement.

EVIDENCE

The reported diagnostic yield of rEBUS is variable. Meta-analyses report a diagnostic yield between 71% and 73%.[5,6] A more recent, multicenter, prospective, randomized trial reported a diagnostic yield of 49%.[7] Larger lesion size, a visible airway on CT leading to the lesion, use of needle aspiration, and concentric ultrasound views have been shown to increase the diagnostic yield of rEBUS.[4,8,9] Using thinner bronchoscopes also increases diagnostic yield, likely due to their ability to reach farther into the periphery of the lung.[3] The combination of rEBUS with evolving technologies such as ultrathin bronchoscopy, electromagnetic navigation, virtual bronchoscopic navigation, and robotic bronchoscopy in addition to different biopsy tools is being actively investigated.

SUMMARY

rEBUS is a safe imaging modality used to confirm the location of peripheral lung lesions in real time. Confirming lesion localization may improve confidence prior to sampling and may improve the diagnostic yield of procedures. rEBUS continues to be explored in combination with additional technologies to potentially further improve the diagnostic yield for peripheral lung lesions.

REFERENCES

1. Rivera MP, Mehta AC, Wahidi MM. Establishing the diagnosis of lung cancer: diagnosis and management of lung cancer, 3rd ed: American College of Chest Physicians evidence-based clinical practice guidelines. *Chest.* 2013;143:142s–165s.

2. Chen AC, Loiselle A, Zhou L, Baty J, Misselhon D. Localization of peripheral pulmonary lesions using a method of computed tomography anatomic correlation and radial probe endobronchial ultrasound confirmation. *Ann Am Thorac Soc.* 2016;13:1586–1592.

3. Oki M, Saka H, Ando M, et al. Ultrathin bronchoscopy with multimodal devices for peripheral pulmonary lesions. *Am J Resp Crit Care Med.* 2015;192:468–476.

4. Chen AC, Chenna P, Loiselle A, Massoni J, Mayse M, Misselhorn D. Radial probe endobronchial ultrasound for peripheral pulmonary lesions: A 5 year institutional experience. *Ann Am Thorac Soc.* 2014;11:578–582.

5. Wang M, Nietert PJ, Silvestri GA. Meta-analysis of guided bronchoscopy for the evaluation of the pulmonary nodule. *Chest.* 2012;142:385–393.

6. Steinfort DP, Khor YH, Manser RL, Irving LB. Radial probe endobronchial ultrasound for the diagnosis of peripheral lung cancer: Systematic review and meta-analysis. *Eur Respir J.* 2011;37:902–910.

7. Tanner NT, Yarmus L, Chen A, et al. Standard bronchoscopy with fluoroscopy vs thin bronchoscopy and radial endobronchial ultrasound for biopsy of pulmonary lesions: A multicenter, prospective, randomized trial. *Chest.* 2018;154:1035–1043.

8. Ali MS, Sethi J, Taneja A, Musani A, Maldonado F. Computed tomography bronchus sign and the diagnostic yield of guided bronchoscopy for peripheral pulmonary lesions. A systematic review and meta-analysis. *Ann Am Thorac Soc.* 2018;8:978–987.

9. Chao TY, Chien MT, Lie CH, Chung YH, Wang JL, Lin MC. Endobronchial ultrasonography-guided transbronchial needle aspiration increases the diagnostic yield of peripheral pulmonary lesions: A randomized trial. *Chest.* 2009;136:229–236.

4

Electromagnetic Navigation Bronchoscopy

Allen Cole Burks and Jason Akulian

INTRODUCTION

Electromagnetic navigation bronchoscopy (ENB) utilizes an electromagnetic field created around the patient to detect and display spatially tracked devices within the magnetic field superimposed over the three-dimensional (3D) virtual bronchoscopic route, i.e., an integrated electromagnetic tracking system within virtual navigational bronchoscopy. The final product is a dynamic, spatially, and temporally tracked virtual representation of the device within the preplanned, patient-specific anatomic "map."

In the United States, there are two commercially available ENB systems: SPiN Drive (VSPN, Veran Medical Technologies, St. Louis, MO, USA), and superDimension/ILLUMISITE (iSD, Medtronic, Minneapolis, MN, USA). Both systems require thin-cut computed tomography (CT) imaging with a specific protocol to plan biopsy targets and overlay/match the magnetic field to CT scan anatomy. There are three primary differences between the systems. The first is the VSPN system's use of inspiratory and expiratory CT images to add respiratory gating versus a static inspiratory breath hold (SD). The second is which devices are tracked during ENB (iSD—locatable guide [LG] via an extended working channel [EWC]; VSPN—tip-tracked biopsy instruments). The SD LG is similar to a tracked probe that passes through the EWC. The EWC is offered with various tip angles (45, 90, and 180 degrees), which allows for steerability during navigation. Once the lesion is reached, the EWC is locked in place and the LG is removed, allowing peripheral biopsy instruments to be used to sample the lesion in question and/or radial probe endobronchial ultrasound (rEBUS) is used for real-time confirmation of the target lesion. Though the VSPN system has recently introduced their own version of an LG/EWC combination, the platform's performance is predicated on the use of "always-on" tipped track biopsy instruments (forceps, brush, and needle) allowing for continuous direct bronchoscopic navigation of the biopsy instrument. The third difference between the systems is a percutaneous approach option provided by the VSPN not found on the iSD system. The percutaneous modality uses a preplanned chest wall entry point to allow for passage of a tracked needle through the chest wall and into the peripheral lung parenchyma/target lesion. Both platforms use similar planning systems and computer software to generate 4D reconstructions of the patient's chest CT and allowing for peripheral lesion targeting and pathway building.

PREPROCEDURAL PREPARATION

Guidelines recommend that nonsurgical biopsy be performed in patients who have an indeterminate nodule >8 mm in diameter in the following situations[1]:

- When clinical pretest probability of malignancy and imaging results are discordant.
- When the overall probability of malignancy is low to moderate (~10%–60%).
- Suspicion of a benign diagnosis, in which diagnostic confirmation would affect management decisions.
- In high-malignancy risk-patients who desire biopsy of proof of malignancy prior to undergoing surgery.

- In high-surgical-risk patients, in whom a diagnosis is requested prior to initiation of radiosurgery or other nonsurgical ablative therapies.
- Part-solid nodules >8 mm in diameter, persistent on radiographic follow-up; based on pretest probability, surgical risk factors, and patient preference.

Endoscopic-guided peripheral lung biopsy is generally preferred over transthoracic approaches in low-to-moderate malignancy probability patients with mediastinal or hilar lymphadenopathy measuring ≥1 cm in diameter in the short axis (regardless of fludeoxyglucose [FDG] avidity on positron emission tomography [PET] scan within the lymph nodes) due to the ability to stage the mediastinum with EBUS-guided transbronchial needle aspirations (TBNAs, see Chapter 2) within a single procedure and anesthesia session.

Equipment Needed for Electromagnetic Navigation Bronchoscopy

- Veran SPiN Drive
  - Veran patient tracking pad (vPad) positioned on the chest ipsilateral to the nodule of interest in a T or L shape (Fig. 4.1)
  - CT scan requirements
    - Inspiratory and expiratory images
      - Slice thickness and interval: thickness (0.75 mm), interval (0.5 mm)
  - Planning station computer with SPiN Drive Planning software installed and USB drive
    - Either connected to intranet for DICOM CT scan upload or with CD-ROM/USB reading capabilities

- USB drive for transitioning the procedure plan to the SPiN Drive electromagnetic navigation (EMN) Platform
- Always-On Tip Tracked instruments (Fig. 4.2)
- Bronchoscope with at least a 2-mm working channel
- For SPiN Perc
  - SPiN Perc Kit
    - Always-On Tip Tracked 19 gauge (G) × 105 mm or 155 mm biopsy needle
    - 20 G × 15 cm or 20 cm fine-needle aspiration (FNA) needle
    - 20 G × 15 cm or 20 cm biopsy gun
- superDimension/ILLUMISITE Navigation System
  - CT scan requirements
    - Full inspiratory images
      - Slice thickness and interval: thickness (1.0–1.25 mm), interval (0.8–1.0 mm)
  - Planning station computer with iSD Planning software installed and USB drive
    - Either connected to intranet for DICOM CT scan upload or with CD-ROM/USB reading capabilities
  - USB drive for transitioning the procedure plan to the ILLUMISITE platform
  - iSD electromagnetic generator and board
  - Bronchoscope with at least a 2.6-mm working channel
  - ILLUMISITE extended working channel (IEWC—0-, 45-, 90-, and 180-degree angulation) (Fig. 4.3)
  - Biopsy instruments
  - For fluoroscopic navigation technology
    - Fiducial board

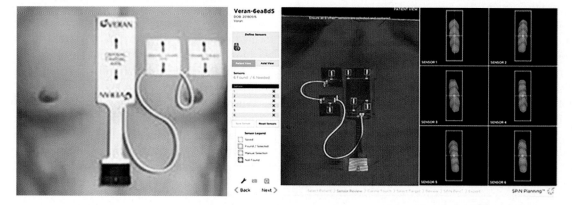

Fig. 4.1 Example of Veran patient tracking pad (vPad) placements and confirmation.

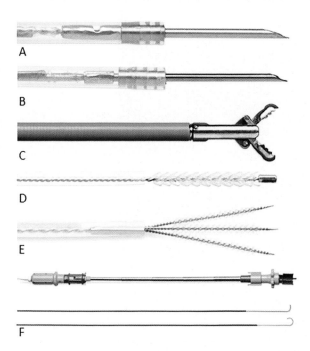

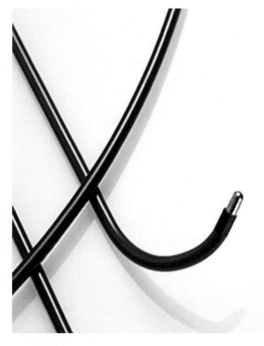

Fig. 4.2 Veran Always-On Tip Tracked tools. (A) Always-On Tip Tracked 21-G ANSO cytology needle. (B) Always-On Tip Tracked 22-G SPiN Flex ANSO nitinol needle. (C) Always-On Tip Tracked forceps. (D) Always-On Tip Tracked brush. (E) Always-On Tip Tracked triple needle brush. (F) SPiN access catheter.

Fig. 4.3 superDimension ILLUMISITE locatable extended working channel.

- For Veran SPiN:
  - Always-On Tip Tracked cytology brush, or
  - SPiN EWC/access catheter with Always-On Tip Tracked guidewire

Staff

- Bronchoscopy technician/nurse for equipment assistance and sample handling
- Anesthesia staff

PROCEDURAL TECHNIQUES

Veran SPiN System

Planning

With the vPad patient trackers appropriately positioned in a T or L configuration, the patient undergoes a non-contrasted CT scan of the chest during end inspiration and expiration. The patient must remain supine until completion of the scan to decrease registration error. Once uploaded to the planning station, the identification of 6 vPad sensors is confirmed (Fig. 4.1). Then the main and secondary carinas ipsilateral to the lesion of interest are marked virtually by right-clicking on the

- A qualified C-arm fluoroscope for use with the navigation system (determined by Medtronic technical service representative)
  - Creates a fluoroscope configuration file installed on the navigation system that corrects fluoroscopic image distortion, allowing recreation of the 3D volume. Each file is specific to the geometric properties of the individual fluoroscope used.
- ENB-guided fiducial placement
  - Fiducial markers (for examples, see Fig. 4.4)
    - SuperLock—0.8 × 3.5 mm gold seed with an attached 4-mm nitinol wire (Medtronic, Dublin, Ireland)
    - Visicoil—0.5 × 5-mm linear gold wire (IBA Dosimetry, Bartlett, TN, USA)
  - Bone wax or surgical lube
  - For iSD:
    - iSD Marker Delivery Kit, or
    - Cytology brush

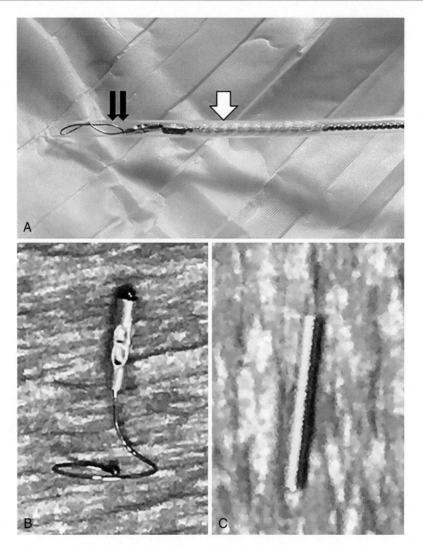

Fig. 4.4 Preparation for endobronchial fiducial marker placement. (A) Fiducial marker *(double black arrows)* loaded into a cytology brush *(white arrow)*. (B) SuperLock nitinol coil fiducial marker. (C) Visicoil fiducial marker.

corresponding carina in the program's generated airway map. The lesion of interest is then chosen by right-clicking, holding, and dragging across the largest diameter of the lesion and clicking save. The software then segments the target lesion and airways creating a high-definition virtual airway map with a proposed pathway to the lesion. Following this, the user will confirm registration by evaluating the overlay of the planned navigation over the expiratory images. If there is significant divergence between the planned route and expiratory images,

this is rectified by selecting the "refine airways" button, aligning the inspiratory and expiratory images side by side, and dropping a point on the main carina on the expiratory images by right-clicking, and then placing a second point on the lesion of interest on expiratory images with a right-click. The software then adjusts the overlay, which the user confirms once appropriate. The next screen is the SPiN Perc planning stage, which can be skipped if desired or the target location is not amenable to percutaneous sampling.

If the nodule is in the peripheral one-third of the lung parenchyma and located in an anterolateral position, then electromagnetic-guided transthoracic needle aspiration/biopsy (EMTTNA) can be considered. When planning for EMTTNA, a needle insertion site is selected by right-clicking at the level of the skin such that a needle entry path is created that is the shortest distance from visceral pleura to target and avoids overlying bony structures, pleural fissures, and is less than 10.5 to 15.5 cm from insertion site to targeted lesion (the working distance of the available SPiN Perc Always-On Tip Tracked TTNA needles). The plan then is uploaded to a USB drive, taken to the SPiN Drive navigation platform and uploaded.

Registration

Once the patient is appropriately sedated and anesthetized, position the magnetic field generator over the vPads such that all six markers are recognized by the system. Using one of the Tip Tracked instruments, place the tip of the instrument on the main carina and confirm by clicking "set main carina." The registration is confirmed by placing the tip of the instrument on the selected secondary carina and affirming that the system is appropriately sensing its location within the virtual map. If there is significant error in the location of the instrument in relation to the secondary or main carina, a point cloud should be created by clicking "create point cloud" and passing the instrument sequentially throughout the right lung, left lung, and trachea. The system collects points in expiration and overlays them on the virtual map; once a system-determined threshold of accuracy is met, the checkmark turns green. Once all three checkmarks have turned green, click "stop collecting," accept registration, and then reassess accuracy by placing the tip of the instrument physically on the respective carinas and confirming their location within the virtual image.

Navigation and Biopsy

Once airway registration is confirmed, the navigation phase of the procedure begins (Fig. 4.5). Using a Tip Tracked needle positioned at the end of the bronchoscope working channel, the proceduralist drives the bronchoscope according to the virtual route and proceduralist's knowledge of the anatomic location of the target lesion. The target will appear purple until the instrument is within 1 cm of the lesion and is aligned such that the lesion is within the throw of the needle, at which point

it will turn orange. The lesion will turn green when the tip of the needle is virtually within the target. An assisting physician, technician, or nurse extends the needle during expiration. Once the needle is deployed, suction can be applied as the needle is agitated within the lesion during expiration—"green on green" (when the tip of the tool is virtually within the lesion and the system senses that the respiratory cycle is in expiration). After approximately 10 agitations, remove suction and retract the needle. Remove the instrument from the working channel and process the sample by institutional protocols. When using the Always-On Tip Tracked biopsy forceps, we recommend opening the forceps at the proximal edge of the virtual representation of the lesion (while the lesion appears orange), advancing the open forceps during expiration into the lesion and closing the jaws of the forceps during "green on green." Transbronchial brushing can be performed in a similar manner.

Alternatively, navigation can be performed through a lockable SPiN access catheter with an Always-On Tip Tracked guidewire. Target lesion location confirmation can then be performed with rEBUS, prior to insertion of the biopsy tools through the catheter.

EMTTNA

First, confirm presence of lung slide and b-lines (vertical hyperechoic ultrasound reverberations that move in sync with lung parenchymal sliding) with ultrasound to rule out a pneumothorax complicating the ENB-guided TBNA and biopsies. Recheck registration of the main and secondary carinas prior to EMTTNA, in order to ensure accuracy of the procedure. Using a nonsterile Tip Tracked TTNA needle, identify the insertion site on the patient with the use of the SPiN Perc software. Mark the insertion site and prepare the site in a sterile fashion. Carefully insert the sterile Tip Tracked TTNA needle into the skin, maintaining the trajectory of the needle by ensuring a green circle within a green square in the heads-up display (HUD) and that the needle trajectory lines transect the target lesion in both oblique and oblique-90 degree views (Fig. 4.6). Once at the virtual pleural edge, an expiratory hold is performed and a single needle insertion is performed across the pleura, then advanced to the proximal edge of the lesion. At this point, it is vitally important to keep the trocar stationary while removing the Tip Tracked stylet. The FNA needle and/or core needle gun is then introduced through the trocar. When performing needle aspirates, the depth of needle throw can be set up

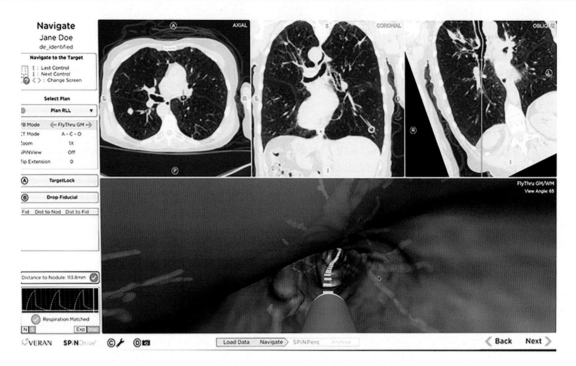

Fig. 4.5 VSPN navigation screen.

to 2 cm with the spring-loaded marker prior to the procedure. Aspirate and agitate within the nodule approximately 10 times (with or without suction), then process the sample according to institutional protocols. Between aspirations, we replace the Tip Tracked stylet to reconfirm location of the trocar's position as it relates to the target lesion. After the last FNA pass, reconfirm trocar location and replace the stylet with the 19-G core needle gun set at the appropriate depth (1–2 cm) based on lesion size and location. Fire the core needle four consecutive times, orienting the needle edge 90 degrees from each prior pass after processing each sample and confirming location of the trocar tip and lesion between fires. Once all needle and core passes have been obtained, 2–4 mL of warm saline or patient's own blood is injected, starting at the proximal edge of the nodule while the needle is withdrawn, to deposit saline or blood throughout the needle tract in an attempt to decrease risk of pneumothorax.

superDimension Navigation System
Planning

A preprocedure, same-day thin-slice noncontrasted CT scan with full inspiratory and expiratory phases is preferred for the iSD system. Once obtained, the CT scan is uploaded to the iSD or ILLUMISITE planning station, where it appears in a patient list. The operator then chooses the patient of interest to create a new plan. This generates a 3D-segmented airway map of the patient's airways. The user then evaluates the automated 3D map for the appropriate number of subsegment divisions, especially in the region of interest. The segmented airways should extend to within 2.5–5 cm of the target. If this is the case, the user clicks "Accept 3D map." In the event the map lacks the desired number of airway segmentations, the user declines the automated map by clicking "Decline map." The system will then prompt the user to complete a series of steps to select the main carina, trachea, and secondary carinas; then click "Generate map." Based on these user inputs, the system then regenerates the segmented airway map. Once the user is satisfied and the map is accepted, the planning station will prompt the user to select (right-click) the target of interest. After target selection, the user will select "Add target"—preferentially selecting the peripheral versus central target buttons based on the target's location in either the outer two-third of the lung parenchyma or within the inner one-third. The user will then

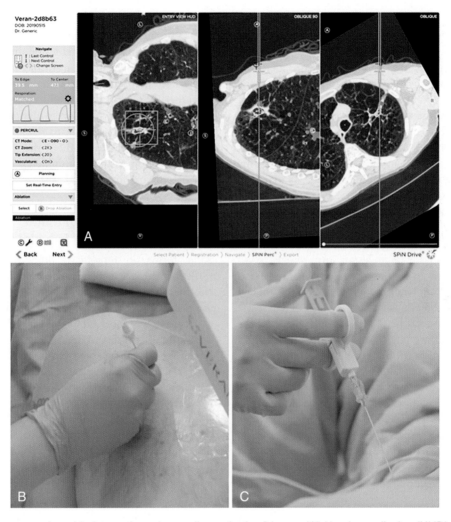

Fig. 4.6 Electromagnetic-guided transthoracic needle aspiration/biopsy. (A) Heads-up display (HUD) example with planned needle track. (B) Identification of insertion site with nonsterile tip-tracked needle. (C) Core needle biopsy.

proceed to "draw" a pathway back to the distal-most recognized airway, generating a virtual airway navigation pathway, which is then reviewed and compared to user's preprocedure expected pathway based on detailed CT review and CT-anatomic correlation. Once complete, the plan is exported to a USB drive and uploaded onto the iSD navigation platform.

Procedural Registration

Prior to anesthesia, the patient is positioned atop the iSD electromagnetic generator and location board (if fluoroscopic navigation is being used, an iSD fiducial board is secured to the location board prior to patient positioning). After appropriate sedation/anesthesia and airway placement, the patient plan is selected on the procedural platform and the plan is activated. The bronchoscope with the IEWC inserted is then driven to the main carina where the EWC is extended 0.5–1 cm. The iSD software in combination with the EWC then "automatically" registers the airways while the proceduralist drives the scope and EWC into each lobar airway. In the event there is significant registration error or CT-patient divergence, manual registration is performed by touching the iSD EWC to each of the preselected registration points.

Navigation, Local Reregistration With Fluoroscopic Navigation Technology, and Biopsy

The navigation phase of the procedure begins after registration by following the virtual pathway through the airways to the "take-off" lobar bronchus. The bronchoscope is wedged into that distal-most airway and EWC is manually advanced and turned (as needed) down the virtual path to the target lesion (Fig. 4.7). The navigation phase can be displayed in up to six different views by the procedural platform including all three standard CT views (axial, sagittal, and coronal), 3D views (virtual—static and dynamic, CT map), and tip view based on user preference.

Following initial airway registration and navigation to within 2.5 cm of the target lesion, local reregistration can be performed using fluoroscopic navigation technology. A series of 2D fluoroscopic images of the fiducial markers within the fiducial board are captured across a 50-degree rotation of the C-arm in an arc around the region of interest, which is marked by the physician on screen. An algorithm within the iSD system then generates a tight cross-sectional, 3D volume by determining the various angles of the C-arm based on the angle of the fiducial grid within the images and automatically removing overlying structural and metal artifacts to improve contrast (Fig. 4.8). This process takes 3–4 min. Using the updated local registration, the EWC is repositioned according to the new virtual map, and reconfirmed with fluoroscopy and/or rEBUS imaging.

At this point, the LG is removed from the EWC and the rEBUS probe is inserted. Upon rEBUS confirmation of EWC relationship with target lesion, the EWC is locked in place, and TBNA and transbronchial biopsy (TBBx) forceps of the proceduralist's choice are then inserted into the EWC and FNAs and forceps biopsies are acquired in a similar fashion to that described earlier. This system allows the EWC to remain locked in place between biopsy passes (without the need for repeated tool navigation with each biopsy), and proprietary biopsy tools are not required.

Electromagnetic Navigational Bronchoscopy-Guided Fiducial Placement

Some forms of stereotactic body radiation therapy (SBRT) require the placement of two to three fiducial markers to allow for lesion tracking throughout the respiratory cycle. Both EMN systems can be used to accurately place fiducials for SBRT simulation and nodule tracking. When using the VSPN, the tip-tracked brush can be employed for deployment of fiducials in and around the target lesion. With the brush completely retracted, the fiducial marker of choice is inserted into the empty tip of the brush catheter (Fig. 4.4). A small amount of bone wax or surgical lubricant is inserted over the fiducial to secure it in place during transit through the bronchoscope working channel and airways. The iSD system has a catheter specifically designed for fiducial marker placement

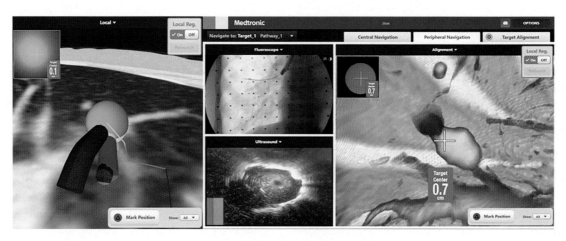

Fig. 4.7 superDimension navigation system. (A) Navigation pane for superDimension. (B) Local registration with fluoroscopic navigation technology and radial endobronchial ultrasound (EBUS) integration.

with a soft tip into which a marker (SuperLock fiducial, Medtronic, Dublin, Ireland) is loaded. Once loaded, the catheter is placed through the EWC to the predetermined placement location, and a deployment wire is used to push the marker out into the lung parenchyma. Alternatively, a cytology brush can be used to deploy markers into the parenchyma via the EWC, similar to the method described earlier for the VSPN, with the main difference being the use of the EWC compared to an electromagnetically tracked brush. Similarly, VSPN system also has available SPiN access catheters that can be used as an EWC through which a marker-loaded brush can be directed to the desired location.

Once the fiducial is loaded in the deployment tool of choice, the tool is then navigated in a similar fashion as mentioned earlier for the specific system being used, with the caveat that the goal is to leave at least two fiducials within 2–5 cm of each other and in relation to the lesion itself. We often will use the original navigation plan to place the first fiducial as close to, or within, the lesion as possible. The tool is navigated to the target lesion and then extended just to the end of the catheter, thus pushing the fiducial into the parenchyma. The bronchoscope technician/nurse simultaneously marks the virtual location of the fiducial with the navigation software. The tool is then retracted and reloaded with the second fiducial. The second fiducial is then navigated in a similar fashion, choosing an alternative distal airway that places the tip of the tool within 2–5 cm of the lesion and/or the first fiducial. Again the tool is deployed

just enough to cause the fiducial to exit the catheter into the parenchyma. A third or more fiducials can be placed in a similar fashion depending on institutional radiation oncology preferences.

PRECAUTIONS AND CAVEATS

- Same-day planning CT scan is recommended to improve registration; however, it should always be compared to the referral CT scan, as the incidence of nodules that decrease in size or resolve between referral CT scan and day-of-procedure scan is significant and can prevent unnecessary procedures.[2]
- We recommend using CT-anatomic correlation in conjunction with ENB, as we find this decreases the time to selection of the correct airway and first biopsy attempt.[3]
- Under anesthesia, atelectasis increases with length of procedure and can affect registration. Positive end-expiratory pressure and muscle relaxants have been used in an attempt to reduce this effect; however, data are limited on their effect on diagnostic yield or procedural success.
- The use of radial ultrasound (see Chapter 3) via a guide sheath or EWC as confirmation of target nodule and proximity to navigation has been shown to increase the diagnostic yield of peripheral bronchoscopy.[4,5]
- The VSPN software provides a virtual tooltip extension. Be aware that this does not represent the tip of the tool; however, the anticipated throw of the tool is based on the depth entered into the software (1–2-cm

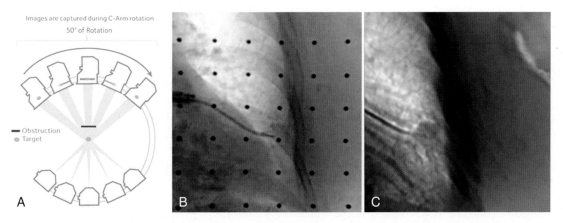

Fig. 4.8 Fluoroscopic navigation technology. (A) A 50-degree arc of images is obtained around the target region. (B) Fluoroscopic image with fiducial board and extended working channel (EWC) before superDimension enhanced visualization. (C) Fluoroscopic image after superDimension enhanced visualization.

throws). When the tool is aligned with the target and the target is within range of that throw, it will appear orange in color.

- Confirm lack of pneumothorax prior to proceeding with EMTTNA either with ultrasound, fluoroscopy, or chest x-ray.
- When performing EMTTNA, do not remove the trocar from the parenchyma once placed.
- Avoid more than one visceral pleural puncture as multiple punctures of the visceral pleura are associated with an increased risk of pneumothorax.[6–9]
- Injection of 2–4 mL of warmed saline or patient's own blood throughout the tract as the trocar is withdrawn during an expiratory hold can decrease rate of pneumothorax during transthoracic biopsy by 3–6-fold.[10]
- When advancing the iSD EWC and utilizing "tip view," keep the target lesion centered in the ring/tip. Follow the arrows' instruction to turn the EWC appropriately to maintain the central relationship.
- When advancing the iSD EWC using the 3D CT view, keep the purple ribbon/pathway "bright" and to the right of the virtual catheter.

COMPLICATIONS

- Pneumothorax
  - 2%–7% with peripheral TBNA and TBBx[5,11–13]
  - 10%–20% with EMTTNA[14]
  - 50% of the pneumothoraces require intervention (hospitalization or tube thoracostomy)[11,12]
- Hemorrhage
  - <1%–2.5%[5,13]
- Hypoxemia/respiratory failure
  - <1%[5,13]

EVIDENCE

A plethora of studies have sought to define the clinical effectiveness of ENB in peripheral lung lesion sampling and reported diagnostic yields have ranged from 39% to 94%.[5,11] Two meta-analyses have been done on ENB for peripheral pulmonary nodules—both of which included many studies of poor methodologic quality. Gex et al. found the pooled diagnostic yield of ENB to be 64.9% (95% confidence interval [CI], 59.2–70.3) and a negative predictive value of 52.1% (95% CI, 43.5–60.6), while Zhang et al. reported the pooled sensitivity, specificity, positive- and negative-likelihood ratios to be

82%, 100%, 19.36, and 0.23, respectively, indicating a prohibitively high false-negative rate when attempting to rule out malignant disease.[11,12] The largest prospective randomized controlled trial with three arms comparing ENB, rEBUS, and combined ENB with rEBUS found similar results for ENB and rEBUS with diagnostic yields of 59% and 69%, respectively. However, the combined technology arm had a significant increase in diagnostic yield (88%) when compared to either rEBUS or ENB alone.[4] A recent prospective, multicenter trial utilizing the iSD platform with rate of pneumothorax as the primary outcome measured a 12-month follow-up of 1157 patients at 37 institutions with a median lesion size of 20.0 mm. The authors reported a 4.3% pneumothorax rate (2.9% requiring hospitalization or intervention), a 2.5% hemorrhage rate (1.5% grade 2 or greater), and 0.7% grade 4 or greater respiratory failure rate—comparable to prior data. Although this study included a large proportion of high pretest probability nodules, a high number of patients had stage II–IV non–small cell lung cancer (NSCLC), and was not powered for diagnostic yield as the primary outcome, however; it reported a 73% diagnostic yield at 12 months and a sensitivity, specificity, positive, and negative predictive values of 69%, 100%, 100%, and 56%, respectively.[13,15] Overall, these data add to the growing body of literature speaking to the safety of ENB. To date, there have been no multicenter prospective trials of ENB with the Veran platform published; however, one such study has completed enrollment and is currently undergoing data review at the time of this publication (ClinicalTrials.gov ID NCT03338049). ENB has a comparable risk profile to that of peripheral lung biopsy using a standard FB and is superior to CT needle biopsy in regard to incidence of pneumothorax.[11–13,16,17]

Several factors have been identified that may positively influence ENB yield: (1) target location in the upper or middle lobe, (2) presence of a bronchus sign on CT imaging, (3) combined use of rEBUS, (4) catheter suctioning as a sampling technique, (5) lower registration error, (6) deep sedation, and (7) larger lesion size (>2 cm).[12,18] Of note, nodule size has been a consistent determinant of biopsy success, with a significant decrement in diagnostic yield reproducibility seen in lesions <20 mm.[19–21]

Regarding the feasibility and utility of ENB-placed fiducial markers for SBRT, a single-center study of ENB-guided fiducial marker placement reported a retention rate of 98.1%, accompanied by a low (6%) pneumo-thorax rate. Over the course of a five-fraction SBRT treatment, fiducial migration was <7 mm in 98% of the fiducials.[22] In a more recent, retrospective review of ENB-placed fiducial markers, 133 markers were placed in 65 patients, with 132 (99%) confirmed durable on follow-up imaging/resection.[23]

The clinical utility of the same-day planning CT scan in reducing unnecessary procedures is illustrated by a study that showed, in the lung cancer screening population, up to 7.7% of nodules will decrease in size or resolve on follow-up.[24] In a subsequent single-center, prospective case series, 6.9% of patients undergoing same-day planning CT scan for ENB of a peripheral lesion reported a decrease in nodule size or resolution leading to procedure cancellation. The study further reported the number needed to screen was 15, with mean time between referral scan and procedure day of 53 days.[2]

▌ SUMMARY

ENB presents additional guidance to the chest physician and has been shown to hold potential advantage over conventional bronchoscopy. While ENB has been associated with improved peripheral lung diagnostic yields, there remains a significant need for practical, affordable, real-time imaging confirmation of tool localization within the target lesion. Given the learning curve associated with ENB-guided peripheral lung biopsy, this practical guide outlines methods and tips for maximizing the use of readily available ENB systems. Arguably, the single most important tip for maximization of diagnostic yield is proper patient selection. Intermediate- to high-risk patients who are poor surgical candidates or prefer a tissue diagnosis prior to surgery are the preferred population, as a higher pretest probability will affect overall diagnostic yield by increasing the incidence of cancer in the procedural population group. Centrally located nodules greater than 2 cm with a clear bronchus ending within the lesion have further been shown as predictors of successful biopsy. Alternatively, peripherally located nodules less than 2 cm in size without radiographic evidence of mediastinal lymphadenopathy should be considered for primary resection or percutaneous needle biopsy.[25] Such thoughtful screening of patients being considered for ENB can serve to ensure proper guideline-directed workup of CT-detected lung abnormalities

and maximize initial first-test evaluation diagnostic yield, possibly avoiding unnecessary procedures and delays in diagnosis.

REFERENCES

1. Gould MK, Donington J, Lynch WR, et al. Evaluation of individuals with pulmonary nodules: when is it lung cancer? Diagnosis and management of lung cancer, 3rd ed: American College of Chest Physicians evidence-based clinical practice guidelines. *Chest*. 2013;143(5 Suppl):e93 S–e120S.
2. Semaan RW, Lee HJ, Feller-Kopman D, et al. Same-day computed tomographic chest imaging for pulmonary nodule targeting with electromagnetic navigation bronchoscopy may decrease unnecessary procedures. *Ann Am Thorac Soc*. 2016;13(12):2223–2228.
3. Chen AC, Loiselle A, Zhou L, Baty J, Misselhorn D. Localization of peripheral pulmonary lesions using a method of computed tomography-anatomic correlation and radial probe endobronchial ultrasound confirmation. *Ann Am Thorac Soc*. 2016;13(9):1586–1592.
4. Eberhardt R, Anantham D, Ernst A, Feller-Kopman D, Herth F. Multimodality bronchoscopic diagnosis of peripheral lung lesions: a randomized controlled trial. *Am J Respir Crit Care Med*. 2007;176(1):36–41.
5. Ost DE, Ernst A, Lei X, et al. Diagnostic yield and complications of bronchoscopy for peripheral lung lesions. Results of the AQuIRE Registry. *Am J Respir Crit Care Med*. 2016;193(1):68–77.
6. Covey AM, Gandhi R, Brody LA, Getrajdman G, Thaler HT, Brown KT. Factors associated with pneumothorax and pneumothorax requiring treatment after percutaneous lung biopsy in 443 consecutive patients. *J Vasc Interv Radiol*. 2004;15(5):479–483.
7. Khan MF, Straub R, Moghaddam SR, et al. Variables affecting the risk of pneumothorax and intrapulmonal hemorrhage in CT-guided transthoracic biopsy. *Eur Radiol*. 2008;18(7):1356–1363.
8. Saji H, Nakamura H, Tsuchida T, et al. The incidence and the risk of pneumothorax and chest tube placement after percutaneous CT-guided lung biopsy: the angle of the needle trajectory is a novel predictor. *Chest*. 2002;121(5):1521–1526.
9. Hiraki T, Mimura H, Gobara H, et al. Incidence of and risk factors for pneumothorax and chest tube placement after CT fluoroscopy-guided percutaneous lung biopsy: retrospective analysis of the procedures conducted over a 9-year period. *AJR Am J Roentgenol*. 2010;194(3):809–814.
10. Huo YR, Chan MV, Habib AR, Lui I, Ridley L. Post-biopsy manoeuvres to reduce pneumothorax incidence

in CT-guided transthoracic lung biopsies: a systematic review and meta-analysis. *Cardiovasc Intervent Radiol.* 2019;42(8):1062–1072.

11. Zhang W, Chen S, Dong X, Lei P. Meta-analysis of the diagnostic yield and safety of electromagnetic navigation bronchoscopy for lung nodules. *J Thorac Dis.* 2015;7(5):799–809.

12. Gex G, Pralong JA, Combescure C, Seijo L, Rochat T, Soccal PM. Diagnostic yield and safety of electromagnetic navigation bronchoscopy for lung nodules: a systematic review and meta-analysis. *Respiration.* 2014;87(2): 165–176.

13. Folch EE, Pritchett MA, Nead MA, et al. Electromagnetic navigation bronchoscopy for peripheral pulmonary lesions: one-year results of the prospective, multicenter NAVIGATE study. *J Thorac Oncol.* 2019;14(3):445–458.

14. Mallow C, Lee H, Oberg C, et al. Safety and diagnostic performance of pulmonologists performing electromagnetic guided percutaneous lung biopsy (SPiNperc). *Respirology.* 2019;24(5):453–458.

15. Thiboutot J, Yarmus LB, Lee HJ, Rivera MP, Ost DE, Feller-Kopman D. Real-world application of the NAVIGATE trial. *J Thorac Oncol.* 2019;14(7):e146–e147.

16. Leong S, Ju H, Marshall H, et al. Electromagnetic navigation bronchoscopy: a descriptive analysis. *J Thorac Dis.* 2012;4(2):173–185.

17. Wilson DS, Bartlett RJ. Improved diagnostic yield of bronchoscopy in a community practice: combination of electromagnetic navigation system and rapid on-site evaluation. *J Bronchol.* 2007;14(4):227–232.

18. Seijo LM, de Torres JP, Lozano MD, et al. Diagnostic yield of electromagnetic navigation bronchoscopy is highly dependent on the presence of a bronchus sign on CT imaging: results from a prospective study. *Chest.* 2010;138(6):1316–1321.

19. Savage C, Morrison RJ, Zwischenberger JB. Bronchoscopic diagnosis and staging of lung cancer. *Chest Surg Clin N Am.* 2001;11(4):701–721. vii-viii.

20. Schreiber G, McCrory DC. Performance characteristics of different modalities for diagnosis of suspected lung cancer: summary of published evidence. *Chest.* 2003;123(1 Suppl):115S–128S.

21. Wang Memoli JS, Nietert PJ, Silvestri GA. Meta-analysis of guided bronchoscopy for the evaluation of the pulmonary nodule. *Chest.* 2012;142(2):385–393.

22. Nabavizadeh N, Zhang J, Elliott DA, et al. Electromagnetic navigational bronchoscopy-guided fiducial markers for lung stereotactic body radiation therapy: analysis of safety, feasibility, and interfraction stability. *J Bronchology Interv Pulmonol.* 2014;21(2):123–130.

23. Belanger AR, Burks AC, Chambers DM, et al. Peripheral lung nodule diagnosis and fiducial marker placement using a novel tip-tracked electromagnetic navigation bronchoscopy system. *J Bronchology Interv Pulmonol.* 2019;26(1):41–48.

24. Zhao YR, Heuvelmans MA, Dorrius MD, et al. Features of resolving and nonresolving indeterminate pulmonary nodules at follow-up CT: the NELSON study. *Radiology.* 2014;270(3):872–879.

25. Gao SJ, Kim AW, Puchalski JT, et al. Indications for invasive mediastinal staging in patients with early non-small cell lung cancer staged with PET-CT. *Lung Cancer.* 2017;109:36–41.

5

Transbronchial Cryobiopsy for Diffuse Lung Diseases

Fabien Maldonado, Otis B. Rickman and Matthew Aboudara

INTRODUCTION

Transbronchial cryobiopsy (TBCB) is a relatively new technique in the diagnosis of diffuse parenchymal lung disease (DPLD). The basic rationale for development of TBCB is based on the inferiority of standard forceps transbronchial biopsies (TBBx) for diagnosis of DLPD as compared to surgical lung biopsies (SLBs). This is due to the small specimen sizes and resultant sampling error with TBBx. As a result, it is recommended that TBBx not be performed in the diagnostic evaluation of usual interstitial pneumonia (UIP), the pathologic correlate to idiopathic pulmonary fibrosis (IPF).[1] In addition, it has been increasingly recognized that SLB carries a risk of morbidity and mortality that may be unacceptable to both clinicians and patients.[2,3] TBCB was developed with three objectives in mind: (1) obtain large enough tissues samples that would be representative of the underlying disease process and positively influence the diagnostic decision-making of a multidisciplinary discussion (MDD), (2) provide diagnostic accuracy approaching that of SLB, and (3) carry less complications than SLB.

The procedure has grown in popularity, with recent data suggesting a good correlation with SLB.[4,5] It has recently been recommended as a suggested diagnostic test in the evaluation of fibrotic hypersensitivity pneumonitis.[6]

TBCB is a procedure performed via either flexible or rigid bronchoscopy under general anesthesia in which a flexible cryoprobe is advanced to preplanned diseased locations within the lung based on the high-resolution computed tomography (HRCT) scan. The cryoprobe is then frozen for 3–5 s (sometimes longer depending on the time taken to generate a 5-mm ice ball at the tip of the cryoprobe) and adherent tissue is extracted en bloc with the cryoprobe. This method has allowed for consistently larger and more intact samples without crush artifact than traditional TBBx forceps (Fig. 5.1).[7]

Guidelines have been recently developed to facilitate standardization of TBCB to ensure patient safety and optimize diagnostic yield.[8,9]

PREPROCEDURE PREPARATION

General principles for performing TBCB consist of (1) appropriate training in the technique, (2) appropriate patient selection, (3) general anesthesia with either an endotracheal tube (ETT) or rigid bronchoscopy, (4) a prophylactic balloon blocker placement, and (5) fluoroscopic guidance.

The importance of proper training in the technique, either within a dedicated interventional pulmonology fellowship or with mentoring over several procedures by an experienced bronchoscopist, cannot be overemphasized. In order to safely perform this procedure and maintain a complication rate that is comparable to that reported in the peer-reviewed literature, bronchoscopy teams should have expertise in the management of life-threatening airway hemorrhage and tension pneumothorax. Familiarity with balloon bronchial blockers is mandatory, as well as expertise with rigid bronchoscopy.

Patient Selection

While no specific criteria exist for patient selection in evaluating someone for TBCB, in general, patient selection should mirror that followed for SLB. Developing a

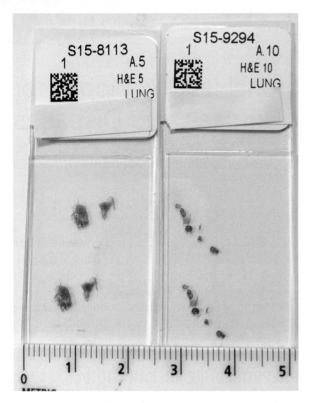

Fig. 5.1 Size difference between transbronchial cryobiopsy and transbronchial biopsy specimens. Specimens prepared on hematoxylin and eosin slide. Transbronchial cryobiopsy specimens on *left*; standard transbronchial biopsy on *right*.

TABLE 5.1	Patient Selection Checklist		
Patient Criteria		**Yes**	**No**
Clinical stability (outpatient status and not hospitalized or with signs/symptoms consistent with worsening of lung disease)			
Anticoagulant and antiplatelet therapy			
Laboratory data: 1. INR <1.5 2. Platelets >50, 000 Th/µL 3. BUN <45 mg/dL[17]			
Pulmonary function data: 1. DLCO >35% 2. FVC >50% 3. TLC >50%			
Hypoxia (≤2 L by nasal cannula): 1. Pao$_2$ >55–60 mmHg 2. Spo$_2$ >90%			
BMI <35 kg/m^2			
Pulmonary hypertension (PASP <50 mmHg by echocardiogram)			
Comorbidities: 1. Uncontrolled hypertension 2. Congestive heart failure 3. Ischemic heart disease 4. End-stage renal disease on dialysis 5. Severe aortic stenosis 6. Bullous lung disease or significant emphysema in the area of biopsy 7. Thromboembolic disease and unable to stop anticoagulation			

BUN, Blood urea nitrogen; *D*LCO, diffusing capacity for carbon monoxide; *FVC*, forced vital capacity; *INR*, International normalized ratio; *PASP*, pulmonary artery systolic pressure; *TLC*, total lung capacity.

simple preprocedure evaluation checklist will help ensure proper patient selection and patient safety (Table 5.1):

1. Clinical stability: A general rule of thumb is that if a patient is unsuitable for SLB, then they are probably unsuitable for TBCB. If the patient has clinical signs or symptoms consistent with worsening DPLD, particularly if an acute exacerbation of IPF is suspected, then the procedure should be canceled. Worsening dyspnea, progressive or rapid decline in diffusing capacity for carbon monoxide (DLCO), or signs of progressive groundglass opacities are all suggestive of worsening disease process.[10,11] While TBCB has been performed in patients on mechanical ventilation, we suggest that in the absence of data demonstrating improved patient outcomes, this should not be considered.[12]

2. Medications: Anticoagulants, clopidogrel, ticagrelor, other antiplatelet drugs, aspirin, and herbal supplements that increase bleeding should be stopped.
3. Laboratory data: International normalized ratio (INR) should be <1.5 and platelet count >50,000. No specific cut-off value for creatinine and blood urea nitrogen has been established, but it is prudent to avoid TBCB in patients with end-stage renal disease (ESRD) on dialysis until more data are available.

4. Pulmonary function tests: D_{LCO} should be >35%, forced vital capacity (FVC) > 50%, and total lung capacity (TLC) > 50% predicated.[4] A D_{LCO} of <35% increases the probability of adverse outcomes and mortality at 30 and 90 days.[13]

5. Hypoxia: Pao_2 > 55–60 or an Spo_2 > 90% while on 2 L of oxygen via nasal cannula is considered a requirement by some, while others consider any use of supplement oxygen a contraindication. Intraprocedural techniques to assess the patient's ability to safely tolerate transient peribiopsy hypoxia are detailed later.[4,14]

6. Obesity: There should be no significant abdominal obesity. A BMI <35–40 kg/m² is considered by some to be a reasonable cut-off value. Significant abdominal obesity may make it difficult to complete the procedure due to the rapid development of atelectasis and increased risk of periprocedural hypoxemia.

7. Pulmonary hypertension: A transthoracic echocardiogram is usually sufficient and is recommended to obtain before the procedure as many patients with DPLD may have coexistent pulmonary arterial hypertension. Pulmonary artery systolic pressure less than 50 mmHg with normal right ventricular function is recommended.[8,9,15] Some centers use BNP as a surrogate marker to exclude significant pulmonary hypertension.[16]

8. Comorbid medical conditions: Uncontrolled hypertension, congestive heart failure, ischemic heart disease, ESRD on dialysis, severe aortic stenosis, significant centrilobular emphysema or bullous lung disease in the area of biopsy, and thromboembolic disease unable to stop anticoagulation or with significant right heart dysfunction are considered contraindications to TBCB.[4]

Equipment

1. 1.9 mm or 2.4 ERBE cryoprobe (ERBE, Marietta, GA, USA)
2. ERBE cryo machine with CO_2 or N_2O gas
3. Flexible bronchoscope with minimum 2.8-mm working channel for 2.4-mm probe (larger working channel recommended for greater suction capacity if not using rigid bronchoscopy)
4. Rigid bronchoscope (operator dependent)
5. Rigid suction catheter (operator dependent)
6. Bronchial blocker (Arndt or Fogarty balloon; Arndt 7 or 9 French; the balloon should be large enough that, when inflated, it obstructs the segmental or mainstem bronchi proximal to the site of the biopsy)

7. Endotracheal tube (standard or wire-reinforced)
8. C-arm fluoroscopy machine
9. Basin with normal saline
10. Formalin specimen collection containers
11. Iced saline or other vasoconstrictor agent

Staff

1. Bronchoscopist
2. Second bronchoscopist or trained bronchoscopy technician to assist with prophylactic balloon inflation
3. Bronchoscopy technician to assist with specimen collection
4. Anesthesia provider
5. Bronchoscopy nurse to administer sedative medications and monitor the patient, if required

Setting

Location suitable for general anesthesia (bronchoscopy suite or operator room).

PROCEDURAL TECHNIQUES

Flexible Bronchoscopy Approach

- *Anesthesia, ventilation, and airway*

  General anesthesia, with or without neuromuscular blockade with placement of an ETT, provides a secure airway in the event of massive airway hemorrhage. By eliminating the cough reflex, risk of malposition of the cryoprobe during the procedure with the unintended consequence of moving the probe either too far into the periphery or too proximal in the chest is reduced. Positive end-expiratory pressure should be kept at a minimum (maximum 5 cmH₂O).

  One of the benefits of using an ETT is the appropriate placement of an endobronchial balloon blocker. There are two methods for placement of the endobronchial blocker in relation to the ETT: (1) within the ETT or (2) external to the ETT. If the endobronchial blocker is passed within the ETT, the patient is first intubated in the standard manner. An Arndt endobronchial blocker is passed through the ETT connector and secured to the tip of the flexible bronchoscope. The connector with the endobronchial blocker attached to the bronchoscope is then attached to the ETT and the balloon blocker is guided through the ETT and positioned proximal to the

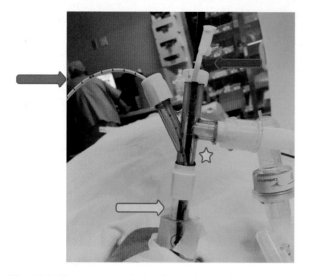

Fig. 5.2 Placement of Arndt endobronchial balloon blocker. The Arndt balloon blocker kit comes with an endotracheal tube (ETT) connector *(yellow star)* that attaches to the ETT. The endobronchial balloon blocker is passed through the connector *(blue arrow)* and meets the bronchoscope that was passed through the connector *(red arrow)*. The blocker is secured to the tip of the bronchoscope *(yellow arrow)*. The entire apparatus is then attached to the ETT.

airway segments being biopsied (Figs. 5.2 and 5.3). One potential limitation to this approach is that the balloon may cause partial obstruction of the ETT and impair removal of the bronchoscope and cryoprobe following biopsy, raising the risk of balloon dislodgement. Alternatively, the endobronchial blocker may be external to the ETT. With this method, the patient is fiberoptically intubated (either awake fiberoptic intubation, followed by total intravenous anesthesia [TIVA] once the tube has been secured or fiberoptic intubation following induction with anesthesia) with an Arndt endobronchial blocker positioned "piggyback" alongside the ETT (Fig. 5.4). This allows ease of placement of the balloon blocker at time of anesthesia induction without obstructing the ETT (Fig. 5.5).[18] One potential advantage of the ETT with an external blocker technique is the ability to selectively intubate the contralateral lung in the setting of severe hemorrhage while leaving the balloon in place on the bleeding side. If the balloon is placed in the lumen of the ETT, the balloon would have to be deflated and retracted in order to pass the ETT into the contralateral mainstem bronchi. A flexible spiral, wire-reinforced ETT (Fig. 5.6) is useful in these circumstances and facilitates easy insertion into the more angulated

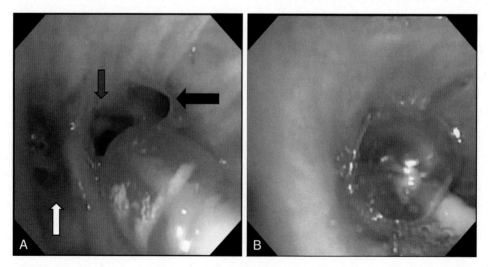

Fig. 5.3 Position of the bronchial blocker in the bronchus intermedius. (A) Correct positioning of the bronchial blocker in the bronchus intermedius. Right middle lobe *(white arrow)*, superior segment *(black arrow)*, remaining right lower lobe segments *(red arrow)*. (B) Fully inflated balloon occluding all segments. This is a test inflation for (1) balloon integrity and (2) assessment of patient's physiologic response to balloon occlusion. If the patient becomes hypoxic with this maneuver, the procedure is aborted.

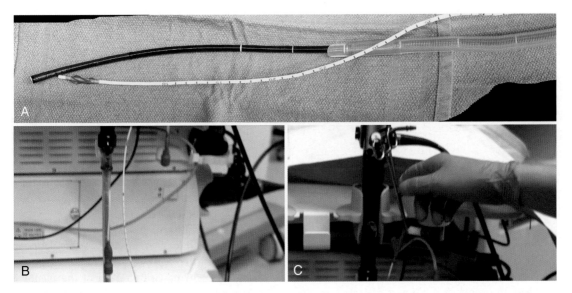

Fig. 5.4 Configuration of bronchial blocker external to the tube. (A) The bronchial blocker secured at the distal end of the bronchoscope. (B) Endotracheal tube loaded on bronchoscope and secured with tape. (C) Bronchial blocker attached to suction apparatus on bronchoscope with hemostat. Hemostat maintains cinch attachment of blocker to bronchoscope.

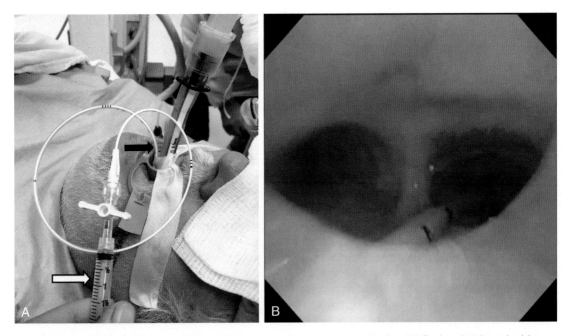

Fig. 5.5 Bronchial blocker positioned external to the endotracheal tube. (A) Patient intubated with endotracheal tube. Bronchial blocker is passing external to the endotracheal tube *(black arrow)*. Syringe attached to blocker to inflate the balloon *(white arrow)*. (B) Bronchoscopic view of distal end of endotracheal tube. Yellow bronchial blocker catheter is passing external to the endotracheal tube and is directed into the right mainstem.

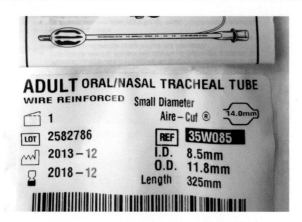

Fig. 5.6 Spiral wire reinforced endotracheal tube. An 8.5-mm internal diameter endotracheal tube.

left mainstem bronchus if biopsies are taken in the right lung and massive bleeding is encountered.

- *Use of prophylactic balloon blocker and bleeding prevention*
  Bleeding is a major concern with this procedure and prevention and expertise in controlling airway hemorrhage is of primary importance. Once appropriate patient selection has been done and the airway secured with either an ETT or rigid bronchoscope, the prophylactic endobronchial blocker is positioned proximal to the segment to be biopsied (Fig. 5.3). The use of a bronchial blocker (Arndt or Fogarty balloon) is considered mandatory by guidelines. Because the large size of the biopsy specimens requires the bronchoscope and cryoprobe to be removed en bloc after a biopsy is taken, the airway remains unprotected and without a bronchial blocker in the airway at the start of the procedure, valuable seconds are lost as blood rapidly fills the anatomic dead space with risk of asphyxiation and death. It is important to test the balloon prior to airway insertion to detect defects that would prevent proper balloon occlusion during the procedure. Once the balloon is in position, a test inflation should be performed to determine the patient's physiologic response to balloon occlusion. If the patient becomes hypoxic during the test inflation, the procedure should be aborted. Once the biopsy is taken, the balloon is then immediately inflated by a second bronchoscopist or trained assistant. After the biopsy is transferred to a saline basin, the bronchoscope is rapidly reinserted into the airway and the balloon is deflated after the scope is positioned in front of the inflated balloon (Fig. 5.7). The specimen is then transferred from the saline basin to the fixative of choice, typically formalin. Mild-to-moderate bleeding can then be controlled with suction, scope tamponade, or iced saline at the discretion of the bronchoscopist. If bleeding is severe and continues with these measures, then the balloon is reinflated to tamponade the bleeding and prevent soiling of additional airways. This technique was originally described with rigid bronchoscopy but then was adopted to allow placement of the balloon external to the ETT as described earlier.[18,19]

The application of fluoroscopy is essential to ensure that biopsies are taken as close to the pleura as possible to ensure representative sampling of diseased lung parenchyma (within 1 cm of the pleura is recommended) while also making sure that the probe is not too proximal so as to avoid large blood vessels and cause severe bleeding. Without the use of fluoroscopy, the stiff cryoprobe may become lodged more proximally than realized due to distorted airways or airway bifurcations if the bronchoscopist solely relies on tactile feedback. Some degree of bleeding should be expected with TBCB but the use of fluoroscopy may help mitigate this risk. Reports of severe bleeding have occurred in situations in which fluoroscopy was not employed.[20]

The use of radial endobronchial ultrasound (rEBUS) has been suggested as a means to reduce bleeding by identifying vessels and thus directed the cryoprobe to lung tissue devoid of vasculature. Currently the data are conflicting on its use in reducing bleeding and this remains an area of active investigation.[21,22]

- *Cryoprobe size and freezing time*
  Once the airway has been secured and the prophylactic balloon blocker has been correctly positioned, the cryoprobe is advanced into the segment of choice under fluoroscopic guidance. The size of cryoprobe used (1.9 mm vs. 2.4 mm) is operator dependent but there may be a higher risk of pneumothorax with the 2.4-mm probe.[23] No significant differences in diagnostic yield have been identified. Current guidelines recommend use of the 1.9-mm probe for this reason.[9] The smaller size may provide easier tactile feedback when the probe makes contact with the pleura.

The size of the sample will depend on the surface area of the probe and the duration of probe activation. As a general rule, the longer the activation time,

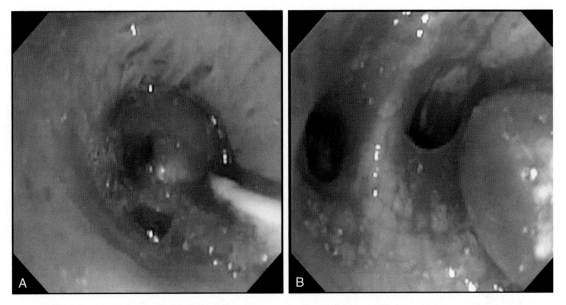

Fig. 5.7 Prophylactic bronchial blocker inflated immediately after biopsy. (A) Fully inflated bronchial blocker immediately after biopsy was taken from the right lower lobe. (B) Balloon is deflated once the bronchoscope is repositioned in the airway and careful inspection can be performed. Suctioning, scope tamponade, administration of vasoconstrictor agents, or immediate reinflation of the balloon can be performed for bleeding control if needed.

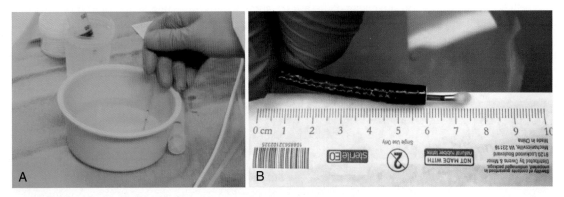

Fig. 5.8 Test freezing the cryoprobe. (A) Test freezing the cryoprobe. (B) Freeze ball should be approximately 5 mm in size. Freezing times vary to achieve this size.

the greater the sample size. Most freezing times are between 4 and 7 s with wide ranges of tissue sample sizes (9–64.2 mm).[7]

An often forgotten but important step before the first biopsy is taken is to test the time it takes for the probe to generate a 5-mm ice ball (Fig. 5.8). Because the pressure of the gas (CO_2 or N_2O) in the cylinder directly impacts the rapidity with which the tip of

the probe freezes, it is not uncommon for a full CO_2 tank to form a large ice ball within 3–4 s. If the probe freeze time is up to 7 s in this situation, a substantially larger specimen than anticipated may be obtained, increasing risk of complications.

- *Cryoprobe distance to pleura*
  Once the patient has a secure airway, the prophylactic balloon blocker is in place, and the fluoroscopy

C-arm is in position, the cryoprobe is advanced through the working channel of the therapeutic bronchoscope, into the target segment and directed close to the edge of the pleura under fluoroscopic guidance. The optimal distance between the probe and the pleura is essential for both safety and diagnostic yield, as samples <1 cm from the pleura significantly increase pneumothorax rates approaching 30%.[19,23,24] Adjusting the cryoprobe within 2 cm of the pleura has the added advantage of sampling small airways and with potential good success in diagnosing constrictive bronchiolitis.[25] The optimal distance of cryoprobe that is currently recommended is 1 cm from the pleura. Lateral airways are preferable whenever possible to assist with accurate positioning of the probe to the pleura. Under direct fluoroscopic guidance, the cryoprobe should be advanced until resistance is felt (considered to be in contact with the pleura). Once the edge of the pleura has been reached, the probe is retracted 1 cm, which can be estimated from the length of the metallic tip of the cryoprobe, which measures 1 cm (Fig. 5.9).

- *Location and number of biopsies*
The location of the biopsy will vary between patients and is dependent on the location and extent of disease as well as technical factors in advancement of the cryoprobe and position of the balloon blocker. It is recommended that biopsies be taken from two different sites: either a different segment within the same lobe or a different ipsilateral lobe. This parallels video-assisted thoracoscopic surgery (VATS)-SLB technique.[26] It also reduces chances of misdiagnosis since two different histologic diagnoses may be seen in different lobes.[27,28] It should be kept in mind that the risk of pneumothorax may increase if two different sites are chosen.

The number of biopsies per segment or lobe is not standardized and is generally operator dependent. However, it is recommended that three to five biopsies be obtained.[8]

- *Processing and collection of the specimen*
The TBCB samples should be handled with care to prevent crush artifact and allow pattern recognition. Once the biopsy is taken and the scope is removed from the airway en bloc, the cryoprobe with the sample attached is placed into saline. The biopsy is then moved gently from saline and placed into formalin (Fig. 5.10). The biopsy should then be embedded and oriented into paraffin to maximize surface area on the slides.

Rigid Bronchoscopy Approach

In general, the principles for each component of the procedure as detailed earlier for the flexible bronchoscopy approach are the same as for rigid bronchoscopy with the exception of some details as it relates to ventilation and balloon blocker. The potential advantages to the rigid bronchoscopy approach include the addition of a large suction device in the event of severe bleeding and

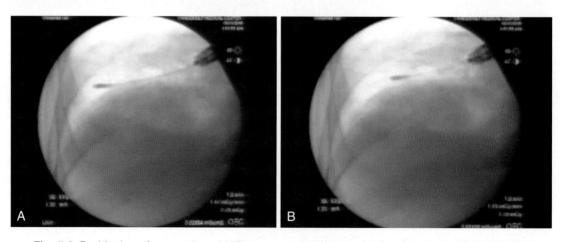

Fig. 5.9 Positioning of cryoprobe with fluoroscopy. (A) Cryoprobe is advanced until the pleural edge is reached. (B) The probe is pulled back 1 cm from the pleural edge. This is estimated based upon the metallic tip of the cryoprobe being 1 cm in length. This is the location where the biopsy is taken.

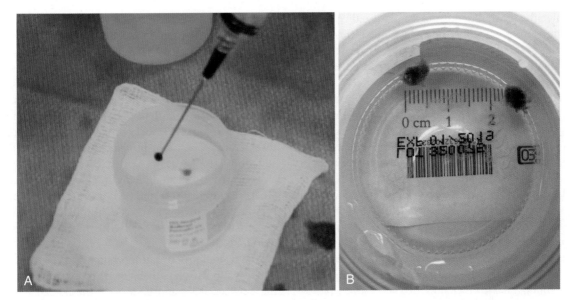

Fig. 5.10 Collection of cryobiopsy specimen. (A) Transfer of cryobiopsy specimen from saline container to formalin with blunt tip needle and syringe. (B) Freshly obtained cryobiopsy specimens.

a large ventilating lumen that allows passage of a therapeutic bronchoscope, endobronchial bronchial blocker, and suction.

- *Anesthesia, ventilation, and airway*
  With the rigid bronchoscopy approach, the patient should be intubated as per institutional standard operating procedures. Sanders' jet ventilation has most often been reported in the literature as this allows for an open system and permits rapid entry into and out of the airway, which is critical with this procedure. Sedation is achieved with TIVA and administration of paralytics. It is important to allow for adequate exhalation time in order to prevent accumulation of positive pressure, thus increasing the risk for pneumothorax. Biopsies should be taken between breaths if possible to reduce this risk as well. If conventional ventilation is used with rigid bronchoscopy, then the same ventilatory principles apply as for flexible bronchoscopy.
- *Use of prophylactic balloon blocker and bleeding prevention*
  A prophylactic balloon blocker is still required with rigid bronchoscopy. An endobronchial balloon blocker can be passed down the lumen of the rigid scope and positioned proximal to the segment to be

biopsied. The same procedures for test inflation and balloon inflation postbiopsy are the same as detailed earlier.

- *Performing biopsies*
  The cryoprobe is tested for the exact freeze time to achieve a 5-mm ice ball. The cryoprobe is then advanced through the lumen of a therapeutic flexible bronchoscope. The flexible scope is then advanced through the rigid bronchoscope and to the segment to be biopsied. The cryobiopsies are performed under fluoroscopic guidance and the flexible scope with the cryoprobe and specimen is removed en bloc through the rigid bronchoscope. The specimen is freed from the cryoprobe in saline and then transferred to formalin. The flexible bronchoscope is then passed through the rigid bronchoscope, placed immediately in front of the inflated balloon, and then the balloon is deflated and evidence for bleeding is observed. Bleeding may then be controlled with suction, flexible scope tamponade, or reinflation of the balloon if bleeding is brisk.

COMPLICATIONS

The safety of cryobiopsy has been a contentious issue with high reports of complication rates seen in situations in which the procedure was not standardized. With the introduction of guideline statements underscoring key elements to standardize the technique to improve safety, this should become less of a hindrance to performing the procedure.

In total, complications occur in roughly 25% of cases, with the most common being bleeding and pneumothorax (Table 5.2).[29] Some degree of bleeding is expected with TBCB and lack of a uniform bleeding severity score, differences in performing the procedure, and differences in size of the cryoprobe used have made it problematic in determining its precise prevalence and associated risk factors. Moderate bleeding, as defined by control of bleeding with endobronchial blocker or administration of iced saline, occurs in approximately 9%–14% of subjects; severe bleeding (hemodynamic compromise, ICU admission, surgical intervention, or active tamponade interventions) has an incidence of 1%.[9,29] Severe bleeding is felt to be more likely when biopsies are taken in the central zones due to the size of adjacent bronchial arteries. From a practical standpoint, however, it can be difficult to determine the exact location of the cryoprobe in the hemithorax on a two-dimensional (2D) fluoroscopy C-arm depending on the lobe and segment being biopsied and the orientation of the C-arm to the thorax.

Pneumothorax occurs in 9% of patients. The rate appears to be related to (1) the number of samples taken, (2) proximity of the probe to the pleura, (3) use of a 1.9-mm or 2.4-mm cryoprobe, (4) UIP pattern on histopathology, (5) fibrotic reticulation on HRCT, and (6) whether the biopsy was in the upper or lower lobes. The 2.4-mm probe, more than one biopsy site, and biopsy of the lower lobes is associated with a higher pneumothorax rate.[23] Chest tube placement is common in these situations (70%).

Exacerbation of underlying interstitial lung disease (ILD) occurs in 0.3% of TBCB and is probably more prevalent in individuals who are hospitalized due to an exacerbation of their ILD.[13,24] This rate remains lower than for SLB (3%).

The overall procedural mortality rate has been consistently reported less than 1% with pooled rates varying between 0.3% and 0.5%.[5,29–32] The 30- and 90-day mortality rate may approach 2.0%, with at-risk individuals being those who are hospitalized and/or had a worsening of their disease before biopsy, severe intraprocedural hemorrhage, and a D_{LCO} of less than 35%.[13] With good patient selection, this mortality rate should improve.

Rare complications include cavitary abscess, pneumomediastinum, bronchial laceration, and seizures.[24,33–35]

TABLE 5.2   Complications of Transbronchial Cryobiopsy

Complication	Rate
Moderate bleeding	9%[a]
Severe bleeding	1%[a]
Pneumothorax	9.4%
Exacerbation of IPF	0.3%
Prolonged air leak	0.3%
Transient respiratory failure	0.7%
Seizures	0.7%
Pneumomediastinum	One case reported
Cavitary abscess	Three cases reported
Bronchial laceration	One case reported
Death	0.5%

[a]Highly variable and dependent on bleeding classification used; one meta-analysis found rate of combined moderate and severe bleeding of 14%.[29]

IPF, Idiopathic pulmonary fibrosis.

EVIDENCE

Overall Pooled Diagnostic Yield of Transbronchial Cryobiopsy

Diagnostic yield is variable between studies ranging from 44% to 90% and is dependent on whether diagnosis was confirmed by histopathology or MDD.[23,36] In general, the pooled diagnostic yield is 72%.[29] The contribution of the MDD cannot be overstated as definite diagnosis may improve by as much as 24% when input from an MDD is considered (e.g., 44% to 68%).[36] This is critical as the MDD (with all clinical, radiographic, and pathologic data) remains the gold standard for diagnosis and, not infrequently, the histopathologic diagnosis may differ from the final MDD diagnosis.

Transbronchial Cryobiopsy Versus Transbronchial Biopsy

Conventional TBBx has a poor histopathologic concordance with SLB and a relatively low diagnostic yield

(36%) in DPLD.[1,37-39] In the only randomized trial comparing TBCB to TBBx, more histopathologic diagnoses were made in the TBCB group than in the TBBx group (74.4% vs. 34.1%, $P < 0.001$).[14] As such, TBBx is not recommended in the diagnosis of IPF.[1] Tissue specimens were significantly larger with TBCB (mean area size of 14.7 [$\pm$11 mm^2] vs. 3.3 $\pm$ 4.1 mm^2, $P < 0.001$). This larger specimen size with TBCB has been consistently reported across the literature (Fig. 5.1).

Transbronchial Cryobiopsy Versus SLB

The best data to date comparing TBCB to SLB come from a study of 65 patients who were deemed by an MDD to need a tissue sample and who underwent TBCB of two different lobes followed by VATS-SLB biopsy of the same lobes during the same anesthesia.[4] Three pathologists were blinded to the acquisition of the specimens and they were analyzed randomly in a nonsequential manner (a total of 130 slides). They were then discussed by an expert MDD, with all members blinded toward the type of biopsy. They reported a raw histopathologic agreement for guideline-refined patterns of 70.8% between TBCB and SLB ($\check{k}$ = 0.7 [95% CI, 0.55–0.86]). For the final MDD diagnosis, the raw agreement between the two methods was 76.9% ($\check{k}$ = 0.62 [0.47–0.78]). For those that were classified as having a highly confident or definite diagnosis by MDD, 60% (39/65) were by TBC and 74% (48/65) by SLB ($P = 0.09$). Using MDD as the gold standard, the diagnosis was changed from a low confidence to high confidence/definite in 74% (48/65) and 77% (50/65), $P = 0.55$ of TBCB and SLB, respectively, and mostly by changing from an unclassifiable diagnosis to a more specific diagnosis. Interestingly, neither TBCB nor SLB was able to provide additional diagnostic clarification in 12% of cases. These results provide convincing evidence that the addition of TBCB data to an MDD compromised of experts in ILD provides as useful information as SLB and, assuming the safety profile and performance of the procedure can be standardized, make TBCB an attractive and reasonable first-line biopsy technique in the evaluation of ILD.

FUTURE DIRECTIONS

While TBCB holds promise as a nonsurgical alternative in the diagnosis of DPLD, questions remain. Safety of the procedure still remains a concern and the lack of procedural standardization within and across centers remains a problem that guideline statements hope to mitigate. Optimal patient selection, probe size, number of segments and lobes to biopsy, use of REBUS, and training competency also remain areas of active research. It is also unknown what role genomic testing will play in the diagnostic algorithm of UIP/IPF and the interface this will have with biopsy specimens. The development of a cryobiopsy registry is needed to track the outcomes of these procedures and provide quality and safety feedback to centers, bronchoscopists, institutions, and the public. In the meantime, it would be wise for interventional pulmonologists to develop institutional procedural protocols to ensure maximum diagnostic yield and safety.

▌ SUMMARY

TBCB is a relatively new biopsy technique in the diagnosis of DPLD. It provides useful histopathologic information that can be incorporated into the MDD discussion to positively influence a definitive diagnostic outcome. The diagnostic contribution of TBCB is superior to TBBx and is good when compared to SLB. As such, it remains a good initial diagnostic procedure in patients with DPLD. The safety profile of TBCB has been contentious with severe bleeding being the most concern. With the institution of guideline statements that stress the routine use of general anesthesia, ETT or rigid bronchoscopy, fluoroscopy, and a prophylactic balloon blocker, the safety profile is expected to increase.

REFERENCES

1. Raghu G, Remy-Jardin M, Myers JL, et al. Diagnosis of idiopathic pulmonary fibrosis. An Official ATS/ERS/JRS/ALAT Clinical Practice Guideline. *Am J Respir Crit Care Med.* 2018;198(5):e44–e68. https://doi.org/10.1164/rccm.201807-1255ST.
2. Hutchinson JP, Fogarty AW, McKeever TM, Hubbard RB. In-hospital mortality after surgical lung biopsy for interstitial lung disease in the United States. 2000 to 2011. *Am J Respir Crit Care Med.* 2016;193(10):1161–1167. https://doi.org/10.1164/rccm.201508-1632OC.
3. Han Q, Luo Q, Xie JX, et al. Diagnostic yield and postoperative mortality associated with surgical lung biopsy for evaluation of interstitial lung diseases: A systematic review and meta-analysis. *J Thorac Cardiovasc Surg.* 2015;149(5):1394–1401. https://doi.org/10.1016/j.jtcvs.2014.12.057. e1.

4. Troy LK, Grainge C, Corte T, et al. Cryobiopsy versus open lung biopsy in the diagnosis of interstitial lung disease (COLDICE): Protocol of a multicentre study. *BMJ Open Respir Res.* 2019;6(1):e000443. https://doi.org/10.1136/bmjresp-2019-000443.

5. Iftikhar IH, Alghothani L, Sardi A, Berkowitz D, Musani AI. Transbronchial lung cryobiopsy and video-assisted thoracoscopic lung biopsy in the diagnosis of diffuse parenchymal lung disease. A meta-analysis of diagnostic test accuracy. *Ann Am Thorac Soc.* 2017;14(7):1197–1211. https://doi.org/10.1513/AnnalsATS.201701-086SR.

6. Raghu G, Remy-Jardin M, Ryerson CJ, et al. Diagnosis of hypersensitivity pneumonitis in adults. An official ATS/JRS/ALAT Clinical Practice Guideline. *Am J Respir Crit Care Med.* 2020;202(3):e36–e69. https://doi.org/10.1164/rccm.202005-2032ST.

7. Lentz RJ, Argento AC, Colby TV, Rickman OB, Maldonado F. Transbronchial cryobiopsy for diffuse parenchymal lung disease: A state-of-the-art review of procedural techniques, current evidence, and future challenges. *J Thorac Dis.* 2017;9(7):2186–2203. https://doi.org/10.21037/jtd.2017.06.96.

8. Hetzel J, Maldonado F, Ravaglia C, et al. Transbronchial cryobiopsies for the diagnosis of diffuse parenchymal lung diseases: Expert statement from the Cryobiopsy Working Group on Safety and Utility and a Call for Standardization of the Procedure. *Respiration.* 2018;95(3):188–200. https://doi.org/10.1159/000484055.

9. Maldonado F, Danoff SK, Wells AU, et al. Transbronchial cryobiopsy for the diagnosis of interstitial lung diseases: CHEST guideline and Expert Panel Report. *Chest.* 2020;157(4):1030–1042. https://doi.org/10.1016/j.chest.2019.10.048.

10. Fujimoto K, Taniguchi H, Johkoh T, et al. Acute exacerbation of idiopathic pulmonary fibrosis: High-resolution CT scores predict mortality. *Eur Radiol.* 2012;22(1):83–92. https://doi.org/10.1007/s00330-011-2211-6.

11. Latsi PI, du Bois RM, Nicholson AG, et al. Fibrotic idiopathic interstitial pneumonia: The prognostic value of longitudinal functional trends. *Am J Respir Crit Care Med.* 2003;168(5):531–537. https://doi.org/10.1164/rccm.200210-1245OC.

12. Cooley J, Balestra R, Aragaki-Nakahodo AA, et al. Safety of performing transbronchial lung cryobiopsy on hospitalized patients with interstitial lung disease. *Respir Med.* 2018;140:71–76. https://doi.org/10.1016/j.rmed.2018.05.019.

13. Pannu J, Roller LJ, Maldonado F, Lentz RJ, Chen H, Rickman OB. Transbronchial cryobiopsy for diffuse parenchymal lung disease: 30- and 90-day mortality. *Eur Respir J.* 2019;54(4):1900337. https://doi.org/10.1183/13993003.00337-2019.

14. Pajares V, Puzo C, Castillo D, et al. Diagnostic yield of transbronchial cryobiopsy in interstitial lung disease: A randomized trial. *Respirology.* 2014;19(6):900–906. https://doi.org/10.1111/resp.12322.

15. Galiè N, Humbert M, Vachiery JL, et al. 2015 ESC/ERS Guidelines for the Diagnosis and Treatment of Pulmonary Hypertension. *Rev Esp Cardiol (Engl Ed).* 2016;69(2):177. https://doi.org/10.1016/j.rec.2016.01.002.

16. Andersen C, Søren M, Ole H, et al. NT-proBNP< 95 ng/l can exclude pulmonary hypertension on echocardiography at diagnostic workup in patients with interstitial lung disease. *Eur. Clin. Respir. J.* 2016;3(1):32027.

17. Khan I, Bellinger C, Lamb C, Chin R, Conforti J. Bronchoscopy in uremic patients. *Clin Pulm Med.* 2010;17(3):146–148.

18. Hohberger LA, DePew ZS, Utz JP, Edell ES, Maldonado F. Utilizing an endobronchial blocker and a flexible bronchoscope for transbronchial cryobiopsies in diffuse parenchymal lung disease. *Respiration.* 2014;88(6):521–522.

19. Casoni GL, Tomassetti S, Cavazza A, et al. Transbronchial lung cryobiopsy in the diagnosis of fibrotic interstitial lung diseases. *PLoS One.* 2014;9(2):e86716. https://doi.org/10.1371/journal.pone.0086716.

20. DiBardino DM, Haas AR, Lanfranco AR, Litzky LA, Sterman D, Bessich JL. High complication rate after introduction of transbronchial cryobiopsy into clinical practice at an Academic Medical Center. *Ann Am Thorac Soc.* 2017;14(6):851–857. https://doi.org/10.1513/AnnalsATS.201610-829OC.

21. Berim IG, Saeed AI, Awab A, Highley A, Colanta A, Chaudry F. Radial probe ultrasound-guided cryobiopsy. *J Bronchology Interv Pulmonol.* 2017;24(2):170–173. https://doi.org/10.1097/lbr.0000000000000368.

22. Pannu J.K., Roller L.J., Lentz R.J., et al. Cryobiopsy with radial ultrasound guidance (CYRUS): a pilot randomized controlled study. J Bronchology Interv Pulmonol. 2021;28(1):21–28.

23. Ravaglia C, Wells AU, Tomassetti S, et al. Diagnostic yield and risk/benefit analysis of trans-bronchial lung cryobiopsy in diffuse parenchymal lung diseases: A large cohort of 699 patients. *BMC Pulm Med.* 2019;19(1):16. https://doi.org/10.1186/s12890-019-0780-3.

24. Ravaglia C, Bonifazi M, Wells AU, et al. Safety and diagnostic yield of transbronchial lung cryobiopsy in diffuse parenchymal lung diseases: A comparative study versus video-assisted thoracoscopic lung biopsy and a systematic review of the literature. *Respiration.* 2016;91(3):215–227. https://doi.org/10.1159/000444089.

25. Lentz RJ, Fessel JP, Johnson JE, Maldonado F, Miller RF, Rickman OB. Transbronchial cryobiopsy can diagnose constrictive bronchiolitis in veterans of recent conflicts in the Middle East. *Am J Respir Crit Care Med.* 2016;193(7):806–808. https://doi.org/10.1164/rccm.201509-1724LE.

26. Raj R, Raparia K, Lynch DA, Brown KK. Surgical lung biopsy for interstitial lung diseases. *Chest*. 2017;151(5):1131–1140. https://doi.org/10.1016/j.chest.2016.06.019.

27. Flaherty KR, Travis WD, Colby TV, et al. Histopathologic variability in usual and nonspecific interstitial pneumonias. *Am J Respir Crit Care Med*. 2001;164(9):1722–1727. https://doi.org/10.1164/ajrccm.164.9.2103074.

28. Monaghan H, Wells AU, Colby TV, du Bois RM, Hansell DM, Nicholson AG. Prognostic implications of histologic patterns in multiple surgical lung biopsies from patients with idiopathic interstitial pneumonias. *Chest*. 2004;125(2):522–526. https://doi.org/10.1378/chest.125.2.522.

29. Sethi J, Ali MS, Mohananey D, Nanchal R, Maldonado F, Musani A. Are transbronchial cryobiopsies ready for prime time? A systematic review and meta-analysis. *J Bronchology Interv Pulmonol*. 2019;26(1):22–32. https://doi.org/10.1097/lbr.0000000000000519.

30. Sharp C, McCabe M, Adamali H, Medford AR. Use of transbronchial cryobiopsy in the diagnosis of interstitial lung disease-a systematic review and cost analysis. *QJM*. 2017;110(4):207–214. https://doi.org/10.1093/qjmed/hcw142.

31. Dhooria S, Sehgal IS, Aggarwal AN, Behera D, Agarwal R. Diagnostic yield and safety of cryoprobe transbronchial lung biopsy in diffuse parenchymal lung diseases: Systematic review and meta-analysis. *Respir Care*. 2016;61(5):700–712. https://doi.org/10.4187/respcare.04488.

32. Johannson KA, Marcoux VS, Ronksley PE, Ryerson CJ. Diagnostic yield and complications of transbronchial lung cryobiopsy for interstitial lung disease. A systematic review and metaanalysis. *Ann Am Thorac Soc*. 2016;13(10):1828–1838. https://doi.org/10.1513/AnnalsATS.201606-461SR.

33. Skalski JH, Kern RM, Midthun DE, Edell ES, Maldonado F. Pulmonary abscess as a complication of transbronchial lung cryobiopsy. *J Bronchology Interv Pulmonol*. 2016;23(1):63–66. https://doi.org/10.1097/lbr.0000000000000182.

34. Barisione E, Bianchi R, Fiocca R, Salio M. Pneumomediastinum after transbronchial cryobiopsy. *Monaldi Arch Chest Dis*. 2018;88(2):909. https://doi.org/10.4081/monaldi.2018.909.

35. Machado D, Vaz D, Neves S, Campainha S. Bronchial laceration as a complication of transbronchial lung cryobiopsy. *Arch Bronconeumol*. 2018;54(6):348–350. https://doi.org/10.1016/j.arbres.2018.01.027.

36. Lentz RJ, Taylor TM, Kropski JA, et al. Utility of flexible bronchoscopic cryobiopsy for diagnosis of diffuse parenchymal lung diseases. *J Bronchology Interv Pulmonol*. 2018;25(2):88–96. https://doi.org/10.1097/lbr.0000000000000401.

37. Tomassetti S, Cavazza A, Colby TV, et al. Transbronchial biopsy is useful in predicting UIP pattern. *Respir Res*. 2012;13(1):96. https://doi.org/10.1186/1465-9921-13-96.

38. Berbescu EA, Katzenstein AL, Snow JL, Zisman DA. Transbronchial biopsy in usual interstitial pneumonia. *Chest*. 2006;129(5):1126–1131. https://doi.org/10.1378/chest.129.5.1126.

39. Sheth JS, Belperio JA, Fishbein MC, et al. Utility of transbronchial vs surgical lung biopsy in the diagnosis of suspected fibrotic interstitial lung disease. *Chest*. 2017;151(2):389–399. https://doi.org/10.1016/j.chest.2016.09.028.

Therapeutic Bronchoscopy Procedures

6

Rigid Bronchoscopy

Coral X. Giovacchini and Kamran Mahmood

RIGID BRONCHOSCOPY

Background

Rigid bronchoscopy has seen a recent resurgence, primarily for therapeutic indications, in management of patients with complex airway disorders.[1] The rigid bronchoscope owes its conceptualization to Gustav Killian, a German otolaryngologist, who adapted an esophagoscope for evaluation of the trachea and mainstem bronchi,[2,3] and performed the first documented successful removal of an airway foreign body, a pork bone fragment, in 1897.[4] Since then, evolution in bronchoscope technology and advancements of flexible bronchoscopic techniques have catapulted bronchoscopy into the mainstream for the general practicing pulmonologist; however, the rigid bronchoscope retains several specific indications and skills that will be discussed in this chapter.

Indications

Evaluation of the airways via bronchoscopy serves two primary purposes: diagnostic evaluation and therapeutic intervention. While there have been numerous technological advances in the flexible bronchoscope and many instruments adapted for use with it, the rigid bronchoscope remains the tool of choice for therapeutic interventions as it simultaneously provides a large conduit for ventilation and instruments.[3,5,6] Specifically, the primary indications for rigid bronchoscopy include therapeutic intervention for benign and malignant central airway obstruction (CAO), including applications such as cryotherapy, heat ablative therapies, stent deployment, foreign body removal, management of massive hemoptysis, and large diagnostic tissue biopsy

(Box 6.1). The use of the rigid bronchoscope is generally combined with the flexible bronchoscope, allowing for simultaneous therapeutic intervention in the large, central airways as well as smaller, distal airways.

Preprocedural Planning

Patient Assessment

A thorough history and physical examination is paramount when evaluating a patient for rigid bronchoscopy to review the indication, plan the procedure, and assess and mitigate risks. Patients undergoing rigid bronchoscopy may carry significant cardiopulmonary comorbidities that can adversely affect procedural outcomes if not carefully considered.[3] It is recommended that rigid bronchoscopy be performed under general anesthesia, and thus all patients being considered for the procedure should undergo a standard cardiopulmonary preoperative assessment and optimization as the clinical situation allows.[3,6] Basic laboratory tests including a complete blood count, chemistries, and coagulation studies may be considered prior to the procedure.

During the physical examination, special attention should be paid to the following upper airway examination parameters (Box 6.2):
- Oral cavity and Mallampati score
- Degree of mouth opening
- Thyromental distance
- Neck mobility
- Teeth and dentures.

Limitations in mouth opening, neck mobility, or a high Mallampati score should alert the proceduralist to the potential for a more challenging intubation with the rigid bronchoscope. The patient should be evaluated

---

BOX 6.1   Indications for Rigid Bronchoscopy

Therapeutic Management of Malignant Central Airway Obstruction

Debridement

Core debulking using rigid bronchoscope

Forceps debulking

Microdebrider

Heat ablative therapies

Argon plasma coagulation

Electrocautery

Laser therapies

Cryotherapy/cryodebridement

Stent deployment, especially silicone stents

Therapeutic Intervention for Benign Central Airway Obstruction

Direct and balloon airway dilation

Heat ablative therapies or cryotherapy

Stent deployment, especially silicone stent

Complex Foreign Body Removal

Management of Massive Hemoptysis

Direct tissue tamponade

Airway isolation

Large Diagnostic Tissue Biopsy

BOX 6.2   Preprocedure Upper Airway Assessment

Modified Mallampati Score

(Assessed by asking the patient, preferably in a sitting posture, to open the mouth and protrude the tongue as much as possible, without phonation)

Class 1: Soft palate, uvula, fauces, pillars visible

Class 2: Soft palate, uvula, fauces visible

Class 3: Soft palate, base of uvula visible

Class 4: Only hard palate visible

Mouth Opening

(Distance between incisors)

Normal: Three or more fingers

Narrow: Less than three fingers

Thyromental Distance

(Measured from the thyroid notch to the tip of the jaw with the head extended and mouth closed)

Normal: Equal or more than three fingers' breadth

Limited: Less than three fingers' breadth

Neck Range of Motion

Normal (>90 degrees)

Limited (<90 degrees)

Teeth

Full

Absent

Missing/loose

Buck teeth *(Prominent upper incisors/upper incisors protrude >0.5 cm from the lower incisors when teeth put together)*

---

for any loose teeth and removal of any dentures or other removable dental apparatus. In addition, all patients being considered for rigid bronchoscopy require an evaluation of neck mobility, both flexion and extension as well as lateral head movements, as appropriate positioning during both the initial rigid bronchoscope intubation and subsequent maneuvering of the rigid bronchoscope into the right and left mainstem requires neck hyperextension and lateral rotational movements of the head, respectively. This is easily accomplished by asking the patient to touch their chin to chest, then raise the chin to extend the neck back as far as possible, and finally to return the chin to a neutral position and rotate the head 90 degrees to look toward each shoulder. Should a patient demonstrate severe limitations in neck mobility, or cervical spine instability is suspected, as with rheumatoid arthritis or cervical spine trauma, rigid bronchoscopy should be avoided in favor of alternative techniques. If a patient's examination is concerning for a higher risk intubation, these issues as well as possible alternative plans for airway management and intubation should be discussed with the anesthesiologist prior to the procedure.

Equipment

The rigid bronchoscope is a rather simple but versatile tool, not having changed much in basic design from the time of its original design in the early 20th century.[2,3] While there are several manufacturers of rigid bronchoscopes, the three essential components of the rigid bronchoscope remain consistent: the barrel; the multifunctional head connector(s); and the rigid telescope, light source, and/or video optics (Box 6.3). Numerous additional tools and accessories have been developed to work within the working channel of the rigid bronchoscope during the procedure:

- *Barrel*: Barrels are manufactured in two general lengths: shorter rigid tracheoscopes and longer rigid bronchoscopes (Figs. 6.1 and 6.2). While the tracheoscope is made to simply intubate to the mid to distal trachea, the longer rigid bronchoscope allows access for intubation of the right or

BOX 6.3 Equipment for Rigid Bronchoscopy

Rigid Barrel(s)
    Consider different sizes and lengths depending on indication
Multifunctional Head Connector(s)
Rigid Telescope
Light Source and Video Optics
Tooth Guard
Adjunct Tools
    Rigid or flexible suction catheter
    Rigid forceps
    Stent deployer
    Airway stents
    Cryoprobe
    Electrocautery
    Argon plasma coagulation
    Microdebrider
Ventilation Equipment
    Traditional or jet ventilator
    Gauze for airway packing
    Silicone caps for rigid bronchoscope
    Self-inflating bag-valve-mask for manual ventilation

left mainstem and has fenestrations in the distal portion of the barrel to allow for contralateral lung ventilation during the procedure. Rigid bronchoscopes typically range in outer diameter from 7 mm to 14 mm for general adult applications, with a wall thickness of 1–2 mm and, due to variations between manufacturers, lengths will vary typically between 33 and 43 cm.[3,5] Some companies color code the size of the barrels making it easier for the proceduralist to identify the size on basic inspection. The barrel itself is essentially a hollow metal tube with a beveled distal tip, which helps with lifting the tongue and epiglottis, and atraumatic passage between the vocal cords during intubation. Further, the beveled tip itself can be used for coring the endobronchial central airway tumors. The proximal end of the rigid barrel can connect to the multifunctional head, allowing for ventilation connections, passage of instruments, and support for the light source and video optics. Selection of the appropriately sized barrel(s) is critical, as different-sized barrels will accommodate different needs and instruments, and multiple-sized barrels may be necessary for a single case. For example, a smaller barrel may be necessary in the case of initially securing the airway during the management of a severe tracheal stenosis; however, a larger barrel will be necessary later if silicone stent placement is planned.

- *Multifunctional head connectors:* The head is a small, separate piece that attaches to the proximal end of the barrel and generally houses multiple ports (Figs. 6.1 and 6.2). The side port allows for attachment of a standard ventilator or self-inflating ventilation bag while still accommodating for passage of multiple tools through the main working channel. Most head connectors include an additional port for a jet ventilator attachment.[6] Silicone caps can be attached to the proximal end of the head connectors to minimize the leak in the system and have ports for passage of tools and a light source.

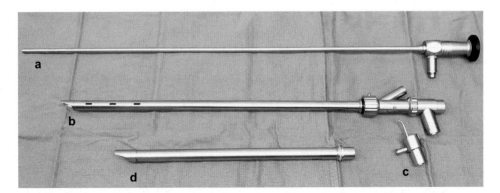

Fig. 6.1 Rigid telescope *(a)*. Rigid bronchoscope with side fenestrations attached to the head connector *(b)*. Jet ventilator connector *(c)*. Rigid tracheoscope *(d)*.

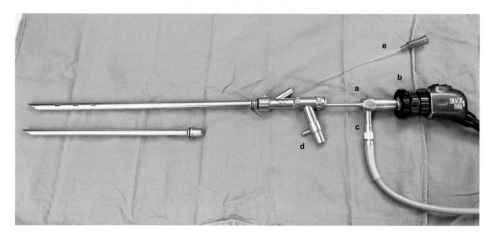

Fig. 6.2 Rigid telescope *(a)* connected to camera head *(b)* and light source *(c)* inserted in the rigid bronchoscope. Jet ventilator connector *(d)* and suction catheter *(e)* are attached to the rigid bronchoscope.

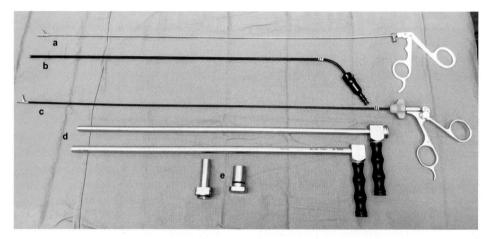

Fig. 6.3 Instruments that are used during rigid bronchoscopy. Rigid forceps *(a)*. Rigid electrocautery *(b)*. Rigid forceps with rotatable jaws *(c)*. Silicone stent deployers *(d)*. Silicone stent loaders *(e)*.

- *Light source and optics:* Most modern rigid bronchoscopes use a long, rigid telescope with a camera head attached proximally, and the image is displayed on a video monitor (Figs. 6.1 and 6.2). Several integrated rigid bronchoscopes have more recently been developed that include optics embedded in the distal end of the rigid bronchoscope barrel. Further during the procedure, visualization can be accomplished using a host of alternative visualization tools including a flexible bronchoscope, optical forceps, etc.
- *Additional tools and accessories:* Numerous additional tools and accessories have been developed to work

within the rigid bronchoscope to aid in the procedure, including rigid forceps, dilators, graspers, scissors, suction catheters, stents and stent deployers, and many others limited only by the imagination of the proceduralist (Fig. 6.3). All equipment for any anticipated adjunct procedures including cryotherapy, heat therapies, and stents should be available at the time of the procedure. We would suggest including a flexible bronchoscope in this arsenal to complement the rigid bronchoscope during the procedure. Gathering and assembling all necessary equipment prior to induction of anesthesia and beginning the procedure will allow for optimization of the procedure for both the proceduralist and the patient (Box 6.3).

STAFFING AND PROCEDURAL SETTING

While rigid bronchoscopy can be performed in an endoscopy suite equipped with appropriate staff, anesthesia support, and maximum monitoring capabilities, the vast majority of rigid bronchoscopies are performed in the operating room as this allows for the most control around the procedure, staffing, and appropriate management of any complications.[7] Staff for the rigid bronchoscopy procedure should include the bronchoscopist, an anesthesiologist, or certified nurse anesthetist comfortable with comanagement of the airway during rigid bronchoscopy, and a trained bronchoscopy assistant knowledgeable in rigid bronchoscopy equipment, tools, accessories, and the procedure itself.

Beyond staffing, the procedural setting should include monitors capable of providing adequate visualization of the bronchoscope optics used during the procedure, as well as real-time data for appropriate patient vital sign monitoring including blood pressure, heart rate, and peripheral pulse oximetry.

ANESTHESIA AND VENTILATION

Anesthetics

Due to the nature of the rigid bronchoscope's largely open system and significant air leak even when silicone-capped systems are utilized, total intravenous anesthesia (TIVA) is preferred for sedation during the procedure and the use of volatile gases should be avoided.[6] We recommend that the bronchoscopist be physically in the procedure room and present at the time of anesthesia induction, and good communication between the bronchoscopist and anesthesiologist prior to and during the procedure is critical. Deep sedation at a minimum is required for patient tolerance of rigid bronchoscope intubation; however, the addition of a short-acting neuromuscular blocking agent may optimize conditions for rigid intubation and allow for a more balanced anesthetic approach and lower doses of short-acting hypnotic agents.[6] Further, in a large database of patients undergoing rigid bronchoscopy for CAO, general anesthesia was associated with a lower rate of complications when compared to deep or moderate sedation.[8] As the majority of rigid bronchoscopy procedures are able to be completed within approximately 60–90 min, rapid onset and reversible agents should be considered in patients undergoing rigid bronchoscopy.

Conventional Ventilation

Ventilation during rigid bronchoscopy can be accomplished using a variety of methods via conventional ventilation or jet ventilation, each with their own advantages and disadvantages.

Conventional ventilation methods include assisted spontaneous ventilation or anesthetist-controlled ventilation. During assisted spontaneous ventilation, the level of sedation is carefully titrated by the anesthesiologist to allow for ongoing patient spontaneous respirations, while supplemental oxygen and assisted breaths are provided by the anesthetist as needed throughout the procedure via the side port of the rigid bronchoscope.[6] While this method can be effective, it requires a high level of involvement by the anesthesia practitioners and neuromuscular blockade should be avoided, potentially making rigid bronchoscope intubation and the procedure itself more challenging due to airway movement. Controlled conventional ventilation can be accomplished by allowing the rigid bronchoscope to act like an endotracheal tube and attaching the ventilator side port to a conventional ventilator or a self-inflating ventilation bag for manual ventilation. While this method allows for utilization of equipment already housed in the operating room, it can be challenging in that one has to overcome system leaks, by packing the mouth and nose of the patient, as well as using a silicone cap over the proximal end of the rigid bronchoscope. Despite the most thorough packing attempts, leaks in this system are common due to the uncuffed rigid bronchoscope; thus measurement and delivery of supplemental oxygen, consistent tidal volumes, and airway pressures can be inaccurate.[6] Some operators have described passing the rigid bronchoscope alongside a small endotracheal tube to allow for a small cuff in the upper trachea and minimize the system leaks. Importantly, during any conventional ventilation strategy, visualization of chest rise during ventilation and monitoring of pulse oximetry is essential.

Jet Ventilation

Jet ventilation, by either a manual or automated system, provides an alternative to conventional ventilation strategies and allows the airway circuit to remain open for procedural manipulation during the entirety of the rigid bronchoscopy procedure while providing adequate ventilation. In this mode, high-pressure oxygen is delivered to the airway. As the system is open, room air is entrained with the gas jet via Venturi effect. During high-frequency jet ventilation (HFJV), tidal volumes fall below dead space volume and instead of bulk flow, there is laminar air flow, direct alveolar ventilation, longitudinal dispersion, pendelluft, and molecular diffusion near the alveolar capillary membrane.[6,9] In both manual and automated jet ventilation techniques, the operator attaches the ventilator to one of the rigid bronchoscope side ports, typically via a luer-lock mechanism, determining a respiratory rate, ventilator driving pressures, inspiratory time, and supplemental FIO_2.[6] Each jet ventilator (Fig. 6.4) carries a different range of manufacturer-recommended settings that both the bronchoscopist and anesthesiologist should familiarize themselves with. The manual jet ventilation requires intermittent hand-triggered delivery of the high-pressure oxygen at a rate of around 8–10 per minute, allowing for adequate passive exhalation at an appropriate interval. Careful attention must be paid to patient chest rise and recoil when using manual jet ventilation. On the other hand, the automated jet ventilator delivers a respiratory rate of 60–150 per minute. Initial settings of HFJV may include driving pressure of 15–25 pounds per square inch (psi), inspiratory fraction of 30–40% and FIO_2 of 1. Inspiratory fraction is the inspiratory time divided by the sum of inspiratory and expiratory times. Oxygenation can be increased by increasing the driving pressure and inspiratory fraction. Carbon dioxide removal can be facilitated by increasing the

driving pressure and inspiratory fraction as well. During automated jet ventilation, patient chest rise may not be visible due to the rapidity of breaths; however, percussive movements should always be detectable by placing a hand over the patient's chest. Advantages of the automated jet ventilator include ongoing high-frequency ventilation and passive exhalation throughout the case, enabling the anesthesiologist to focus on other aspects of patient management during the case. Compared to conventional ventilation methods, both methods of jet ventilation allow for decreased diaphragmatic excursion, and lower mean and peak airway pressures allowing for greater airway stability during rigid bronchoscopy procedures and possibly shorter procedural duration.[10] However, potential disadvantages include hypercapnia as a function of the lower tidal volumes obtained during jet ventilation. Because end-tidal CO_2 is not reliably assessed in the setting of an open system, the team may elect to serially monitor arterial blood gases to evaluate adequacy of the gas exchange. Hypercapnia can be managed by ensuring an adequate expiratory time and increasing driving pressures with or without decrease in the respiratory rate.[6] Other limitations include the development of atelectasis due to the low tidal volumes and mean airway pressures during jet ventilation. Specific patient populations, including those with restrictive lung physiology, noncompliant chest walls, and obesity, can be challenging to ventilate with a high-frequency jet strategy. Increased airway pressures and respiratory frequency may be necessary to provide adequate oxygenation for these patients.[6] Obese patients can also be placed into the reverse Trendelenburg position, which assists in off-loading the chest by pushing the diaphragm and abdomen down. Nevertheless, manual ventilation with large tidal volumes may be required intermittently in some challenging cases. Prior to the rigid bronchoscopy, the proceduralist and anesthesiologist should discuss any concerns regarding ventilation strategies and possible backup accommodations arranged to optimize patient safety and procedural success.

PROCEDURAL TECHNIQUES

Procedure

All patients should be preoxygenated prior to the induction of anesthesia with 100% oxygen as is typically done prior to any intubation. Once the desired level of sedation is achieved, any oropharyngeal secretions are suctioned, and a tooth guard is placed over the upper

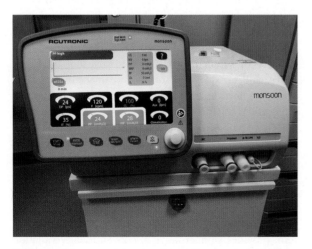

Fig. 6.4 Automated jet ventilator (Acutronic Monsoon Jet Ventilator, Acutronic Medical Systems AG, Hirzel, Switzerland).

teeth. There are a variety of tooth guard devices that can be used, including plastic mouth guards, foam rubber guards, or gauze pads.

Appropriate patient positioning is critical to the success of rigid bronchoscope intubation. The patient is laid in the supine position and the neck is hyperextended carefully by allowing the head of the operating room table to drop (Fig. 6.5A). The patient's head should always be supported and not floating off the bed after alignment is achieved. Each individual patient will have slightly different anatomy and require a slightly different manipulation to achieve optimal positioning.

Rigid bronchoscopy intubation can be achieved using a variety of techniques: direct intubation, laryngoscopy-assisted intubation, intubation alongside a previously placed endotracheal tube, or intubation via a preexisting tracheostomy:

- *Direct intubation*: The most common method is direct intubation, typically accomplished with the assistance of a rigid telescope housed within the rigid bronchoscope barrel. The rigid bronchoscope should never be blindly advanced. Utilizing this technique, the operator stands directly behind the head of the bed of the supine patient. The assembled rigid bronchoscope should be held with the bevel up in the dominant hand of the bronchoscopist while bracing the rigid telescope within the barrel so that any unnecessary movements are avoided, appropriate orientation of the optics is maintained, and the entirety of the distal rim of the rigid bronchoscope barrel is visible. The nondominant hand is used to brace open the patient's mouth and protect the upper and lower lips and teeth (Fig. 6.5B). The nondominant thumb in particular should be placed over the upper teeth as an additional shield from the rigid bronchoscope during intubation. The rigid bronchoscope is then introduced into the patient's mouth at a 90-degree angle and perpendicular to the bed, maintaining the rigid barrel bevel in the anterior position (Fig. 6.5B and C). The rigid bronchoscope should then be advanced along the upper airway, following the median sulcus of the tongue and the uvula, taking care to maintain a midline position within the airway. As the rigid bronchoscope is advanced, the operator slowly drops the angle of the rigid bronchoscope making it almost parallel to the bed, using the nondominant thumb as a fulcrum pressure point for the rigid bronchoscope barrel, taking care to maintain protection of the upper teeth. After passing the uvula and base of the tongue, the epiglottis will come into view. The bevel of the rigid bronchoscope should be used to gently lift the epiglottis so that the barrel of the bronchoscope glides as it advances along the airway, taking care to avoid trauma to the posterior wall of the pharynx. Once the epiglottis is elevated, a full view of the vocal cords can be obtained. With the vocal cords in view, the rigid bronchoscope is advanced while rotating the bevel of the rigid bronchoscope barrel by

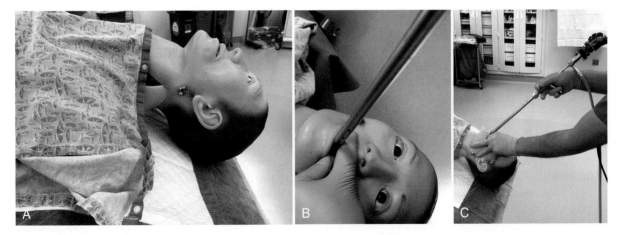

Fig. 6.5 Rigid bronchoscopic intubation. (A) Neck is hyperextended. (B) Lips and upper teeth are protected by the thumb of the nondominant hand, while the fingers move the tongue away from the bronchoscope. (C) Bronchoscope is held by the dominant hand and advanced into the airways.

90 degrees, allowing the bevel of the rigid broncho-scope to pass through the airway parallel to the vocal cords so as to minimize any trauma. As the barrel passes through the vocal cords, the operator should be aware of the location of the arytenoids inferiorly and avoid any damage to these while advancing the rigid bronchoscope through the airway, as the bev-eled edge of the rigid bronchoscope barrel can eas-ily induce injury with a cutting edge in this position. Once the vocal cords and arytenoids have been safely bypassed, the operator should rotate the barrel of the bronchoscope another 90 degrees so that the bevel turns posteriorly and ultimately comes to rest along the posterior tracheal membrane. Care should be exercised to advance the bronchoscope in midline and avoid contact with the airway wall. The bron-choscopist should ensure that the distal lateral venti-lation ports of the rigid bronchoscope barrel are well within the airway prior to connecting the proximal head connector side ports to the ventilation method of choice. Ultimately positioning the rigid barrel in the mid to distal trachea at the completion of the intubation should easily accomplish this appropriate positioning. In the case of upper tracheal masses that would limit appropriate positioning of the distal rigid bronchoscope ventilation ports, the bronchoscopist should use a rigid tracheoscope, with a shorter barrel that allows for a higher resting positioning within the airway. Please access Video 6.1 (Rigid Bronchoscope Intubation) online

- *Laryngoscopy-assisted intubation*: Some operators may be more comfortable obtaining a view of the vocal cords with a laryngoscope to assist rigid bron-choscope intubation. This method can also be utilized if there is difficulty obtaining an appropriate view of the vocal cords after an attempt at direct intubation with the rigid bronchoscope. For laryngoscopy-as-sisted rigid bronchoscope intubation, the patient is prepared and positioned in the same manner for direct intubation; however, a laryngoscope (either straight or curved) is first placed into the midline of the mouth to achieve a view of the vocal cords. The rigid bronchoscope is then introduced into the airway as described for direct intubation at a slightly lateral position to the laryngoscope. Care should be taken to keep the rigid bronchoscope as centered as possible to avoid any airway wall injury, and a direct view of the distal rim of the rigid barrel should be maintained

at all times during the intubation. The laryngoscope can be removed after the rigid bronchoscope passes the vocal cords, with the operator then relying on the rigid telescope for visualization during advancement of the rigid bronchoscope beyond the subglottic space.

- *Intubation alongside a previously placed endotracheal tube*: Should a patient already have an endotracheal tube in place, it can be used to guide the rigid bron-choscope. Utilizing this method, the operator should advance the rigid bronchoscope to the point of ele-vating the epiglottis and obtaining a clear view of the vocal cords. Once the vocal cords have been visualized, the endotracheal tube cuff can be deflated and tube removed under visualization, while the rigid broncho-scope is advanced through the vocal cords and into the trachea using the same technique as described earlier during direct intubation. In this scenario, the rigid bronchoscope replaces the endotracheal tube as the primary conduit for maintaining the airway (Fig. 6.6).

- *Rigid tracheostomy intubation*: Rigid bronchoscope intubation via a preexisting tracheostomy is a rather simple modified intubation technique. In this setting, the bronchoscopist may find it easier to stand to one side of the patient's head so as to approach the air-way laterally. Topical lidocaine can be applied to the tracheostomy stoma to minimize any postprocedural pain after manipulation with the rigid bronchoscope. The rigid bronchoscope is then passed into the stoma at a 90-degree angle with the bevel maintained in the anterior position, as is the case during direct oral intu-bation. Due to the short distance from the stoma to the posterior wall of the trachea, the operator should be prepared to quickly lower the angle of the rigid bronchoscope barrel in transition toward the parallel position, taking care to maintain visualization of the entire distal portion of the rigid bronchoscope bar-rel and avoiding contact with the posterior tracheal lumen during the intubation. Once the trachea has been intubated the bevel can be rotated to rest along the posterior tracheal membrane.

Once the rigid intubation has successfully occurred with the distal portion of the barrel resting in the mid to distal trachea and the proximal head connected to the ventilation method of choice, the rigid bronchoscope can be advanced to the lower central tracheobron-chial tree as needed. Because the rigid bronchoscope is an inflexible tool and limited by linear movements along the airway, the more distal lobar bronchi are not

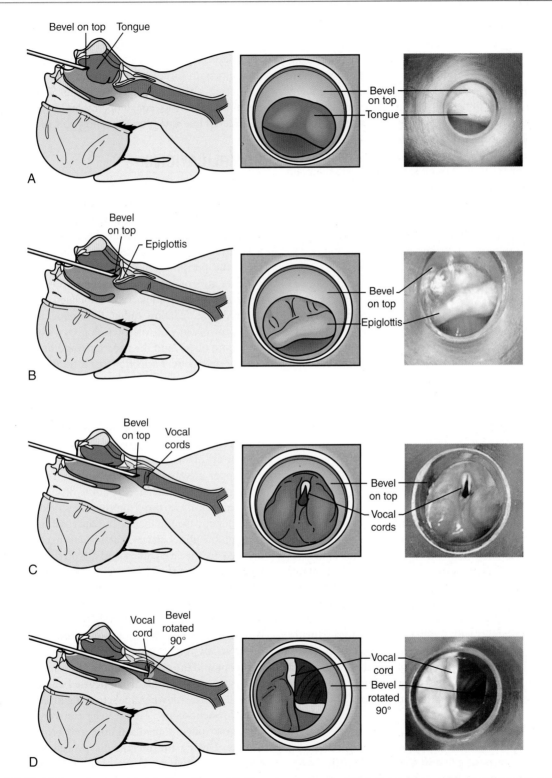

Fig. 6.6 Rigid Bronchoscopy Intubation Steps (A) Bronchoscope elevating the tongue with bevel on the top (B) Epiglottis came into view (C) Vocal cords came into view (D) Rotation of bevel to 90 degrees for introducing bronchoscope through the vocal cords.

accessible; however, the right mainstem, left mainstem bronchi, and bronchus intermedius can be traversed with the rigid bronchoscope with some maneuvering. For intubation of the right mainstem, the patient's head should be turned to the left, straightening the alignment from the trachea to the right mainstem. Similarly, turning the patient's head to the right allows access for the rigid bronchoscope to traverse the left mainstem bronchus. Regardless of the direction the rigid bronchoscope is advanced, the bronchoscopist should always maintain a clear view of the distal end of the rigid bronchoscope barrel and avoid contact with the airway walls. Loss of visualization, appropriate orientation, and contact with the airway walls while the rigid bronchoscope is advanced can result in serious airway injury and potential perforation.

Adjunct Procedures

As discussed, the rigid bronchoscope can function as a conduit for numerous other common tools and instruments that may need to be deployed during the procedure including but not limited to flexible bronchoscope, cryotherapy, electrocautery, argon plasma coagulation (APC), laser, microdebrider, and airway stent deployment. These therapeutic modalities are discussed in depth in other chapters.

PRECAUTIONS AND CAVEATS

Contraindications

There are very few absolute contraindications for rigid bronchoscopy; however, as with any procedure, the proceduralist should be familiar with these prior to considering rigid bronchoscopy. Absolute contraindications include unstable facial fractures, facial malformations, laryngeal disease or upper airway obstructions that would preclude passage of the rigid instruments, cervical spine instability with trauma or rheumatoid arthritis, prior cervical spine fusion, severe cervical spondylosis, or other limited cervical neck mobility that would limit hyperextension of the neck required for appropriate positioning and successful rigid intubation.[1,6]

Other Considerations

Because rigid bronchoscopy is performed generally for therapeutic purposes often in a vulnerable patient population, the goals of the procedure and potential benefits should be weighed carefully against the risks. There is a risk of respiratory failure with rigid bronchoscopy and anesthesia, and it should be contemplated against the predictors of successful therapeutic outcomes before subjecting a patient to the procedure. Similarly, other cardiovascular risks, coagulopathy, and so on, should be considered like any other bronchoscopic procedure.

COMPLICATIONS

Complications during rigid bronchoscopy are relatively rare, cumulatively reported between 3.9% and 13.4% depending on the series[5,8]; however, these can occur at any time during the procedure including intubation, as a function of adjunct procedure during the case, and/or in the periprocedural setting. Overall mortality of patients undergoing rigid bronchoscopy is <1%,[5,8] with increased complication risk associated with the use of moderate sedation rather than general anesthesia, American Society of Anesthesiologists (ASA) classification score of >3, and the need for re-do bronchoscopy.[8] Appropriate patient selection, team training, and development of expertise in rigid bronchoscopy are essential to mitigate these complications.

The most common complication after rigid bronchoscopy is a sore throat, but more serious complications can occur. Specifically, poor technique during intubation or an inadequate assessment of the teeth, mouth, and upper airway prior to the procedure can result in damage to the lips, teeth (including dislodgement), and oropharyngeal mucosa if appropriate shielding and care is not taken when maneuvering the rigid bronchoscope through the upper airway. Further, laryngeal edema and damage to the arytenoids and vocal cords can occur when traversing the larynx. Cervical spine injuries and paralysis can occur due to hyperextension of the neck in patients with severe cervical stenosis, unstable cervical spine or even with limited mobility in severe osteoporosis. Lacerations and perforation of the airway wall can occur at any time during navigation of the rigid bronchoscope and the operator should always have appropriate visualization of the distal, beveled end of the barrel to reduce this risk when maneuvering or advancing the rigid bronchoscope. Airway tear can result in pneumothorax, pneumomediastinum, and bronchovascular fistulae. During the therapeutic procedure, the bronchoscopist should be aware of the potential for bronchospasm, airway bleeding, airway trauma, and any additional specific complications that may be encountered by the use of adjunct procedures and tools.

Finally, the bronchoscopist should always be aware of the need for shared airway management with the anesthesiologist. Hypoxemia and hypercapnia can easily develop during rigid bronchoscopy and should be managed promptly. Adequate communication between the bronchoscopist and the anesthesiologist is needed at all times during the procedure to ensure appropriate strategic airway management and minimize the risks of any procedure under general anesthesia including respiratory failure, myocardial infarction, cerebrovascular accident, or death.

EVIDENCE

Benign and Malignant Central Airway Obstruction

We prospectively assessed 53 patients who underwent rigid bronchoscopy for management of malignant and benign CAO.[7] Flexible bronchoscopy was used as an adjunct in all the procedures. Airway debulking, heat ablative therapies, balloon dilation, and airway stent placement were performed as needed for the underlying disease process. Therapeutic bronchoscopy improved spirometry, dyspnea, and quality of life. The airway patency was achieved in 83% patients. The survival was better in patients with malignant airway obstruction in whom airway patency was successfully achieved. Complications from the bronchoscopy were rare, including airway tear, pneumothorax, and transient hypoxemia. Similar experience was reported by Ong and colleagues, who showed, in patients with malignant CAO who underwent therapeutic bronchoscopy, primarily using rigid and flexible bronchoscope, improvement in dyspnea and quality of life last long term.[11] While the flexible bronchoscope can be used to place various stents, the silicone stents cannot be deployed without a rigid bronchoscope.[12]

Management of Massive Hemoptysis

The rigid bronchoscope can offer many advantages when managing massive hemoptysis.[13] It can be used to intubate the mainstem bronchus of the lung from where the bleeding is originating, while the contralateral lung is ventilated with the side ports of the rigid scope. Various instruments, including flexible bronchoscope, large suction catheters, heat ablative modalities, endobronchial blockers, and so on, can then be introduced into the airway to manage the bleeding.

Foreign Body Removal

Removal of a foreign body was the first indication of rigid bronchoscopy,[2] and it dramatically decreased the mortality of foreign body aspiration. However, with the advent of the flexible bronchoscope in 1970s, most of the foreign bodies are now removed via flexible bronchoscopy.[14] However, the rigid bronchoscope can provide a larger conduit for foreign body removal, while maintaining the airway and ventilation. It has been used as a rescue procedure when flexible bronchoscopy failed.[15]

RIGID BRONCHOSCOPY TRAINING

Formal rigid bronchoscopy training is generally limited to interventional pulmonary fellowships and thoracic surgery training programs. Rigid bronchoscopy experience is only offered in around 4.4% of general pulmonology training programs, as flexible bronchoscopy has largely replaced the rigid bronchoscope as the tool of choice for general pulmonologists.[5] Several governing bodies including the American Thoracic Society (ATS), European Respiratory Society (ERS), and the American College of Chest Physicians (ACCP) have published guidelines regarding recommended training and suggested minimum procedural numbers for a proceduralist to obtain and maintain competence in performing rigid bronchoscopy. The 2002 ATS/ERS-combined statement suggests that all proceduralists performing rigid bronchoscopy possess prior "extensive experience" in both flexible bronchoscopy and endotracheal intubation and perform at least 20 rigid bronchoscopies while supervised in a training setting prior to independent practice, and at least 10–15 additional rigid bronchoscopies annually thereafter to maintain procedural competency.[1] Similarly, the ACCP agrees with these guidelines as a minimum for rigid bronchoscopy skill acquisition, but further emphasizes the importance of ongoing training, lifelong learning, and continuous periodic reassessment of skills and opportunities for improvement during the practice of rigid bronchoscopy.[16] As such, recommendations for training and evaluation of procedural competency have been moving away from simple number-based threshold towards skill proficiency assessments. One such tool, the RIGID-TASC, developed as a 23-point checklist scored on a 0–100-point scale by an independent examiner observing a trainee performing rigid bronchoscopy intubation and airway navigation, has demonstrated validity and reliability as an assessment of rigid bronchoscopy skills and ability to classify operators into novice, intermediate, and expert categories.[17] RIGID-TASC can be used for both initial assessment and ongoing periodic appraisal of rigid bronchoscopy procedural skills. Further, incorporating simulation-based training and skills assessments can also provide improved learning outcomes and additional competency in rigid bronchoscopy skills, and is recommended as a part of a multimodal training program.[1,5,16,18]

▌ SUMMARY

Rigid bronchoscopy remains an essential tool in the arsenal of the properly trained interventional pulmonologist or thoracic surgeon offering the advantage of maintaining a secure airway and effective ventilation while allowing for multiple rigid and flexible instruments introduced into the airway for therapeutic indications. Numerous adjunct techniques, including cryotherapy, heat therapies, and stent deployment, are optimized when utilized in tandem with the rigid bronchoscope. Prior to performing rigid bronchoscopy, the proceduralists should ensure appropriate patient evaluation, optimize comorbidities, maintain good communication with the supporting anesthesiology team, and acquire and maintain competency of the skills required to perform rigid bronchoscopy safely and effectively.

ACKNOWLEDGMENT

Hope Johnson, RRT, RCP and Wendy Curry, RRT for their assistance with figures.

REFERENCES

1. Bolliger CT, Mathur PN, Beamis JF, et al. ERS/ATS statement on interventional pulmonology. European Respiratory Society/American Thoracic Society. *Eur Respir J*. 2002;19(2):356–373.
2. Panchabhai TS, Mehta AC. Historical perspectives of bronchoscopy. Connecting the dots. *Ann Am Thorac Soc*. 2015;12(5):631–641.
3. Dutau H, Vandemoortele T, Breen DP. Rigid bronchoscopy. *Clin Chest Med*. 2013;34(3):427–435.
4. Prowse SJ, Makura Z. Gustav Killian: beyond his dehiscence. *J Laryngol Otol*. 2012;126(11):1164–1168.
5. Alraiyes AH, Machuzak MS. Rigid bronchoscopy. *Semin Respir Crit Care Med*. 2014;35(6):671–680.
6. Pathak V, Welsby I, Mahmood K, Wahidi M, MacIntyre N, Shofer S. Ventilation and anesthetic approaches for rigid bronchoscopy. *Ann Am Thorac Soc*. 2014;11(4):628–634.
7. Mahmood K, Wahidi MM, Thomas S, et al. Therapeutic bronchoscopy improves spirometry, quality of life, and survival in central airway obstruction. *Respiration*. 2015;89(5):404–413.
8. Ost DE, Ernst A, Grosu HB, et al. Complications following therapeutic bronchoscopy for malignant central airway obstruction: results of the AQuIRE Registry. *Chest*. 2015;148(2):450–471.
9. Sklar MC, Fan E, Goligher EC. High-frequency oscillatory ventilation in adults with ARDS: past, present, and future. *Chest*. 2017;152(6):1306–1317.
10. Pawlowski J. Anesthetic considerations for interventional pulmonary procedures. *Curr Opin Anaesthesiol*. 2013;26(1):6–12.
11. Ong P, Grosu HB, Debiane L, et al. Long-term quality-adjusted survival following therapeutic bronchoscopy for malignant central airway obstruction. *Thorax*. 2019;74(2):141–156.
12. Dumon JF. A dedicated tracheobronchial stent. *Chest*. 1990;97(2):328–332.
13. Davidson K, Shojaee S. Managing massive hemoptysis. *Chest*. 2020;157(1):77–88.
14. Hewlett JC, Rickman OB, Lentz RJ, Prakash UB, Maldonado F. Foreign body aspiration in adult airways: therapeutic approach. *J Thorac Dis*. 2017;9(9):3398–3409.
15. Limper AH, Prakash UB. Tracheobronchial foreign bodies in adults. *Ann Intern Med*. 1990;112(8):604–609.
16. Ernst A, Wahidi MM, Read CA, et al. Adult bronchoscopy training: current state and suggestions for the future: CHEST Expert Panel Report. *Chest*. 2015;148(2):321–332.
17. Mahmood K, Wahidi MM, Osann KE, et al. Development of a tool to assess basic competency in the performance of rigid bronchoscopy. *Ann Am Thorac Soc*. 2016;13(4):502–511.
18. Kennedy CC, Maldonado F, Cook DA. Simulation-based bronchoscopy training: systematic review and meta-analysis. *Chest*. 2013;144(1):183–192.

7

Mechanical Debridement

Russell Jason Miller and Lakshmi Mudambi

MANDATORY DOD DISCLAIMER

INTRODUCTION TO MECHANICAL DEBRIDEMENT

Mechanical debridement of the airways is the method of using tools to manually remove benign or malignant obstructive lesions. In principle, mechanical debridement of endotracheal or endobronchial lesions is one step in a very complex and intricate approach to the management of central airway obstruction (Fig. 7.1). The characteristics of the patient, the lesion, and the tools must be considered when choosing one method or modality of debulking over another. Additionally, what may be considered a basic bronchoscopic procedure can have significant risks if there is inadequate preparation or access to the equipment and skill sets needed to manage complications.

There are two major advantages of mechanical debulking. First, some of these tools (rigid coring, rigid dilatation, microdebrider) provide the ability to rapidly debulk tumors. This is important in lesions that are causing critical stenosis, especially in the trachea. Second, all these tools can be used in patients who have high oxygen requirements, whereas thermal tools are contraindicated due to the risk of fire. Still, it is important to remember that coagulation of a tumor prior to mechanical debulking remains a foundational principle of endobronchial therapeutic interventions.

RIGID CORING

Role of Instrument

Rigid coring can be used in the management of endobronchial obstruction from benign or malignant disorders. Typically, mechanical coring is used to debulk endobronchial obstructive tumors following devascularization with thermal therapies. Its unique benefit, however, is in the situation of life-threatening obstruction when rapid tumor removal is necessary to avoid asphyxiation, when there is insufficient time to use other modalities. The severe, life-threatening obstruction necessitating this technique is usually apparent at presentation, but occasionally an unexpected degree of obstruction and hypoxia will follow anesthetic induction and muscle relaxation. As such, it is an important skill that the proceduralist should be prepared to rapidly employ.

Equipment Details

As discussed in other sections of this book, the rigid scope is a hollow metal tube with a beveled distal tip. Rigid coring is the technique of using the beveled tip of a rigid ventilating bronchoscope or tracheoscope to debulk an exophytic endotracheal or endobronchial tumor. It is most useful to remove exophytic lesions that are pedunculated with a narrow-based stalk. It can also be used to debulk sessile tumors in pieces. This method allows resection of the tumor from the airway, but removal of the resected tumor requires the use of other equipment.

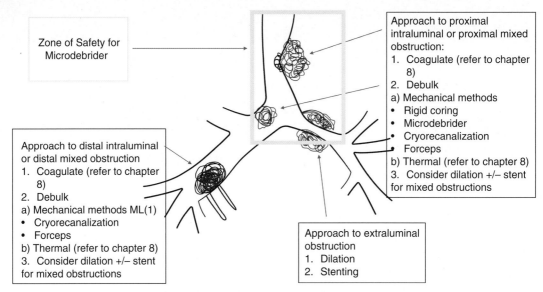

Zone of Safety for
Microdebrider

Approach to proximal
intraluminal or proximal mixed
obstruction:
1. Coagulate (refer to chapter
   8)
2. Debulk
a) Mechanical methods
   • Rigid coring
   • Microdebrider
   • Cryorecanalization
   • Forceps
b) Thermal (refer to chapter 8)
3. Consider dilation +/− stent
   for mixed obstructions

Approach to distal intraluminal
or distal mixed obstruction
1. Coagulate (refer to chapter
   8)
2. Debulk
a) Mechanical methods ML(1)
   • Cryorecanalization
   • Forceps
b) Thermal (refer to chapter 8)
3. Consider dilation +/− stent
   for mixed obstructions

Approach to extraluminal
obstruction
1. Dilation
2. Stenting

This diagram describes the technical approach to central airway obstruction. It does not explain the indications for intervention (see Chapter 8 for decision-making in central airway obstruction).

Fig. 7.1 Approach to central airway obstruction.

Method of Use

The beveled tip of the rigid scope is maneuvered gently to the proximal base of the exophytic lesion under direct visualization with a 0-degree rigid telescope. The plane of dissection is along the tract between the lesion and the mucosal wall of the airway. The rigid scope is corkscrewed gently across the entire base of the tumor while applying pressure along the plane of dissection toward the distal end of the tumor. Alternatively, rigid forceps can be used to stabilize the exophytic lesion while using the rigid scope to dissect it under direct visualization. The airway axis needs to be defined prior to coring, and the bronchoscope should remain parallel to the longitudinal axis of the airway to avoid accidental airway perforation. The use of tactile feedback is valuable to inform the physician as dissection occurs, ensuring that the airway wall and airway cartilage are not being perforated. This can help confirm that indeed the longitudinal axis of the airway is being followed when visualization is compromised.[1] The use of in-line large-volume suction catheters (rigid or flexible) is extremely helpful during coring to aspirate blood that can obstruct viewing and to collect detached tumor. Additionally, as there can be temporary worsening of obstruction during coring and

tumor removal, using suction to remove as much of the secretions, debris, and mucus surrounding the tumor as possible prior to coring will improve visualization and respiratory reserve during the intervention. Use of thermal therapies to devascularize the lesion prior to coring is strongly suggested to reduce the likelihood of bleeding. If devascularization is not possible or if there is significant bleeding, the rigid bronchoscope should be slightly advanced to cover and tampon the base for at least 3 min before evaluating the resection base for evidence of hemostatic control.

Pitfalls

While this technique is useful for debulking central airway tumors, it is also one of the most dangerous in inexperienced hands, especially in the setting of active clinical deterioration requiring rapid tumor removal or during active bleeding that compromises visualization. While the beveled tip feels blunt, one must always remember that when excessive force is used or airway planes are not respected, collateral damage such as mucosal tears, full-thickness perforation, and catastrophic injury to vascular structures can occur.

AIRWAY DILATATION (BALLOON OR RIGID)

Role of Instrument

Airway dilatation can be performed for both benign strictures as well as malignant obstruction and can be accomplished with airway balloons or serial rigid bronchoscopes, as well as serial insertion of tapered bougies. In malignant obstruction, the effects of airway dilatation are typically temporary, and it is typically used to expand the airway to allow for stent implantation or passage of other debulking instruments. Dilatation can occasionally be used alone in malignant disease, as a sizable minority of patients can have more than a transient effect, with one study showing short-term benefit with 43% of patients having sustained response at 7 days postdilatation.[2] Thus, when no other options are available, balloon dilatation can be occasionally used alone to briefly palliate symptoms or to facilitate extubation.

Dilatation can have long-lasting effects for benign strictures that are secondary to fibrotic weblike stenotic lesions.[3,4] However, complicated stenosis with cartilage involvement or in the setting of inflammation or calcified lesions (such as in fibrosing mediastinitis) usually does not respond to balloon dilatation alone.[5] The use of laser or electrocautery knife to create radial incisions into stenotic webs is advocated, prior to dilatation, to reduce the amount of uncontrolled mucosal tearing by generating controlled points for tearing and hence reducing local injury that can contribute to recurrence of stenosis.[6–8]

When choosing between balloon dilatation and rigid bronchoscopic dilatation, generally balloons are preferable, as they do not cause longitudinal sheering, which increases the degree of mucosal injury and risk of fibrosis and restenosis, since the balloon is expanded after insertion through the stenotic segment. In contrast, longitudinal mucosal injury is unavoidable with the forward insertion of rigid bronchoscopes or bougie dilators.[9] One advantage of the rigid dilatational method over balloon dilatation is that the tactile feedback provided by the rigid scope facilitates assessment of airway stiffness and resistance to dilatation, possibly reducing the risk of perforation when used by experienced operators. Another advantage of the rigid system is in patients with tracheal obstruction who have minimal respiratory reserve and cannot tolerate complete airway occlusion for the appropriate amount of time necessary to dilate with a balloon. In this situation the rigid dilatational method allows constant ventilation during the procedure.[10] By contrast, balloon dilatation requires 30–60-s periods of airway obstruction while the balloon is inflated. Jackson dilators are tapered bougies that can be serially inserted through an airway obstruction to dilate the airway lumen. They have been largely replaced by balloon dilatation systems, as they work similarly but require rigid bronchoscopy for insertion, obscure the distal view during insertion, and are difficult to use in the distal trachea, as the distal tip will angulate to either the left or right as it passes the carina.[10]

Equipment Details

Dilatational bronchoplasty balloons are designed to pass through the working channel of the therapeutic bronchoscope and are composed of high-pressure, low-compliance inflatable thermoplastic polymers that, when expanded by injection through a pressure-regulated water system filled with either saline or occasionally radiopaque contrast medium, inflate in a uniform manner to a specified diameter. There are a variety of disposable and reusable inflation devices available.[11] Balloons come as either single-phase dilatational balloons that expand to one specific diameter or multiphase balloons that expand to multiple different diameters depending on the specific manometrically monitored expansible pressure induced when fluid is injected. Originally airway dilatation was performed with 5.5-cm long balloons designed for esophageal dilatation; however, shorter balloons are now available that have been specifically designed for the airway.[12] Typically, the balloons can be wire-guided, but this is usually only necessary in rare cases where balloon dilatation is performed using fluoroscopy without bronchoscopic guidance.

Vascular cutting balloons work in a similar fashion to standard dilatational balloons; however, they have three to four longitudinally oriented microsurgical blades attached that, during dilatation, produce incisions that reduce uncontrolled mucosal tears. Cutting balloons have traditionally only been placed over a guidewire using fluoroscopic guidance, due to the high risk of bronchoscope damage. This has made them a generally unattractive option for bronchoscopic dilatation; however, reports of these balloons being used in the management of airway obstruction do exist, and there are few situations where cutting balloons might have unique advantages over other dilatational methods.[13,14] The first is in extremely tight long-segment stenosis or when hypoxia exists that precludes safe usage of the electrocautery knife or laser for creation of mucosal incisions, and the second is in children where only small-caliber bronchoscopes, which do not allow the insertion of cutting instruments, are required. Although rarely used in the airways, the role of cutting balloons might gain new attention, since bronchoscopic insertion could be performed through disposable bronchoscopes that are now widely available. Malleable, high-volume, low-pressure, vascular latex Fogarty balloons are traditionally considered an emergency tool to rapidly occlude a hemorrhagic airway, but they also can have an occasional role in dilatation, which we will discuss further within this section.

Serial insertion of standard rigid bronchoscopes of increasing size is also an effective tool for airway dilatation. The ability to perform rigid dilatation, however, does depend on the rigid system that is being used. The Jackson rigid bronchoscope, which is no longer produced, was considered ideal for airway dilatation due to the presence of a blunt and more rounded tip that allowed for safer passage through the obstruction when compared with the modern rigid bronchoscopes.[15] Serial rigid dilatation is much more practical with modular rigid bronchoscopic systems with detachable universal bases than systems where the base is fused to the barrel of the bronchoscope. By first inserting a large-caliber tracheoscope, detaching the base, and then inserting smaller-diameter but longer-ventilating rigid bronchoscopes, serial dilatation can be achieved without the need to reintubate the patient every time.

Methods of Use

Rigid bronchoscopic dilatation requires general anesthesia, whereas balloon dilatation with conscious sedation is an option for disease distal to the main carina. Some patients can tolerate tracheal dilatation under moderate sedation; however, often general anesthesia may be necessary with prolonged dilatation, as a sense of asphyxiation may result in considerable distress to the patient.

As mentioned previously, radial incisions with either the electrocautery knife or with laser can reduce the amount of uncontrolled tearing and fibrin production, hence decreasing the likelihood of restenosis. The electrocautery knife is a reusable instrument that is employed

through the working channel of a flexible bronchoscope. Selection of a laser with cutting properties (carbon dioxide, holmium:yttrium aluminum garnet, or diode) provides the best option to produce precise radial incisions without inciting an inflammatory response or deeper tissue damage.[16] Three 1–2-mm incisions mimicking the Mercedes emblem (12, 4, 8 o'clock) are made along the stenosis.[7] Following radial incision, balloon bronchoplasty is typically performed.

For balloon bronchoplasty, the size of the balloon selected depends on consideration the size of the stenotic airway as well as consideration of the normal adjacent airways that are contiguous with the lesion. When balloons are oversized relative to the stenosis, the improvement of diameter will be greater, but the risk of airway perforation will also be higher. Small incremental dilatations should be performed beginning with a balloon that only slightly expands the airway. Dilatation is continued serially with balloons of increasing size until target dilatation is achieved. The literature varies in regard to the optimal inflation time and repetitions, but typically two to three dilatations with inflation periods of 30 to 90 s per dilatational stage are sufficient.[7,9,10]

The specifications of balloon and inflation device preparation vary based on manufacturer. It is important to refer to the user manual, as an in-depth description of each of these devices is beyond the scope of this chapter. There is a tag on each balloon that correlates specific manometric pressures to balloon inflation diameter. Lubricating the tip of the deflated balloon can help pass the instrument more easily through the working channel of a flexible bronchoscope. The balloon must be completely out of the working channel prior to inflation to prevent scope damage. The uninflated balloon should be passed into the stenotic segment with at least 0.5 cm of the balloon proximal to the level of the stenosis, as it can easily slide out of place if too proximal or distal.[9] Retraction of the balloon to make contact with the tip of the flexible bronchoscope while simultaneously inflating it can fix the balloon in place across the stenosis. A 360-degree view through the balloon can be obtained by applying suction to the fluid-filled balloon, which allows the operator to visualize developing airway tears, indicating potential for perforation (see Fig. 7.2). Once the dilatation cycles are complete, the balloon can be deflated and removed from the working channel. Repeated reinsertion results in reduced catheter tip strength, which can make it impossible to reinsert the balloon. This is

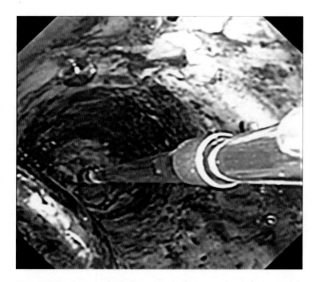

Fig. 7.2 Balloon dilatation of malignant obstruction with airway view through the balloon.

The major risk of inflating a balloon catheter beyond the visible field is airway injury or rupture; however, this is much less likely with the soft malleable Fogarty balloon. This technique is useful in segmental airways, at acute angles where stiffer flexible instruments such as the cryoprobe or forceps prevent adequate scope flexion required to engage the target tissue.

For rigid bronchoscopic dilatation, it is ideal to insert a large tracheoscope and detach the universal base, which will allow insertion of smaller rigid bronchoscopes in a serial fashion without requiring repeated reintubations. In tight stenosis the use of neonatal/pediatric bronchoscopes during the initial phases of dilatation is sometimes necessary. The rigid bronchoscopes are inserted through the stenotic lesion using a twisting motion similar to the apple-coring motion used for mechanically debulking tumors. As ventilation can be maintained with this technique, dilatation can be performed for longer periods than with balloon dilatation.

Pitfalls

It is important to consider the patient's ability to tolerate periods of hypoxia and hypoventilation during dilatation, especially with tracheal involvement or in patients with contralateral disease when dilatation is performed beyond the main carina. In addition to inability to tolerate long tracheal dilatation periods, symptoms consistent with negative pressure pulmonary edema have also been reported following long periods of tracheal dilatation in the spontaneously breathing patient.[21] Barotrauma resulting in pneumothorax or pneumomediastinum can theoretically occur when jet ventilation is used beyond a tight stenosis, especially with higher respiratory rates or with accidental occlusion of the proximal ports. If the patient can tolerate it, holding ventilation during balloon inflation periods is reasonable. To minimize the risk of accidental expiratory occlusion, caution should be used if instrumentation is performed through the rigid bronchoscope during dilatation, and simultaneous insertion of multiple instruments should be avoided.

Overinflation of dilatational balloons can result in airway lacerations, bleeding, and perforation.[9,22] It is important to vigilantly monitor the airway mucosa through the inflated balloon for signs of developing airway tears and to use gentle incremental dilatations instead of dilating to a maximum or near-maximum diameter immediately. A potential source for accidental

less of a problem with some of the newer inflation balloons that are designed to allow multiple passes through the working channel of the scope.

Wire-guided balloon dilatation with fluoroscopy without bronchoscopic visualization is an alternative method to direct bronchoscopic visualization of balloon dilatation, which is performed in a similar manner to fluoroscopic-guided insertion of self-expandable metallic stents. This method might be considered in children or patients intubated with smaller endotracheal tubes that cannot accommodate the therapeutic bronchoscope.[17] The major disadvantage of this technique is the inability to visually monitor for complications such as evidence of impending airway rupture or hemorrhage. For this procedure the balloon is filled with a nonionic water-soluble contrast material such as iohexol diluted at least 50% in case of accidental balloon rupture, as hypertonic solutions can result in serious bronchospasm.[9,18]

Fogarty balloons can be useful adjuncts to standard balloon dilatation, especially in the smaller airways. When the larger, more rigid dilating balloons cannot safely pass an obstruction, the soft malleable Fogarty catheter can be extended beyond the obstruction prior to inflating, and then the catheter can be withdrawn in a retrograde fashion.[19] This technique can be used to compress an obstructive tumor against the airway walls or for extraction of debris, clots, or foreign bodies.[9,20]

overinflation is related to miscommunications between bronchoscopist and technician, as the pressure in standard atmospheres (atm) required to inflate the balloon to a specific diameter in millimeters falls in similar ranges. For example, a balloon might require 8 atm to inflate to 12 mm. If the technician interprets the instruction of "inflate to 12" to mean atm, balloon rupture could occur. Closed-loop communication can help mitigate this risk.

Aggressive dilatation of highly vascular lesions, mixed obstructive tumors involving vasculature adjacent to the airway, or those with fragile mucosa or ulceration can lead to significant hemorrhage. Balloon dilatation should usually be avoided when visualization is impaired beyond the stenosis, but very gentle dilatation with the tip of the balloon is safe even in tight stenosis to allow distal visualization.

RIGID FORCEPS

Role of Instrument

The rigid forceps are indispensable and possibly the most useful instruments available to the rigid bronchoscopist. Competence with the forceps is a mandatory skill for anyone who performs rigid bronchoscopic procedures. They are the primary modality for removing detached tissue, foreign bodies, and stents from the airways but also play an important role in the debulking of endobronchial obstructive lesions.

Equipment Details

The rigid forceps are available in several different configurations similar to the flexible forceps: cupped, alligator, pointed serrated, and peanut grasping. Forceps are broadly classified as either single action or double action based on whether only one jaw or both move with opening (see Fig. 7.3). Typical rigid forceps open in a superior and inferior orientation; however, forceps are available that allow rotation of the tip while the operator maintains the hand in a neutral position, as well as backward grasping forceps which open proximally. While most forcep handles are nonratcheting, allowing for free opening and closing, ratcheted forceps are also available that allow the operator freedom to release the handle grip. The rigid cupped forceps have a smooth tip and are appropriate for obtaining biopsies. They produce minimal trauma to the mucosa and surrounding normal tissue. The rigid alligator forceps have a sharp tip

and serrated teeth, making them appropriate for grasping large tumors, foreign bodies, and stents for removal through the rigid bronchoscope.[23] The rigid optical forceps are forceps that are coupled with a channel through which the telescope is secured. They are available in several configurations as well.

Method of Use

For tumor debulking, the beveled tip of the rigid bronchoscope is maneuvered to the proximal end of the tumor in the airway. The rigid forceps are passed through the rigid bronchoscope just distal to but parallel with the rigid telescope so that the tip is always visible. The forceps are opened, and pieces of the tumor are grasped and removed under direct visualization by moving the telescope and forceps as a single unit. If using the rigid optical forceps, the telescope is inserted into the channel and locked in place before inserting the forceps into the rigid bronchoscope. The optical forceps allow for direct viewing during grasping; however, they are less maneuverable, cannot be inserted through smaller rigid bronchoscopes, and cannot access tissue that extends more than a short distance beyond the reach of the rigid telescope. Familiarity with both optical and nonoptical instruments is necessary.

Pitfalls

The rigid forceps can cause mucosal tears and perforations if used incorrectly. When working in tight spaces, the rigid forceps can often extend to a diameter greater than that of the residual airway. When this is done using sharp-tipped forceps, such as the alligator forceps, perforation or mucosal tears can develop. In this scenario the use of single-action forceps with the opening jaw directed toward the lumen can reduce the likelihood of injury. Just as with the other nonthermal therapies that have been discussed, there is no coagulative effect, and use of rigid forceps generally should be performed in conjunction with thermal therapies.

FLEXIBLE FORCEPS

Role of Instrument

Flexible forceps are not designed for tumor debulking but rather as a tool for biopsy. In debulking procedures, flexible forceps can be used to remove debris following thermal treatments such as argon plasma coagulation (APC) or laser, but standard biopsy forceps can also

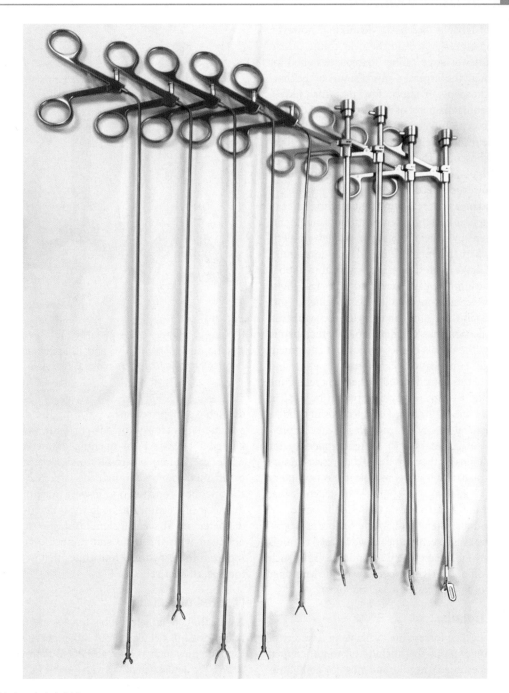

Fig. 7.3 Variety of rigid forceps.

have a role in debulking tumor in small spaces, such as the bronchus intermedius, lobar, or segmental bronchi. They are also useful for necrotic tumors with low propensity for bleeding. Flexible forceps can also be helpful in areas in which precision is needed, such as when debulking recurrent tumor or granulation tissue near metallic stents, which could be damaged with the larger and less precise rigid forceps.

The role of flexible forceps in debulking, however, might develop a greater role in the near future due to the advent of newer large-caliber forceps, designed for insertion through the larger 2.8-mm channel of the therapeutic bronchoscope, or jumbo forceps, which have a maximum opening diameter of nearly twice that of standard biopsy forceps and can be used through a 3.2-mm channel of the recently reintroduced large channel therapeutic bronchoscope. There are no data regarding the role of the large and jumbo flexible forceps for tumor debulking; however, anecdotally they have provided a relatively rapid means of removing tissue debris and can be an effective tool for larger central tumors, augmenting rigid forceps by providing greater maneuverability. An example where this might be useful includes debulking tumors at acute angles, such as just distal to a lobar carina, which cannot be easily accessed with rigid tools.

The use of insulated monopolar electrocautery "hot" forceps, which allow for simultaneous electrocoagulation and tissue collection, has a limited role in therapeutic bronchoscopy. The details of the physics and equipment required to utilize the electrocautery forceps can be found in the chapter of this book devoted to thermal therapeutic devices (Chapter 8). Hot biopsy forceps can be used in similar situations as the standard cold forceps in debulking more peripheral airway obstruction and may be preferable for vascular tumors with a high propensity for bleeding. Additionally, they can be used to resect tumors arising from a stalk that is not amenable to electrocautery snare due to a wide base, or complete obstruction that does not allow the snare to bypass the lesion.[24] Obviously, for tracheal and mainstem lesions, other, more appropriate therapies are available, but when a wide-based tumor is present just beyond an angulated secondary carina, such as at the take-off of the right upper lobe or the left upper lobe proper, hot forceps can be a useful tool.

Equipment Details

The standard flexible forceps are available in a variety of sizes and configurations that include rat tooth, cupped (smooth or fenestrated), needle, and alligator configurations. For the purpose of mechanical debulking, alligator forceps are generally the preferred configuration, as the disadvantage of crush artifact on histology is not an issue.

The most commonly used flexible forceps for both endobronchial biopsy and transbronchial lung biopsy can be inserted through a standard 2.0-mm bronchoscope working channel and have a maximum opening

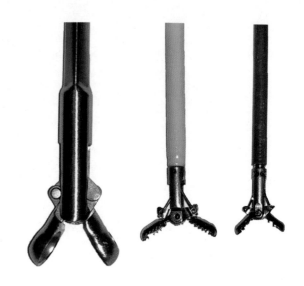

Fig. 7.4 Size comparison between (A) rigid forceps, (B) large biopsy forceps (Boston Scientific Corp., Marlborough, MA, USA), and (C) standard biopsy forceps (Olympus Corp., Shinjuku City, Tokyo, Japan).

diameter of approximately 5.0 mm. The dedicated disposable large biopsy forceps currently available in the United States have an opening diameter of 7.1 mm, while the jumbo gastrointestinal forceps, which can be adapted for use through the large 3.2-mm channel therapeutic bronchoscope, have a maximum opening diameter of 8.8 mm. Although the difference in opening diameter might seem insignificant, the sample volume obtained with the large and jumbo forceps has been reported to be two and four times that of the standard forceps, respectively (see Fig. 7.4).[25,26]

Method of Use

As mentioned earlier, flexible forceps are rarely the primary mode of debulking but rather serve as an adjunct to modalities such as laser or APC to remove coagulated debris. For actual debulking with flexible forceps, the technique is most applicable when tumor is directly in front of the endoscope, whereas when tumor is lying along the airway wall, the "burn and shave" method, using the barrel of the rigid bronchoscope to shave off coagulated debris, is more effective than using flexible forceps.

When using the biopsy forceps, it is helpful to keep the forceps in close proximity to the lesion and advance the scope with the forceps as a unit to increase the depth of tissue collection. After closing the forceps, the forceps and bronchoscope should be retracted as a single unit until the tissue detaches from the primary tumor. This will result in much larger pieces of removed tissue. These pieces are released as detached tissue fragments in the airway until multiple detached fragments have accumulated, which can then be suctioned en bloc from the airway or removed with the assistance of a bronchoscopic basket. This technique saves time and allows the operator to maintain a view of the lesion immediately after sampling.

With the hot forceps, the duration of electrocautery and the wattage used increase the depth of tissue effect. Very short durations of electrocautery, less than 1 s, likely will only result in very superficial electrocoagulation and hence not significantly affect propensity for bleeding. Long pulses of electrocautery can result in excessive depth of penetration and injury to the airway wall. To avoid injury, pulse duration typically should not exceed 2 s, and care should be used to avoid contact with the airway wall.[11] As the purpose is to coagulate to prevent bleeding and not cut tissue, the soft coagulation mode is ideal and the maximum power should not exceed 30 W.[27]

Pitfalls

The major pitfall of flexible forceps is that the size of the tissue debulked is very small. Other modalities provide superior tissue removal and control of bleeding in far shorter time periods. With cold forceps the risk of bleeding is not insignificant. Hot forceps reduce the risk of bleeding but in most cases are less effective tools than the standard thermal therapies discussed elsewhere in this book.

MICRODEBRIDER

Role of Instrument

The microdebrider is a powered instrument that was initially used by otolaryngologists to remove tissue and bone during sinus surgery, but with the advent of an extended blade for use through the rigid bronchoscope, it has also become an extremely useful debulking device both in benign and malignant central airway lesions. The device combines a rotational blade with associated suction to morselize and aspirate endobronchial tissue. As

with the other devices discussed in this chapter, it is nonthermal and thus useful in situations where high oxygen requirements prohibit the use of thermal techniques. The unique advantage of this device compared to other nonthermal techniques is its rapid action combined with instantaneous aspiration of tissue, which removes the tedious and time-consuming step of piecemeal extraction of detached tissue. This feature makes the device ideal for rapid debulking of infiltrative endobronchial tumors that extend over a long length of airway.

Equipment Details

The device consists of an integrated power console suction irrigation system, a rotating cutting blade at the end of a rigid metal suction catheter, a handpiece, and a foot pedal to control the device. The blade tip is angulated at 15 degrees in a hockey stick configuration, and the handpiece is equipped with a control wheel that allows precise 360-degree rotation of the cutting tip.

The power console is used to provide suction, adjust flow rates for irrigation, and set the speed of revolutions for the blade. In the United States, the only commercially available bronchial blade is 4 mm in diameter and 45 mm in length and has a serrated cutting tip. Shorter airway blades are available with other configurations and can be used with suspension laryngoscopy for subglottic and proximal tracheal lesions.

Method of Use

The power console is attached to the handpiece, which is attached to the bronchial blade. The beveled tip of the rigid bronchoscope is maneuvered to the proximal end of the tumor in the airway. The bronchial blade is passed into the rigid bronchoscope just distal to the rigid telescope so that the blade is always visualized. The size of the tissue that is debulked is directly proportional to the pressure applied by the blade on the tumor and inversely proportional to the speed of rotation of the blade. Therefore the blade is gently applied to the surface of the tumor, and the suction draws the tumor into the hollow metal suction catheter (see Fig. 7.5). Very little pressure is applied by the blade onto the tumor. The foot pedal is activated, which causes the blade to rotate and debulk tumor. The device can clear blood and debris while debulking tumor by coupling debulking with suction. This provides a clear view of the target. The recommended operating speed for these blades ranges from 500 to 1200 rpm.[28]

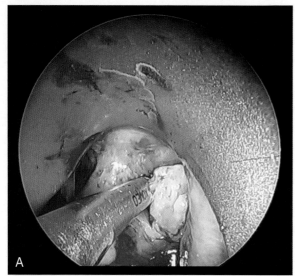

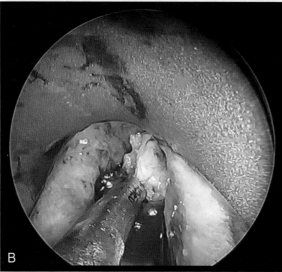

Fig. 7.5 (A) Microdebrider blade brought in proximity to tumor. (B) Suction is used to draw tumor into the catheter tip where tissue is morselized and sucked through the catheter.

Pitfalls

The microdebrider, however, does have its limitations. It is extremely rigid and relatively bulky, which limits mobility when inserted through a standard 12-mm diameter bronchoscope alongside the optical telescope. As a result, it is really only suitable for debulking in the trachea and proximal mainstem bronchi. As with the other nonthermal instruments, the inability to coagulate the tumor or cauterize bleeding does limit its use in vascular tumors. The biggest advantage of the microdebrider is also its biggest risk. The ability to rapidly morselize extensive tumor in a limited time makes the microdebrider extremely useful; however, the device does not discriminate normal from abnormal tissue or respect airway planes. Because of this, in the hands of a novice or distracted proceduralist, catastrophic complications such as perforation of airways and massive hemorrhage, from perforation of large vessels, can easily occur.

CRYORECANALIZATION

Role of Instrument

Cryoprobes can be used for their cytotoxic effects in cryotherapy, which has a delayed response and is not appropriate for severe airway obstruction, or for cryobiopsy of endobronchial or parenchymal tissue. This section, however, will focus specifically on the use of the cryoprobe for cryorecanalization, also known as cryodebulking. Cryorecanalization is performed by freezing a target tissue with the cryoprobe and retracting the frozen tissue en bloc with the probe and the bronchoscope to open the airway. It is most useful in situations where refractory hypoxia does not allow lowering supplemental oxygen to the levels required to utilize thermal techniques. However, it also has significant value even when thermal therapies are not contraindicated, as cryorecanalization allows debulking of large pieces of tissue in a rapid fashion.

The effects of cryotherapy depend on the water content within the tissue. Tumor, mucous membranes, and granulation tissue have high water content and are therefore cryosensitive, whereas cartilage and fibrotic material have low water content and are considered cryoresistant.[29] The optimal target for cryorecanalization is loosely adhesive exophytic airway tumors. Cryorecanalization, however, is not an appropriate method for debulking firmly adhesive tumors or granulation tissue, as the device will not separate the lesion from the underlying normal airway, possibly resulting in hemorrhage or airway rupture.

Cryorecanalization, as a modality for debulking obstructive tumors, should be performed only by physicians with extensive training in the technique who are also capable of managing the associated complications. This differs from cryoadhesion, which is the use of the cryoprobe for removal of obstructive blood clots, mucous plugs, and foreign bodies. Cryoadhesion is a valuable technique in critical care/pulmonology and can be mastered with less training.

Equipment Details

The principle of cryotherapy is based on the Joule-Thomson effect in which a change in temperature of a liquid as it flows from a region of high pressure to that of low pressure results in rapid expansion and dissipation of heat, resulting in rapid temperature drops and thus freezing. The cryotherapy procedure utilizes a dedicated console with a gas cylinder. A transfer line is used to connect the console to the cryoprobe, and a foot pedal is used to initiate the flow of liquid through the probe. The compressed gas coolant is usually either nitrous oxide or carbon dioxide. When delivered through the high-pressure probe to the tip, gas rapidly expands, resulting in cooling to approximately $-89°C$ at the metallic tip. When the probe tip comes in direct contact with the liquid components of tissue, cryoadhesion occurs between the probe and the tissue. Flexible cryotherapy probes are 90 cm in length and available in a variety of diameters for insertion through the working channel of a flexible bronchoscope.[30] Rigid cryoprobes do exist but do not offer any advantages over the more maneuverable flexible probes and likely no longer have a place in bronchoscopic procedures.

Method of Use

When utilizing the cryotherapy probe for debulking, the probe's metallic tip should make direct contact with the lesion and the foot pedal should be activated, at which point visible ice crystals begin to form. The area of tissue adhesion is increased by exerting pressure with the probe on the tumor and with longer cooling durations. Additionally, although cartilage is cryoresistant, the associated normal airway mucosa is quite cryosensitive.[31] Although obtaining large fragments of tissue is desirable, excessive freezing radius or accidental direct contact with the airway mucosa increases the risk of injury to normal airways as well as bleeding. Short freezing duration of 3–6 s is recommended. To prevent injury, the retrograde force used to detach tissue should be constant and gentle. If significant resistance is encountered, pedal activation and retraction should be stopped and the tumor allowed to detach before reattempting at a different attachment point. Slight withdrawal of the probe at the first sign of tissue adhesion, to gently pull the tumor away from the airway wall, before completing the pedal

activation period will reduce the likelihood of adhesion to the adjacent normal airway mucosa. Once the tumor is detached, it should be removed en bloc from the airway to allow the adhered tissue to thaw and detach from the probe (see Fig. 7.6). During this time period, visualization of the airway is lost. Immersing the probe tip in microwaved saline significantly reduced the time needed to remove the specimen and return to the airway.

Pitfalls

Cryorecanalization should be avoided if there is pure extrinsic compression and with strongly adhesive tissue. Extreme care should be taken when debulking tumors along the cartilage-free posterior tracheal wall to prevent airway injury or perforation. Caution should be used, or the technique avoided, in highly vascular tumors or when the tumor involves or invades vasculature adjacent to the target airway, as major hemorrhage can occur.[32] While with most nonthermal mechanical debulking tools, devascularization of the tissue with laser or other thermal therapies prior to debulking is ideal, this is less effective when utilizing the cryoprobe, as the use of thermal therapies reduces the intracellular water content necessary for cryoadhesion. With appropriate target selection, significant bleeding from the residual tumor bed is uncommon; however, slow oozing is frequently encountered.[33] One should always have a plan in place to manage bleeding during this procedure. APC and laser can be helpful for oozing but cannot be used if cryorecanalization is being performed due to the inability to tolerate hypoxemia. Epinephrine, topical tranexamic acid (TXA), and cold saline can be used as adjuncts to control bleeding and should be readily available along with Fogarty balloons or endobronchial blockers to protect the contralateral lung when bleeding develops distal to the main carina. A common misconception among trainees is that because cryorecanalization uses extreme cold, it somehow provides hemostasis. It does not. It is essentially a mechanical debridement technique, and bleeding can and does result.

▌ S U M M A R Y

Mechanical debridement tools are essential components of the interventional pulmonologist's tool kit. While combined usage with thermal therapies is ideal, in the setting of severe hypoxia, these instruments are often the only options available to effectively obtain rapid

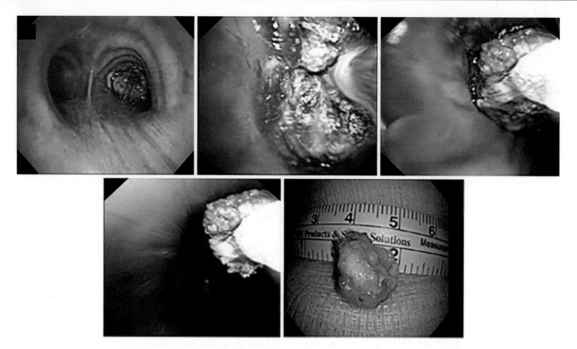

Fig. 7.6 Cryorecanalization of a large exophytic mass within the right mainstem.

recanalization of obstructed airways. As sheer force is required to operate most mechanical instruments, they are inherently less forgiving than their thermal counterparts. One must understand not only the roles of these tools but also the potential risks with these less precise and nonablative tools, such as airway perforation as well as bleeding, and be prepared to manage the complications.

REFERENCES

1. Mathisen DJ, Grillo HC. Endoscopic relief of malignant airway obstruction. *Ann Thorac Surg*. 1989;48(4): 469–473; discussion 473–475.
2. Hautmann H, Gammara F, Pfeifer KJ, Huber RM. Fiberoptic bronchoscopic balloon dilatation in malignant tracheobronchial disease: indications and results. *Chest*. 2001;120(1):43–49.
3. Lee KW, Im JG, Han JK, Kim TK, Park JH, Yeon KM. Tuberculous stenosis of the left main bronchus: results of treatment with balloons and metallic stents. *J Vasc Interv Radiol*. 1999;10(3):352–358.
4. Ferretti G, Jouvan FB, Thony F, Pison C, Coulomb M. Benign noninflammatory bronchial stenosis: treatment with balloon dilation. *Radiology*. 1995;196(3):831–834.
5. Dalar L, Karasulu L, Abul Y, et al. Bronchoscopic treatment in the management of benign tracheal stenosis: choices for simple and complex tracheal stenosis. *Ann Thorac Surg*. 2016;101(4):1310–1317.
6. Shapshay SM, Beamis Jr JF, Hybels RL, Bohigian RK. Endoscopic treatment of subglottic and tracheal stenosis by radial laser incision and dilation. *Ann Otol Rhinol Laryngol*. 1987;96(6):661–664.
7. Tremblay A, Coulter TD, Mehta AC. Modification of a mucosal-sparing technique using electrocautery and balloon dilatation in the endoscopic management of web-like benign airway stenosis. *J Bronchol*. 2003;10(4):268–271.
8. Ossoff RH, Tucker Jr GF, Duncavage JA, Toohill RJ. Efficacy of bronchoscopic carbon dioxide laser surgery for benign strictures of the trachea. *Laryngoscope*. 1985;95(10):1220–1223.
9. McArdle JR, Gildea TR, Mehta AC. Balloon bronchoplasty: its indications, benefits, and complications. *J Bronchol Interv Pulmonol*. 2005;12(2):123–127.
10. Liberman M. Bronchoscopic evaluation of the trachea and dilation of the trachea. *Semin Thorac Cardiovasc Surg*. 2009;21(3):255–262.
11. Sachdeva A, Pickering EM, Lee HJ. From electrocautery, balloon dilatation, neodymium-doped:yttrium-aluminum-garnet (Nd:YAG) laser to argon plasma coagulation and cryotherapy. *J Thorac Dis*. 2015;7(Suppl 4):S363–S379.

12. Mayse ML, Greenheck J, Friedman M, Kovitz KL. Successful bronchoscopic balloon dilation of nonmalignant tracheobronchial obstruction without fluoroscopy. *Chest.* 2004;126(2):634–637.

13. Kim JH, Shin JH, Song H-Y. Cutting balloon treatment for resistant benign bronchial strictures: report of eleven patients. *J Vasc Interv Radiol.* 2010;21(5):748–752.

14. Sakata KK, Midthun DE. Cutting balloon dilation for central airway stricture. *J Bronchol Interv Pulmonol.* 2018;25(3):e29–e30.

15. Stephens Jr KE, Wood DE. Bronchoscopic management of central airway obstruction. *J Thorac Cardiovasc Surg.* 2000;119(2):289–296.

16. Miller RJ, Murgu SD. Bronchoscopic resection of an exophytic endoluminal tracheal mass. *Ann Am Thorac Soc.* 2013;10(6):697–700.

17. Lee WH, Kim JH, Park J-H. Fluoroscopically guided balloon dilation for postintubation tracheal stenosis. *Cardiovasc Intervent Radiol.* 2013;36(5):1350–1354.

18. Alraiyes AH, Kumar A, Gildea TR. Peering beyond an occluded airway. *Ann Am Thorac Soc.* 2015;12(1):124–127.

19. Fouty BW, Pomeranz M, Thigpen TP, Martin RJ. Dilatation of bronchial stenoses due to sarcoidosis using a flexible fiberoptic bronchoscope. *Chest.* 1994;106(3):677–680.

20. Mehta AC, Rafanan AL. Extraction of airway foreign body in adults. *J Bronchol Interv Pulmonol.* 2001;8(2):123–131.

21. Morales-Estrella JL, Machuzak M, Pichurko B, Inaty H, Mehta AC. Suffocation from balloon bronchoplasty. *J Bronchol Interv Pulmonol.* 2018;25(2):156–160.

22. Kim YH, Sung DJ, Cho SB, et al. Deep tracheal laceration after balloon dilation for benign tracheobronchial stenosis: case reports of two patients. *Br J Radiol.* 2006;79(942):529–535.

23. Lund ME. Foreign body removal. In: Ernst A, Herth FJF, eds. *Principles and Practice of Interventional Pulmonology.* Springer; 2013:477–488.

24. Ugajin M, Kani H. Successful treatment of carcinomatous central airway obstruction with bronchoscopic electrocautery using hot biopsy forceps during mechanical ventilation. *Case Rep Oncol Med.* 2017;2017:5378583.

25. Matsuo Y, Yasuda H, Nakano H, et al. Successful endoscopic fragmentation of large hardened fecaloma using jumbo forceps. *World J Gastrointest Endosc.* 2017;9(2):91.

26. Rubio ER, Le SR, Whatley RE, Boyd MB. Cryobiopsy: should this be used in place of endobronchial forceps biopsies? *Biomed Res Int.* 2013;2013:730574.

27. Horinouchi H, Miyazawa T, Takada K, et al. Safety study of endobronchial electrosurgery for tracheobronchial lesions: multicenter prospective study. *J Bronchol Interv Pulmonol.* 2008;15(4):228–232.

28. Casal RF, Iribarren J, Eapen G, et al. Safety and effectiveness of microdebrider bronchoscopy for the management of central airway obstruction. *Respirology.* 2013;18(6):1011–1015.

29. Mazur P. The role of intracellular freezing in the death of cells cooled at supraoptimal rates. *Cryobiology.* 1977;14(3):251–272.

30. Sunna R. Cryotherapy and cryodebridement. In: Ernst A, Herth FJF, eds. *Principles and Practice of Interventional Pulmonology.* Springer; 2013:343–350.

31. Hetzel M, Hetzel J, Schumann C, Marx N, Babiak A. Cryorecanalization: a new approach for the immediate management of acute airway obstruction. *J Thorac Cardiovasc Surg.* 2004;127(5):1427–1431.

32. Schumann C, Hetzel M, Babiak AJ, et al. Endobronchial tumor debulking with a flexible cryoprobe for immediate treatment of malignant stenosis. *J Thorac Cardiovasc Surg.* 2010;139(4):997–1000.

33. Yılmaz A, Aktaş Z, Alici IO, Çağlar A, Sazak H, Ulus F. Cryorecanalization: keys to success. *Surg Endosc.* 2012;26(10):2969–2974.

8

Rapid Ablative Techniques

Donald R. Lazarus

INTRODUCTION

Rapid ablative techniques refer to various thermal therapies used to treat endobronchial diseases which have their effect almost immediately. They include laser, electrocautery, and argon plasma coagulation (APC). They are most appropriate for lesions within the airway lumen causing obstruction or hemoptysis. Rapid ablative techniques can be used alone or in combination with delayed ablative techniques and mechanical debridement. This chapter will briefly discuss general indications and technical considerations for the rapid ablative techniques and then provide more detailed information about each of the three commonly used rapid ablative methods. Mechanical debridement and delayed ablative techniques will be reviewed elsewhere in this book.

GENERAL CONSIDERATIONS FOR RAPID ABLATIVE TECHNIQUES

General Indications

Rapid ablative techniques are primarily indicated for palliative treatment of endoluminal lesions of the central airways. They are effective for obstruction caused by both malignant and benign lesions as long as the obstruction is caused by endoluminal disease. Rapid ablative techniques are not indicated to treat central airway obstruction (CAO) caused primarily by extrinsic compression. Complex lesions with both extrinsic compression and endoluminal obstruction are optimally treated with multimodality therapy including rapid ablative techniques for the endoluminal component followed by mechanical dilation or stenting for

residual obstruction after the endoluminal portion of the lesion has been ablated. Rapid ablative techniques are also very effective for hemoptysis arising from a central endoluminal source. Rapid ablative techniques have also been used for local control of minimally invasive endobronchial tumors when more established and definitive therapies such as surgery or radiotherapy are contraindicated.[1]

General Technical Considerations

Several anatomic characteristics of endobronchial lesions predict their suitability for treatment with rapid ablative techniques. The most important of these is a predominant endoluminal component. The presence of normal lung distal to the obstructing lesion with an intact distal blood supply is also important. Pedunculated or polypoid lesions are better candidates for rapid ablative techniques than sessile ones. It should also be recognized that lesions of the central airways are most amenable to rapid ablation, and conversely lesions present in the upper lobes are more difficult to treat with these methods.[1,2]

Rapid ablative techniques can be used with both rigid and flexible bronchoscopes. Advantages of ablation through the rigid bronchoscope include better control of the airway, availability of additional therapeutic options, better suction, and the ability to isolate a bleeding area while ventilating the contralateral lung. Advantages of ablation with the flexible bronchoscope include familiarity to most pulmonologists, ease of use, better access to distal airways and the upper lobes, and the ability to intervene through an endotracheal tube when required. In practice introducing the flexible bronchoscope through the rigid instrument allows the interventional bronchoscopist to enjoy the advantages of both techniques when rigid bronchoscopic intubation is utilized as the initial therapeutic modality.

Because all of the rapid ablative therapies discussed here use thermal energy to destroy endobronchial lesions and achieve hemostasis, the fraction of inspired oxygen (FIO_2) must be reduced to 40% or less to reduce the risk of airway fire. In addition to reducing the FIO_2, frequent venting or suctioning of the gases produced by thermal destruction of tissue is recommended as the gases may be volatile and ignite if allowed to persist in high concentrations. Additionally the electric current utilized for ablation with electrocautery and APC requires grounding and may affect the function of implanted medical devices. Laser may be preferred in patients with such devices if feasible. Staffing for therapeutic bronchoscopy requiring ablative techniques should include at minimum a nurse, a technician, and the bronchoscopist. It is usually prudent to perform complex cases with anesthesia support if the need for ablation is recognized beforehand. Therapeutic bronchoscopy for malignant CAO using moderate sedation is associated with a higher complication rate than therapeutic bronchoscopy using general anesthesia.

LASER

General Principles of Laser Bronchoscopy

Laser is an acronym for light amplification by stimulated emission of radiation. There are three properties of laser light that make it useful in medicine. First, it is monochromatic—of a single wavelength and color. Laser is also coherent, indicating a tightly focused beam. Finally, laser is collimated, meaning that the beam stays narrow over distance.[3] Laser light may interact with tissue in a variety of ways. These include conversion into thermal energy, the stimulation of biochemical reactions within tissue, and being reflected or scattered at the surface of the tissue. The wavelength of the laser determines which of these effects is predominant, and most lasers used in bronchoscopy are those which produce a thermal effect on tissue resulting in cutting, coagulation, and vaporization.[1,3]

For a laser to be useful in bronchoscopy a delivery system that allows it to be used within the airway is needed. Most of the lasers used in bronchoscopy can be delivered via optical fibers, and both rigid and flexible probes are available. The ratio of absorption and scattering coefficients in soft tissue also determines the effect of a given laser. Increased absorption relative to scattering produces cutting effects, while increased scattering leads to more coagulation. The tissue effect is also determined by the power, duration of exposure, and distance from the tissue of the laser fiber.[1,3] The CO_2 laser was the first used in medicine and remains popular in otolaryngology due to its ability to cut with great precision. However, its utility in bronchoscopy is limited since it is not suitable for transmission by optical fibers and requires a rigid delivery system and it is also poor at achieving hemostasis because of its very shallow depth of penetration. The neodymium:yttrium aluminum garnet (Nd:YAG) laser is the most commonly used and studied in bronchoscopy. It is able to achieve excellent coagulation and even vaporization of tissue, and its shorter wavelength is suitable for transmission through flexible optical fibers.[1,3] Other lasers used in bronchoscopy include neodymium:yttrium aluminum perovskite (Nd:YAP), holmium:yttrium aluminum garnet (Ho:YAG), argon, thulium, and diode lasers. Each has distinct tissue effects determined by the wavelength of light used and the way it interacts with tissues. Characteristics of some commonly used medical lasers are summarized in Table 8.1.[3-5]

Preprocedural Preparation

As discussed earlier, selection of patients for bronchoscopic laser ablation should begin with an assessment of the lesion. Raised endoluminal lesions of the central airways are ideal. The respiratory status of the patient should also be assessed to determine whether or not the patient can tolerate hypoxemia since the safe use of laser requires that the FIO_2 be reduced to 40% or less. Because lasers deliver thermal energy by light and not electricity, laser is safe for use in patients with pacemakers or other implanted cardiac devices.

Equipment:
- Laser console with foot pedal to activate the laser
- Reusable or disposable optical fiber to carry the beam (both rigid and flexible fibers are available, as are contact and noncontact probes)
- Safety glasses for the specific wavelength of light used by the laser.

Technique of Laser Bronchoscopy

When planning a laser procedure it is of critical importance for the bronchoscopist to know the patient's anatomy and maintain good orientation in the airway at all

Type of Laser	Wavelength (nm)	Coagulation	Cutting and Vaporization	Depth of Penetration (mm)	Typical Power Settings (W)
CO₂	10, 600	+	+++	<1	4–8
Nd:YAG	1064	++	+++	5–15	20–40
Nd:YAP	1340	+++	+	3–10	20
Ho:YAG	2100	+	+++	<1	10
Argon	516	++	+	1	5
Thulium	2000	++	+++	<1	10
Diode	Variable	++	++	3–10	2–4

TABLE 8-1   Lasers Used in Interventional Bronchoscopy[3]

CO₂, Carbon dioxide; *Ho:YAG,* holmium:yttrium aluminum garnet; *Nd:YAG,* eodymium:yttrium aluminum garnet; *Nd:YAP,* neodymium:yttrium aluminum perovskite.

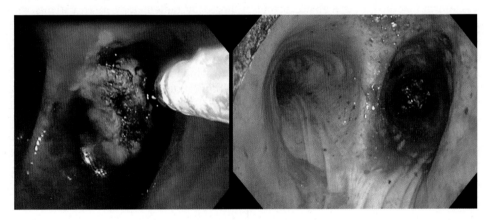

Fig. 8.1 Neodymium:yttrium aluminum perovskite photoresection of non–small cell lung cancer obstructing the right mainstem bronchus. (Photo courtesy the author, used with permission.)

times. The F_{IO_2} should be reduced to 40% or less before activating the laser. All personnel present in the procedure suite must wear safety glasses prior to activating the laser. Typical settings for laser bronchoscopy include power of 20–40 W and a pulse time of 0.4–1 s for the Nd:YAG laser, but exact setting varies based on the type of laser. The bronchoscope is advanced until the target lesion is visualized, and then the fiber is extended beyond the tip of the scope by at least 4 mm. Only then should the assistant arm the laser.

The bronchoscopist should orient the axis of the laser fiber parallel to the long axis of the airway to reduce the risk of perforation. Treatment should begin with the fiber at least 0.4–1 cm away from the target and start with short-duration pulses. The effect of laser on the tissue is then evaluated, and if more effect is desired the fiber can be moved closer to the target lesion or longer pulses can be used. Large obstructing lesions can be coagulated using a lower power setting prior to mechanical debulking (see Fig. 8.1). This method of coagulation using thermal ablation followed by mechanical debulking is repeated in an iterative manner to progressively resect larger tumors. The bronchoscopist is essentially shaving the tumor down by coagulating, then resecting the tumor, and then repeating the process until the airway is open. Smaller or friable tumors can be vaporized using higher power settings. Prolonged firing or firing in an axis other than parallel to the airway increases the risk of perforation with attendant bleeding and respiratory failure and should be avoided.

Complications of Laser

- Hemorrhage (immediate and delayed)
- Respiratory failure/hypoxemia
- Perforation
- Fistula
- Pneumothorax/pneumomediastinum
- Airway fire
- Eye injury
- Gas embolism.

Precautions and Pearls

- Laser can cause airway fire when used in an oxygen-rich environment. The FIO_2 must be decreased to 40% or less when using laser. Clear verbal communication with the procedure assistant or anesthetist is critical to confirm that the FIO_2 is at an acceptable level before activating the laser. Closed-loop communication is recommended, meaning that the bronchoscopist should give an order specifying the FIO_2 desired and the anesthesiologist should repeat and confirm the message once the FIO_2 is adjusted prior to any thermal ablation.
- Laser is best for pedunculated or protruding lesions. Because it delivers energy as light the beam travels straight ahead in the axial plane, so radial firing is not possible. This makes treating sessile mucosal lesions difficult.
- Laser is good for deeper tissue penetration when compared to APC, but this increases the risk of perforation relative to APC. Treatment of the posterior tracheal and mainstem bronchial walls imparts increased risk of perforation and should be considered with caution.
- Laser is preferred over electrocautery and APC in patients with implanted cardiac devices because the light beam transmitting thermal energy does not affect them in the way that electric current does.
- Different lasers have different effects based on the wavelength of their light. Be familiar with the device you are using and its characteristic tissue interactions.

Evidence

Numerous case series demonstrate the effectiveness of laser for CAO and bleeding, although few of these studies have been randomized or controlled. It is also important to remember that most recent studies report data on procedures that are multimodality, using a combinations of thermal techniques (e.g., laser plus electrocautery) with combinations of mechanical debridement techniques (e.g., coring out and forceps) with or without stenting. Effectiveness measures and complications reported are really a reflection of the multimodality approach, and it is difficult to dissect how different parts of the multimodality approach impact outcomes. Given these limitations, Cavaliere and colleagues reported the results of almost 1400 laser procedures in 1000 patients, with 64% having malignant CAO. Significant improvement in airway lumen size or ventilation was seen in over 90% of patients with malignant bronchial tumors, but symptoms were not measured with validated instruments in these early studies.[6] Performance status in similar patients with malignant CAO was also significantly improved by laser treatment.[7] Treatment with Nd:YAG laser followed by radiotherapy in 15 patients with inoperable lung cancer and CAO requiring emergent treatment led to increased survival compared to radiotherapy alone in 11 historical controls.[8] However, when assessing efficacy and complication rates, it is important to recognize that complication rates for therapeutic bronchoscopy vary by indication. Patients with malignant CAO have higher complication rates than those with benign airway disease undergoing therapeutic bronchoscopy.[9] The AQuIRE multicenter registry evaluated 1115 procedures in 947 patients with malignant CAO undergoing therapeutic bronchoscopy using multimodality approaches.[10,11] Laser bronchoscopy was utilized in 24% of cases. They found that 93% of procedures resulted in technical success, defined as significant anatomic improvement in airway obstruction (<50% residual obstruction). Clinically significant improvement in symptoms occurred in 48%. The overall complication rate was 3.9%, but there was significant variation between centers (range 0.9%–11.7%). Risk factors for complications included use of moderate sedation, urgent or emergent procedures, American Society of Anesthesiology score >3, and redo therapeutic bronchoscopy cases. Limited data are available on the impact of therapeutic bronchoscopy on quality adjusted survival.[12] In a prospective observational study of 102 patients with malignant airway obstruction, anatomic technical success was achieved in 90% of cases, resulting in decreased dyspnea at 7 days (mean change in Borg score −1.7) and improved health-related quality of life (HRQOL) (change in utility at 7 days + 0.047 utiles, $\underline{P} = 0.0002$). Improvements in dyspnea and HRQOL were maintained long term. Data on impact of therapeutic bronchoscopy using laser on quality adjusted survival in benign disease are currently lacking. Overall, the data suggest that the efficacy and safety profile of bronchoscopic laser treatment as part of a multimodality airway approach is acceptable in experienced hands, with overall complication rates ranging from 2.3% to 8.4% in the largest series.[10–14]

Summary

Laser is a safe and effective method for relieving CAO and treating bleeding in the airways. It is expensive and requires special eyewear, but does not affect implanted medical devices and has a long track record of safety.

ELECTROCAUTERY

General Principles of Bronchoscopic Electrocautery

Electrocautery uses high-frequency electrical current to generate heat which then coagulates and destroys tissue. Contact between the cautery instrument and the tissue is required for the thermal effect. Because the heat is generated by an electrical current the patient must be grounded to avoid shock and allow the current a safe way to exit the body. The tissue effect is determined by voltage, duration, area of contact, tissue density, and the water content of the tissue.[1,15,16]

Different electrocautery devices are used for different purposes. Common instruments used for electrocautery include a blunt probe, hot forceps, cautery knife, and cautery snare. The flexible blunt probe is used to coagulate and destroy tissue with direct contact. Rigid electrocautery blunt probes function similarly. In addition, there are rigid electrocautery-suction probes that provide the additional benefit of providing electrocautery coagulation and destruction while simultaneously suctioning the airway of blood. The hot forceps are able to deliver heat while a transbronchial or endobronchial biopsy is being taken (see Fig. 8.2). The cautery knife is used to precisely cut through tissue and is particularly good at disrupting benign webs causing airway stenosis (see Fig. 8.3). The cautery snare is used to grasp pedunculated lesions at the base to facilitate rapid removal.[1,2,16]

Preprocedural Preparation

Patient selection for bronchoscopic electrocautery is similar to that for laser and other rapid ablative

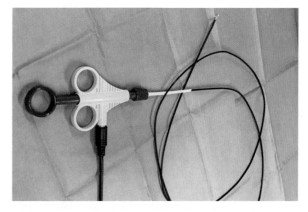

Fig. 8.2 Electrocautery forceps. (Photo courtesy the author, used with permission.)

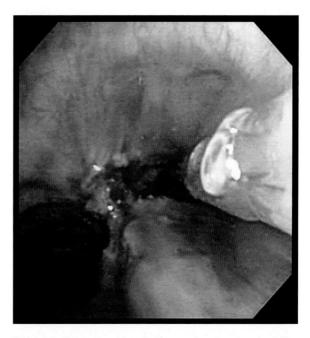

Fig. 8.3 Electrocautery knife cutting benign weblike stricture near the main carina. (Photo courtesy the author, used with permission.)

techniques. The patient must be able to tolerate reduction of the FIO_2 to 40% or less for safe use of electrocautery. Assessment of the lesion to be treated is also critical to allow the selection of the appropriate cautery instrument as outlined earlier.

The electrical current used to generate thermal energy in electrocautery can interfere with the functioning of cardiac pacemakers and other implanted medical devices. Patients with such devices who must undergo procedures in which electrocautery may be used should have the devices placed in asynchronous mode by reprogramming or using a magnet. The devices should then be reevaluated after the procedure to ensure the resumption of normal function.[17] If the patient cannot tolerate pacing with asynchronous mode then electrocautery should not be used.

Equipment:
- Electrocautery console with foot pedal for activation
- Grounding pad for the patient
- Electrocautery instruments:
  - Reusable or disposable electrocautery blunt probe
  - Reusable electrocautery-suction probe
  - Hot electrocautery forceps
  - Electrocautery knife
  - Electrocautery snare.

Electrocautery Technique

As with other rapid ablative techniques the bronchoscopist must be familiar with the patient's anatomy and maintain good orientation in the airway at all times. The F_{IO_2} should be reduced to 40% or less before activating the cautery instrument. A grounding pad must be placed on the patient and connected to the cautery machine to avoid shock. Most cautery machines have two foot pedals—one for cutting and one for coagulation. Depressing the cutting (yellow) pedal generates more energy to destroy tissue quickly but with higher risk of unintended collateral damage and less effective control of bleeding. The coagulation (blue) pedal cauterizes tissue with less energy and so traverses the tissue more superficially and is more effective for hemostasis of bleeding lesions without vaporizing them as effectively.[18] The coagulation mode has somewhat less risk of unintended consequences such as perforation. Some proceduralists alternately activate the cutting and coagulation pedals as they treat the target lesion with the intent to optimize tissue destruction, hemostasis, and safety. Typical settings for bronchoscopic electrocautery include power of 20–60 W, with the coagulation mode set to the lower end and the cutting mode nearer the upper end. Short activations are used to reduce the risk of perforation. The tissue effect of a given electrocautery setting will vary between tumors and patients, so if there is uncertainty it is best to start on the lower side, treat, observe tissue effects, and adjust settings and techniques accordingly based on empiric observation in that individual patient.

Blunt Electrocautery Probe Technique

The operator should advance the bronchoscope until good visualization of the lesion is attained. Then the probe is advanced a sufficient distance beyond the working channel to avoid damage to the tip of the scope. Many probes have a mark on the catheter which designates the minimal safe distance to avoid damage to the scope. Then the tip of the probe is touched to the target tissue from the luminal side and activated using the foot pedal for a very short time, generally no more than 1–2 s.[19] The bronchoscopist should visually reassess the lesion after each activation and deliver additional energy as needed. When the rigid cautery probe is used the technique is the same except that the tip of the probe must be advanced at least 1–2 cm beyond the tip of the rigid bronchoscope to avoid potential shock to the operator.

It is important to avoid prolonged cautery activation to avoid affecting deep layers of tissue and increasing the risk of perforation and other complications. Particular care must be taken when treating sessile lesions on the bronchial wall or any lesion on the posterior tracheal or mainstem bronchial walls.

Hot Forceps

The hot forceps are biopsy forceps augmented with electrical current with the idea of reducing bleeding after biopsies are taken by cauterizing it as the tissue is pulled away. The forceps are advanced from the working channel of the bronchoscope to the target tissue to be removed. Many forceps have a mark on the shaft indicating the minimum safe distance needed to avoid damage to the bronchoscope. Once the forceps are in contact with the target lesion the assistant closes the forceps on the tissue and then the operator activates the electrocautery using the foot pedal for a few seconds. The tissue is then removed by gently pulling the forceps.

While the intent of the hot forceps is to reduce bleeding, studies evaluating its effectiveness for this purpose have not demonstrated a clinically significant reduction in bleeding.[20,21] For this reason this instrument is no longer frequently used in practice.

Electrocautery Knife

The electrocautery knife is not actually sharp, but rather has a small almost needle-shaped tip that is able to cut through tissue like a true knife when activated with energy. It is typically used to cut benign weblike stenotic lesions within the central airways. The sheath is first advanced through the working channel of the scope far enough to avoid damaging the tip. Please access Video 8.1 (Electrocautery Needle Knife) online. Many models have a colored mark on the sheath indicating the minimum safe distance. Then the metal tip is protruded from the sheath. The bronchoscope is then flexed so that the tip of the knife is in contact with the web with very slight pressure to direct the knife. After this the energy is activated with the foot pedal for a very short time— less than a second—causing the desired cut in the tissue. The electrocautery knife is able to cut through the tissue extremely quickly, so it is important to avoid prolonged activations as this may lead to perforation of the airway.

Most operators recommend radial cuts at the 9 o'clock, 12 o'clock, and 3 o'clock positions. The posterior wall of the airway (6 o'clock) is not treated because the lack of cartilaginous support increases the risk of perforation. Mechanical dilation may be used if needed after radial cuts are made (see Fig. 8.4). The electrocautery knife is not recommended for malignant airway lesions since it does not coagulate effectively and is very fast.

Electrocautery Snare

The electrocautery snare is used to remove polypoid or pedunculated lesions within the airway. First the bronchoscopist should try to determine the location of the stalk as accurately as possible. Then the snare sheath is advanced out of the working channel of the bronchoscope to a safe distance, and the snare itself is then advanced from the sheath on the luminal side of the lesion that is open (i.e., opposite to the side with the stalk). Please access Video 8.2 (Electrocautery Snare and APC) online.

[Note: First part of the video covers Electrocautery Snare and the later part covers APC] The snare will open on its own as it is advanced and is positioned to lasso the lesion. The bronchoscope is then moved toward the side of the wall where the stalk originates and used to manipulate the snare around the lesion toward the lesion's base. The assistant then tightens the snare slowly around the base of the lesion until it is completely encircled and some resistance is felt. Then the assistant slowly tightens the snare while the operator activates the energy using the foot pedal. These actions should occur simultaneously until the snare is completely closed around the lesion or cuts through the base and the lesion appears loose in the airway. The snare can be used to remove the lesion if the lesion remains in its grasp. If the stalk is cut through and the lesion falls loose in the airway then forceps, suction, or the cryotherapy probe can be used to remove the tissue (see Fig. 8.5).

Complications Of Electrocautery

- Hemorrhage
- Perforation
- Airway fire
- Snare entrapment
- Shock to patient or operator
- Implanted cardiac device malfunction.

Precautions and Pearls

- Like laser, electrocautery can cause airway fire when used in an environment with a high oxygen concentration. The FIO_2 must be decreased to 40% or less when using electrocautery and good communication with the procedure assistant or anesthetist is

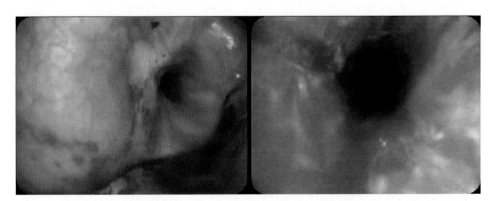

Fig. 8.4 Benign subglottic stricture before and after treatment with radial cuts using the electrocautery knife. (Photo courtesy the author, used with permission.)

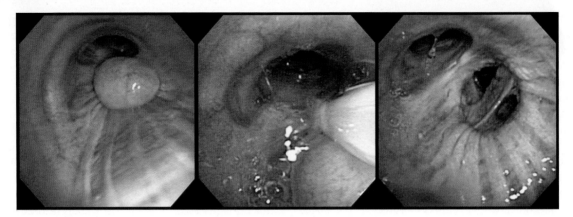

Fig. 8.5 Right lower lobe endobronchial lipoma before, during, and after resection using the cautery snare. (Photo courtesy the author, used with permission.)

critical to confirm that the F_{IO_2} is at an acceptable level before activating the instrument. Closed-loop communication practices should be utilized.

- Contact electrocautery is less effective when there is excessive blood in the area to be treated. This is because the wet surface diffuses the point of contact with the tissue, limiting the effect of the cautery instrument.[18] In this situation the bronchoscopist should either use suction to remove blood and allow effective treatment with cautery or choose a noncontact tool such as APC to control bleeding. Use of the rigid electrocautery-suction instrument to simultaneously suction blood and coagulate the bleeding source can be useful in this context.
- It is important to match the tool to the lesion. Each cautery instrument has a different utility.
- It is often useful to use contact and noncontact modalities together for optimal tissue destruction and hemostasis.
- Electrocautery must be used with caution in patients who have implanted cardiac devices. A magnet should be used to convert pacemakers and automated implanted cardioverter-defibrillators (AICDs) to asynchronous mode, and electrocautery should be avoided in patients who cannot tolerate this. Postprocedure device interrogation is prudent.
- It is often helpful when using the blunt probe or the cautery knife to perform a "dry run" with the instrument without activating the electrocautery to allow the physician to predict the angle and direction of movement before they treat the tissue.

Evidence

When assessing the evidence, as with laser bronchoscopy, it is important to remember that most recent large series use a multimodality approach, combining different thermal techniques, electrocautery among them, with different debridement techniques and sometimes stenting. Complications and outcomes also vary by indication.[1,9,10] As such it can be difficult to dissect out the risk of electrocautery in isolation. A number of small series and trials have demonstrated the effectiveness of bronchoscopic electrocautery to relieve CAO and improve dyspnea and reported a favorable safety profile.[18,22,23] Given this context, Wahidi and colleagues evaluated 94 patients who underwent 117 bronchoscopic electrocautery procedures for both malignant and benign CAO with 94% of patients having significant endoscopic improvement. Seventy-one percent of patients reported improvement in their symptoms, and radiographic improvement by computed tomography (CT) was seen in 78% of patients. Minor complications were seen in 6.8% of cases, with major complications in 0.8% and no periprocedural deaths reported.[24] Bronchoscopic electrocautery has also been shown to be less costly than laser treatment with similar effectiveness.[18,22,23]

Summary

Bronchoscopic electrocautery is a versatile tool especially well suited for relieving benign and malignant CAO. In experienced hands it has an acceptable safety profile. It is less expensive than laser and no protective eyewear is required. It does use electrical current to generate electricity so must be used with caution in patients with implanted medical devices. Airway fire is a risk so FIO_2 must be maintained at 40% or less.

ARGON PLASMA COAGULATION

General Principles of APC

APC is a noncontact form of electrocoagulation in which argon gas is ionized by a high-frequency electrical current and then travels from a catheter to the nearest ground where it is converted to heat, producing coagulation and fulguration of the targeted tissue.[25,26] The nearest ground may not be in the axial plane—firing to the side and even retrograde firing are also possible. APC generally has a superficial depth of penetration, between 2 and 3 mm.[2,26] This happens largely because the electrical resistance of tissue increases as it becomes coagulated and desiccated, limiting further conduction.[2] As resistance increases, the ionized argon gas, which acts as a conductor, will bend toward the path of least resistance, which will be the adjacent nontreated tissue. For this reason vaporization is not typically achieved, but APC has an excellent hemostatic effect and the coagulation produced allows easier mechanical debulking of obstructing lesions.

Preprocedural Preparation

Patient selection for APC is essentially the same as for electrocautery and laser. Appropriate lesions for APC are bleeding or obstructing lesions within the central airways that are visible with the bronchoscope. The patient must be able to tolerate an FIO_2 of 40% or less in order to safely use APC within the airway. Because APC is a monopolar electrical current, the same precautions must be taken as electrocautery for those patients who have implanted cardiac devices. These are summarized earlier, in the section on preprocedural preparation for electrocautery

Equipment:
- APC/electrocautery console with foot pedal for activation
- Grounding pad for the patient
- APC probe:
  - Flexible or rigid
  - Large or small size
  - Axial, side-firing, or circumferential-firing tip.

APC Technique

As with laser and electrocautery the interventionalist must know the patient's anatomy and maintain good orientation in the airway at all times. The FIO_2 should be reduced to 40% or less before activating the APC device. A grounding pad must be placed on the patient and connected to the APC console to avoid shock. Many consoles are used for both contact electrocautery and noncontact APC. Unlike with the contact cautery tools, however, activation of APC is done only with one foot pedal—typically the coagulation (blue) pedal. The operator can choose from large and small size flexible APC probes. The smaller probe is 1.5 mm in diameter and can be used in standard size bronchoscopes with a 2-mm working channel. The larger size probe is 2.3 mm in diameter and requires a therapeutic flexible bronchoscope. The smaller probe is more flexible and better suited for lesions in the upper lobes or more distal airways. The larger probe can accommodate a higher flow of gas and produces a more rapid tissue effect. The different tips direct the flow of ionized gas (current) in different directions.

Most APC consoles have three modes with slightly different effects. Forced APC mode is characterized by a continuous output of high-frequency voltage and has the most tissue effect. It is most useful for hemostasis of diffuse areas of bleeding and rapid devitalization of tissue. In pulsed APC mode the output of energy is discontinuous, with pulses of energy at varying frequencies. Pulsed APC is useful for diffuse bleeding and tissue devitalization in areas that are thermosensitive and when more controlled power output is desired. In both of these modes the tissue effect is determined by adjusting the power settings. Precise APC mode is characterized by continuous output of energy, but the tissue effect is determined by the effect setting rather than power. It is used to treat superficial bleeding or devitalize tissue in thin-walled areas and has a more superficial depth of penetration. Typical settings for APC include power of 20–40 W and gas flows between 0.3 and 1.8 L/min with higher flows used for the larger size probe. For a given probe size, a higher flow rate will result in greater range/reach of the APC.

The bronchoscope is advanced within the airway until the target lesion is visualized, and then the APC probe is extended beyond the tip of the scope by at least 5–10 mm before activation to avoid damaging the bronchoscope (Video 8.1). APC probes have black rings every 10 mm starting from the tip to allow the operator to determine an appropriate distance. Once the probe is sufficiently extended the bronchoscopist should move it closer to the lesion using primarily the movement of the bronchoscope rather than additional independent movement of the probe. This helps prevent the operator from inadvertently withdrawing the tip of the probe too near the scope. Once the tip of the probe is within about 4 mm of the target lesion the operator can activate the APC using the foot pedal. Activation times vary but it is generally prudent to start with activations of 1–3 s before evaluating the effect and then adjusting the distance to the tissue or the duration of activation as needed. The bronchoscopist should also attempt to avoid touching the probe to the tissue in order to reduce risk of gas embolism. For hemostasis APC fulguration alone is usually sufficient (see Fig. 8.6). For debulking of obstructing lesions mechanical techniques are often employed after coagulation to achieve an optimal effect.

Because the monopolar flow of current travels to the nearest ground regardless of direction, the advantages of using the side-firing probe or the circumferential-firing probe are limited. The standard axial-firing probe will also conduct current radially or even retrograde if that is the area of tissue nearest the tip.

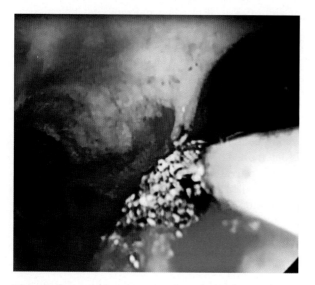

Fig. 8.6 Argon plasma coagulation of bleeding endotracheal papillomatous tumors. Photo courtesy the author, used with permission.

Complications of APC

- Bleeding
- Respiratory failure
- Perforation
- Airway fire
- Gas embolism
- Implanted cardiac device malfunction.

Precautions and Pearls

- Like the other rapid ablative techniques, APC can cause airway fire when used with high F_{IO_2}. The F_{IO_2} should be reduced to 40% or less when using APC. The bronchoscopist must communicate well with the procedure assistant or anesthetist to ensure that the F_{IO_2} is safely reduced before beginning treatment. Closed-loop communication is recommended.
- APC is excellent for hemostasis and coagulation, but it is less effective than laser or electrocautery for tissue destruction. It can often be used as part of multimodality therapy to coagulate obstructing lesion before mechanically debulking it to reduce bleeding risk.
- Desiccation and coagulation increases the resistance of the tissue, leading to a degree of self-limiting depth of penetration and less risk of perforation with APC.
- With APC the operator can fire radially with the axial probe as long as tip is closer to the side wall than the nearest forward ground.
- The ability to side-fire makes APC especially effective for treating sessile or flat lesions.
- The smaller APC probe is better able reach distal lesions and treat lesions within the upper lobes because of its flexibility.
- The flow rate dictates the range/reach of APC. Higher flow results in greater range. In smaller airways lower rates are recommended to avoid unintended collateral damage.
- Do not fire and advance the APC at the same time. If you accidentally impale tissue while firing the APC you can cause an air embolism. Instead, fire the APC and slowly withdraw the bronchoscope to cover larger areas. Then hold fire, reposition distally, and repeat. This will help minimize risk of gas embolism. Limiting activation times to 1–3 s initially and during the procedure will also help mitigate gas embolism risk.

Evidence

Although many case reports describing the use of APC in bronchoscopy have been published, there have been relatively few case series evaluating its role in the airway. Reichle and colleagues reported their experience with 482 procedures in 364 patients, predominantly having malignant disease. For those patients with malignant airway stenosis complete or partial recanalization was reported in 67%, with most of the failures due to absence of viable distal lung. Successful treatment of acute hemoptysis was accomplished with APC in >99% of cases. Complications were rare and seen in only 3.7% of cases with no periprocedural deaths.[25] Morice and colleagues described their experience using APC in 60 patients with hemoptysis, symptomatic airway obstruction, or both. All patients presenting with hemoptysis had good symptom control with APC. Of those patients with bronchial obstruction, the mean degree of obstruction improved from 76% pretreatment to 18% posttreatment with concomitant improvement in symptoms. No complications from the procedures were reported.[26] As with laser and electrocautery, the APC is usually used as part of a multimodality approach, frequently combined with other ablative techniques (e.g., laser or conventional electrocautery) and mechanical debridement (e.g., coring out or forceps) and sometimes stenting for mixed lesions.

Summary

APC is a noncontact form of electrocautery that is particularly well suited for treatment of hemoptysis or bleeding in the central airways. It is also useful in combination with mechanical techniques to devitalize obstructing endobronchial lesions before mechanical debulking, thereby reducing bleeding risk. The depth of penetration for APC is less than laser because the ionized gas will bend toward the path of least resistance. It has a very favorable safety profile.

SUMMARY OF RAPID ABLATIVE TECHNIQUES

Laser, electrocautery, and APC are all excellent modalities for treating endobronchial lesions causing airway obstruction and bleeding. No single method is clearly superior to the others, although each has its particular advantages and drawbacks. The bronchoscopist should choose the rapid ablative technique for a given case based on the nature of the problem and local experience, equipment, and expertise.

REFERENCES

1. Bolliger CT, Sutedja TG, Strausz J, Freitag L. Therapeutic bronchoscopy with immediate effect: laser, electrocautery, argon plasma coagulation, and stents. *Eur Respir J.* 2006;27(6):1258–1271.
2. Ernst A, Feller-Kopman D, Becker HD, Mehta AC. Central airway obstruction. *Am J Respir Crit Care Med.* 2004;169(12):1278–1297.
3. Khemasuwan D, Mehta AC, Wang KP. Past, present, and future of endobronchial laser photoresection. *J Thorac Dis.* 2015;7(Suppl 4):S380–S388.
4. Miller RJ, Murgu SD. Bronchoscopic resection of an exophytic endoluminal tracheal mass. *Ann Am Thorac Soc.* 2013;10(6):697–700.
5. Lee HJ, Malhotra R, Grossman C, Shepherd RW. Initial report of neodymium:yttrium-aluminum-perovskite (Nd:YAP) laser use during bronchoscopy. *J Bronchology Interv Pulmonol.* 2011;18(3):229–232.
6. Cavaliere S, Foccoli P, Farina PL. Nd:YAG laser bronchoscopy: a five-year experience with 1396 applications in 1000 patients. *Chest.* 1988;94(1):15–21.
7. Ross DJ, Mohsenifar Z, Koerner SK. Survival characteristics after neodymium:YAG laser photoresection in advanced stage lung cancer. *Chest.* 1990;98(3):581–585.
8. Desai SJ, Mehta AC, VanderBrug Medendorp S, Golish JA, Ahmad M. Survival experience following Nd:YAG laser photoresection for primary bronchogenic carcinoma. *Chest.* 1988;94(5):939–944.
9. Ernst A, Simoff M, Ost D, Goldman Y, Herth FJF. Prospective risk-adjusted morbidity and mortality outcome analysis after therapeutic bronchoscopic procedures: results of a multi-institutional outcomes database. *Chest.* 2008;134:514–519.
10. Ost DE, Ernst A, Grosu HB, et al. Complications following therapeutic bronchoscopy for malignant central airway obstruction: results of the AQuIRE Registry. *Chest.* 2015;148:450–471.
11. Ost DE, Ernst A, Grosu HB, et al. Therapeutic bronchoscopy for malignant central airway obstruction: success rates and impact on dyspnea and quality of life. *Chest.* 2015;147:1282–1298.
12. Ong P, Grosu HB, Debiane L, et al. Long-term quality-adjusted survival following therapeutic bronchoscopy for malignant central airway obstruction. *Thorax.* 2019;74:141–156.
13. Cavaliere S, Foccoli P, Toninelli C, Feijo S. Nd:YAG laser therapy in lung cancer: an 11-year experience with 2253 applications in 1585 patients. *J Bronchol.* 1994;1(2):105–111.

14. Perin B, Zaric B, Jovanovic S, et al. Patient-related independent risk factors for early complications following Nd:YAG laser resection of lung cancer. *Ann Thorac Med*. 2012;7(4):233–237.

15. Van Boxem TJ, Venmans BJ, Schramel FM, et al. Radiographically occult lung cancer treated with fiberoptic bronchoscopic electrocautery: a pilot study of a simple and inexpensive technique. *Eur Respir J*. 1998;11(1):169–172.

16. Sheski FD, Mathur PN. Endobronchial electrosurgery: argon plasma coagulation and electrocautery. *Semin Respir Crit Care Med*. 2004;25(4):367–374.

17. Stone ME, Salter B, Fischer A. Perioperative management of patients with cardiac implantable electronic devices. *Br J Anaesth*. 2011;107(S1):i16–i26.

18. Coulter TD, Mehta AC. The heat is on: impact of endobronchial electrosurgery on the need for Nd-YAG laser photoresection. *Chest*. 2000;118(2):516–521.

19. Van Boxem TJ, Westerga J, Venmans BJ, Postmus PE, Sutedja TG. Tissue effects of bronchoscopic electrocautery: bronchoscopic appearance and histologic changes of bronchial wall after electrocautery. *Chest*. 2000;117(3):887–891.

20. Tremblay A, Michaud G, Urbanski SJ. Hot biopsy forceps in the diagnosis of endobronchial lesions. *Eur Respir J*. 2007;29(1):108–111.

21. Firoozbakhsh S, Seifirad S, Safavi E, Dinparast R, Taslimi S, Derakhshandeilami G. Comparison of hot versus cold biopsy forceps in the diagnosis of endobronchial lesions. *Arch Bronconeumol*. 2011;47(11):547–551.

22. Van Boxem T, Muller M, Venmans B, Postmus P, Sutedja T. Nd-YAG laser vs bronchoscopic electrocautery for palliation of symptomatic airway obstruction: a cost-effectiveness study. *Chest*. 1999;116(4):1108–1112.

23. Sutedja TG, Van Boxem TJ, Schramel FM, Van Felius C, Postmus PE. Endobronchial electrocautery is an excellent alternative for Nd:YAG laser to treat airway tumors. *J Bronchol*. 1997;4(2):101–105.

24. Wahidi MM, Unroe MA, Adlakha N, Beyea M, Shofer SL. The use of electrocautery as the primary ablation modality for malignant and benign airway obstruction. *J Thorac Oncol*. 2011;6(9):1516–1520.

25. Reichle G, Freitag L, Kullman HJ, Prenzel R, Macha HN, Farin G. Argon plasma coagulation in bronchology: a new method—alternative or complementary? *J Bronchol*. 2000;7(2):109–117.

26. Morice RC, Ece T, Ece F, Keus L. Endobronchial argon plasma coagulation for treatment of hemoptysis and neoplastic airway obstruction. *Chest*. 2001;119(3):781–787.

9

Delayed Ablation Techniques: Photodynamic Therapy and Cryotherapy

Michael Dorry and Jasleen Pannu

PHOTODYNAMIC THERAPY

Introduction

The advent of photodynamic therapy (PDT) was one of the early advances in interventional pulmonology that elevated therapeutic bronchoscopy into the curative arena. First used by Hayata in 1982, PDT has not significantly changed in principle or application.[1] PDT is based on the concept that malignant cells absorb and retain a photosensitive compound and become very sensitive to light.[2] The photosensitizer is then activated with a light wavelength corresponding to the photosensitizer absorption spectrum that takes the singlet basic energy state to the goal excited triplet state.[3] The excited triplet state leads to the generation of reactive oxygen species, which cause cellular damage and apoptosis of tumor cells.

The procedure involves three steps:
- First step: intravenous injection of the photosensitizer agent porfimer sodium (Photofrin, Pinnacle Biologics, Bannockburn, IL, USA) at 2 mg/kg
- Second step: 48 h after injection, performing a bronchoscopy and using a light diffuser through the working channel of scope to expose the sensitized tumor cell to a nonthermal laser light (wavelength of 630 nm)
- Third step: 48 h after index procedure, performing a bronchoscopy to remove sloughed tissue with suctioning, forceps, or cryoprobe. If the intended lesion does not appear to be adequately treated, a second light treatment can be delivered at this session.

PDT can be used with curative intent for patients with carcinoma in situ or as adjunctive therapy or palliative treatment for malignant central airway obstruction.

PREPROCEDURE PREPARATION

Patient Selection

Identifying the appropriate patient for PDT relies on selecting the optimal target lesion. If aiming for curative intent of carcinoma in situ, consider factors such as a lesion size <1.5 cm (<1 cm for optimal results), proximal airway location, and intraluminal disease. It is important to remember that the depth of tissue penetration for PDT is 4–6 mm. The therapeutic effects of PDT are delayed such that its application is limited in critical malignant central airway obstruction.

Injection Encounter

In the United States, Photofrin is the only approved photosensitizer compound available. It is dosed 2 mg/kg 48 h prior to bronchoscopy. After its administration, it is retained in tumor cells and cleared from most healthy issues in 6 h except for the lung, reticuloendothelial tissues, and the skin. The unique properties that allow for Photofrin to accumulate in malignant cells have not been well elucidated. Proposed mechanisms involve elevated numbers of lower-density protein receptors on tumor cells, decreased pH in the tumor microenvironment, and the presence of macrophages.[4]

As mentioned earlier, Photofrin does not just accumulate in malignant cells but is highly concentrated in the spleen, liver, kidney, and orders of magnitude lower in the skin.[5] Given that the spleen, liver, and kidney are protected from light, they are not considered when it comes to PDT. Photofrin can be retained in skin for up to 8 weeks after injection, requiring patients to be cautioned to avoid light. Emphasis should be placed on wearing protective clothing, gloves, and eye protection to avoid burns, which are usually mild in severity and are generally cited as occurring in 5%–28% of cases.[6]

Equipment

- Bronchoscope
- Bronchoscope tower
- Laser system
- Cylindrical diffuser

Staff

- Bronchoscopist
- Bronchoscopy technician/respiratory therapist
- Anesthesia team

Setting

PDT is typically performed in the bronchoscopy suite as an outpatient procedure. It can be done under moderate sedation or general anesthesia. Sedation should be deep enough for the patient as to not disrupt activation of light at the target lesion. Picking the procedural day for PDT is important, as a repeat bronchoscopy must be completed 2 days after the light activation procedure. Depending on staff and bronchoscopy suite scheduling, this usually precludes scheduling PDT on Thursday or Friday. The preprocedural preparation area should keep the lights dimmed to diminish ambient light thereby minimizing potential skin irritation. The same holds true for the bronchoscopy procedure room if possible.

PROCEDURAL TECHNIQUES

Once the patient is sedated, the bronchoscope is introduced for an airway examination to ensure that the lesion has not significantly changed from when PDT was originally offered. A cylindrical diffuser, which comes in both rigid (outer diameter 1.7 mm) and flexible (1.07 mm) fibers, is attached to the diode laser machine. The diffuser fiber length is selected to match the length of the target lesion. Light is distributed in a 360-degree radius from the fiber when activated. Red light (625–630 nm) is the preferred light band, as it penetrates best into tissue, with 800 nm considered the limit to generating a photodynamic reaction. Tissue activation of 200 J/cm is the most commonly selected dose as it is the maximum that can be applied to the airway. The diffuser length is then selected on the calculation menu of the laser machine providing the time needed to deliver the desired light dose.

The diffuser, when introduced through the bronchoscope, is then placed in the middle of the airway across the target lesion. Special glasses are distributed to protect the eyes during energy activation. The bronchoscope is steadied and the catheter is maintained in the airway. While the diffuser is activated, bright light that renders the screen indiscernible occurs. Maintaining diffuser position is important to ensure direct delivery of the light to the target lesion. Once the activation is completed, the bronchoscope is removed and the patient is recovered and given discharge precautions regarding worsening respiratory distress and the importance of returning for repeat bronchoscopy. Reillumination can be offered to patients, as the Photofrin remains biochemically active in malignant cells for an additional 6 to 7 days from injection.[7]

When the patient returns for repeat bronchoscopy 48 h after activation, the airway is inspected and denuded respiratory epithelium is removed. This is accomplished with suctioning and pulmonary forceps in most cases. A cryoprobe may be needed in some cases to remove very adherent or large amount of sloughed tissue. Once the sloughed tissue is removed, the patient is recovered and discharged home. Repeat bronchoscopy 1–3 months after PDT should be performed to assess the treated area is free of disease.

Figs. 9.1–9.5 show bronchoscopic images of a PDT procedure performed to treat a carcinoma in situ in the bronchus intermedius.

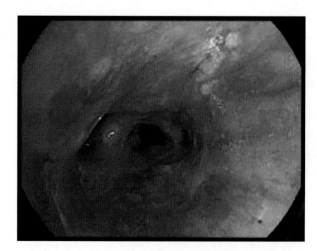

Fig. 9.1 Endobronchial squamous cell carcinoma in situ (white plaques).

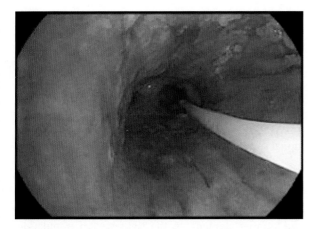

Fig. 9.2 Diffuser positioned in airway adjacent to carcinoma in situ.

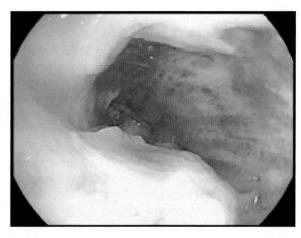

Fig. 9.4 Sloughing of airway 48h following activation.

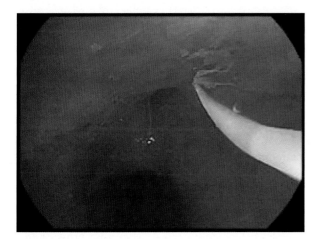

Fig. 9.3 Diffuse activation with red light wavelength.

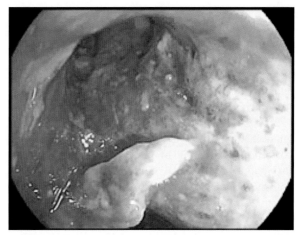

Fig. 9.5 View of airways after removal of sloughed tissue.

COMPLICATIONS

There are some notable complications associated with PDT. Photofrin is retained in the skin for approximately 6–8 weeks following infusion, causing significant photosensitivity. This can lead to significant sunburn that necessitates patients wear protective clothing and eye protection when exposed to sunlight.[8] The tissue death occurring 2 days after treatment necessitates repeat bronchoscopy to remove desiccated tissue. In 7% of cases, tissue sloughing can result in significant airway obstruction causing life-threatening respiratory distress.[2] Therefore a repeat bronchoscopy 48h after PDT

is essential to remove sloughed tissue. Bronchial stenosis has been reported if the treatment area overlaps with normal respiratory mucosa. While extremely rare, life-threatening hemoptysis can occur if the target area is <1cm from a major mediastinal vessel.

EVIDENCE

PDT is employed in two clinical scenarios, one with curative intent for carcinoma in situ and the other for palliation of symptoms in obstructive malignant disease. In a prospective study of 175 lung cancer patients from 1982 to 1996, McCaughan and Williams used PDT to treat 16 patients with stage I disease, 9 patients with stage II disease, 106 with stage III, and 44 patients with stage IV disease.[9] Most patients had squamous cell carcinoma of the airway. The authors applied energy of 400 J/cm diffusing fiber for trachea and main bronchi, 300 J/cm for lobar bronchi, and 200 J/cm for segmental bronchi. The median survival of all patients in the study was 7 months, but when assessing each subgroup, stage I survival was not reached, stage II was 22.5 months, stage IIIA 5.7 months, stage IIIB 5.5 months, and stage IV 5 months. Three patients with squamous cell carcinoma in situ had complete responses (CRs) with no evidence of disease at 8, 74, and 121 months. The disease-free survival for stage I disease was 93%.[9]

In a different study from Japan, a total of 204 patients with 264 centrally located early stage lung cancer lesions underwent PDT between February 1980 and February 2005.[10] Two hundred and fifty-eight of the lesions were squamous cell carcinomas, 185 were clinical stage 0, and 79 were clinical stage I. Tumor dimension was less than 1 cm in 180 lesions, between 1 and 2 cm in 50 lesions, and more than 2 cm in 34 lesions. For the 56 tumors <0.5 cm, CR was 94.6%, lesion 0.5–1 cm CR was 93.5%, 1–2 cm CR 80%, and >2 cm CR 44.1%. The distal margin of the tumor was visible on 203 of the lesions, which corresponded to a CR of 91.6%. Importantly, though, for lesions <1.0 cm the CR of 92.8% corresponded with a 5-year survival rate of 57.9%. The authors of the study attribute this to the study participants' frailty, as they were not deemed surgical candidates and the vast majority of patients died from other diseases associated with their poor cardiopulmonary reserve.

Regarding palliation of symptoms, Moghissi and colleagues recruited 100 patients with advanced inoperable lung cancer (73% stage IIIa, 10% stage IV) between May 1990 and May 1997.[11] The study was set up to record symptoms (dyspnea, cough, and hemoptysis) and performance status using the World Health Organization (WHO) scale. The WHO scale is arranged from 0 (able to carry out all normal activities without restriction) to 4 (completely disabled). Patients (59% squamous, 24% adenocarcinoma) underwent PDT to their airway tumor following Photofrin injection. Follow-up of these patients was completed every 6–8 weeks for 1 year and then in 3–6-month intervals. At these visits data were collected. Pre-PDT treatment, 43 patients had a WHO scale of ≤2 and 54 patients had a WHO scale of ≥2. Six to eight weeks following PDT treatment, 87 patients had a WHO scale of ≤2 and 10 patients had a WHO scale of ≥2. Similarly forced expiratory volume in the first second of expiration (FEV_1) increased by 0.28 L following PDT and forced vital capacity (FVC) increased by 0.43 L. While multivariate analysis demonstrated that only performance status was statistically significant for survival, there was a significant improvement in functional status following treatment with PDT.

SUMMARY

PDT elevated the field of therapeutic bronchoscopy to the curative domain. In the right patient population, particularly patients with <1 cm length squamous cell carcinoma in situ, there is a ~90% chance of CR. While tumors are ideally centrally located, there is increasing interest in using available technology to provide treatment to distal airways.[12] PDT also has applications for malignant central airway obstruction, often used in tandem with other usual treatment modalities such as chemotherapy and radiation. Newer tumor-specific photosensitizers are being developed with fewer side effects and hopefully more efficacy. PDT is a technology that has continued to evolve since 1982 and is anticipated to remain in the armamentarium of interventional pulmonologists worldwide.

CRYOTHERAPY

Introduction

Endobronchial lesions can develop from primary lung cancer or metastatic disease leading to airway obstruction. Most of these patients are not candidates for surgical resection and are likely to experience shortness of breath, hypoxemia, hemoptysis, and recurrent postobstructive pneumonia.[13] Airway obstruction due to benign conditions like mucus plugging, blood clot impaction, foreign body aspiration, and benign strictures can also lead to similar symptoms. The use of cryotherapy for immediate recanalization of the airway by debulking endobronchial lesions is described elsewhere. However, cryotherapy has a vital role as delayed therapy to restore the patency of airways for treatment and palliation purposes. This section summarizes the critical aspects of using cryotherapy as a delayed endobronchial ablative treatment and cryoextraction to remove foreign bodies, mucus plugs, and blood clots obstructing the airways.

The use of severely low temperatures to treat tumors was first described as early as 1851 by James Arnott for a lesion in the breast.[14] Cooper and Lee subsequently introduced the first closed-tip cryoprobe using liquid nitrogen in 1961; its first endobronchial use was by Gage using a rigid cryoprobe.[15,16] A flexible cryoprobe was developed in 1994.[13] The cryoprobe gets cold to extremely low temperatures. It captures the cooling effect of the rapid expansion of a gas that has been liquefied under high pressures. This phenomenon is also known as the Joule-Thomson effect.[17,18] Cryotherapy is applied to tissue through multiple approaches: percutaneous, thoracic, endobronchial, and so on.[19] It has been shown to treat or palliate unresectable cancers and can potentially increase long-term survival.[20,21] Endobronchial cryotherapy is suggested for the treatment of endobronchial tumors and removal of foreign bodies and blood clots obstructing airways in the European Respiratory Society/American Thoracic Society guidelines (2002) and American College of Chest Physician Guidelines in 2003.[22,23]

MECHANISM OF ACTION

Cryotherapy induces tissue destruction through intracellular and extracellular cryocrystallization. Through the specially designed cryoprobe, extremely low temperatures can be applied to a local area leading to the initiation of these destructive events. Intracellular ice crystal formation leads to damage to intracellular organelles like mitochondria and endoplasmic reticulum, whereas extracellular ice crystallization leads to intracellular dehydration and cell death. Mazur described the cell death mechanism by cryotherapy; 90% cell death can be achieved if tissue is cooled quickly to $-40°C$ at the rate of $-100°C$ per minute. Lower temperatures and repeat freeze-thaw cycles contribute incrementally to cell death.[24] Also, cryotherapy leads to microthrombi formation in the surrounding vasculature, hastening cell death and selectively targeting the hypervascular tumor tissue. For the same reason, tissues with higher water content are more sensitive to cryotherapy (granulation tissue, tumor, nerves, endothelium), while bronchial cartilage is relatively spared from tissue destruction, along with fibrosis, nerve sheath, and connective tissue.[25,26]

Immediate relief of an obstructed airway from foreign bodies, blood clots, and mucus plug can also be obtained through cryotherapy and is based on a different mechanism of action. Under bronchoscopic guidance, the cryoprobe is put in direct contact with the culprit obstructing tissue/foreign body and is activated. As the cryoprobe freezes to extremely low temperatures, it adheres to the adjacent tissue. The cryoprobe is then removed en bloc with the bronchoscope. Large fragments of mucus, organized blood clots, and some foreign bodies can be removed with this technique, which may otherwise not have been possible through flexible bronchoscopy alone.

PREPROCEDURAL PREPARATION

Indications and contraindications to performing endobronchial cryoablation or cryoextraction can guide patient selection and should be reviewed before planning these procedures.

Indications

1. Intraluminal tumors of histology-proven malignancies causing endobronchial obstruction.[19]
2. Treatment of low-grade endobronchial malignancies like carcinoid tumors that are otherwise unresectable.[27]
3. Granulation tissue growth leading to airway obstruction.[23]
4. Retrieval of foreign objects from central and segmental airways. Objects with more water content like certain food materials and tissue are more amenable to cryoextraction as opposed to metallic objects, plastics, teeth, bone material, etc.[23]
5. Retrieval of organized blood clot/thrombus and mucus plugs from the airways, not cleared with therapeutic suctioning and causing respiratory compromise or risk of postobstructive pneumonia.[28]

Contraindications

1. Lack of expertise or training in performing endobronchial cryotherapy.
2. Presence of bleeding diathesis, thrombocytopenia $<50 \times 10^9$, use of clopidogrel and newer antiplatelet agents, and anticoagulant therapy would present a high risk of bleeding complications with endobronchial cryotherapy as well as any endobronchial intervention.
3. Any contraindications to undergoing the bronchoscopy procedure itself.

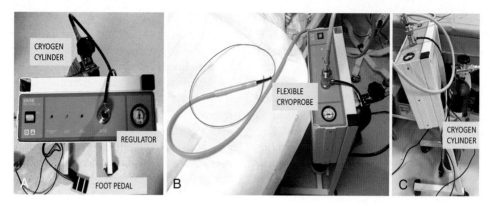

Fig. 9.6 Cryotherapy machine showing the flow regulator, foot pedal for activation, and cylinder with cryogen (A). Cryotherapy machine assembled with cryoprobe attached (B, C).

Equipment

For delivery of cryotherapy for any of the aforementioned indications, a combination of the below three types of equipment is needed (Fig. 9.6):

1. Cryosurgery device or cryoprobe: The flexible cryoprobe comes in two operating diameters: 2.4 mm and 1.9 mm. Its length is 90 cm, and the length of the cooling tip is 7 mm (ERBE USA, Inc.; Marietta, GA, USA).[13] Besides the flexible probe, rigid and semirigid cryoprobes are also available but are less commonly used. The rigid and semirigid cryoprobe can only be used with a rigid bronchoscope. Their advantage is a short thawing phase of the probe leading to a faster procedure; however, this can also decrease the extent of cellular injury achieved, and hence use of the flexible probe may be overall preferred.[26,27]

2. Cryogen or cooling agent: The cryogen is stored in a liquefied state under high pressure in a cylinder on the cryo machine. Nitrous oxide, nitrogen, and carbon dioxide are the most commonly used cryogens. Nitrous oxide is reported to cool the cryoprobe tip to −89°C, whereas the carbon dioxide cools to −79°C within a few seconds.[29] The cylinder connects to the cryoprobe, and, when activated, cryogen is released through a transfer line to the cryoprobe tip. The tip has a chamber for ingress and egress of the gas leading to its rapid freezing.[27] A regulator located on the cryo machine controls the rate of freezing of the cryoprobe by regulating the flow of the cryogen (Fig. 9.6).

3. The delivery device: A flexible fiberoptic bronchoscope or a rigid bronchoscope can be used to deliver endobronchial cryotherapy. Using the flexible bronchoscope does not always require general anesthesia. It can also reach the distal bronchi and upper lobes, which is otherwise difficult with a rigid bronchoscope. Flexible fiberoptic bronchoscopes with a large working channel of 2.8 mm or more allow the cryoprobe to be inserted easily and also leave the ability to apply some suction if needed (Fig. 9.7).

Staff

Physicians with prior training and experience in interventional procedures of the lung with cryotherapy and airway management should lead these procedures. Allied staff including nurses, technicians, and respiratory therapists should be well versed in using the cryotherapy equipment.

Setting

Cryotherapy-assisted ablation and extraction can be performed using standard monitoring in a fully equipped bronchoscopy suite. Equipment should be checked for functionality before the procedure, including the appropriate level of cryogen in the cylinder, freeze time of the cryoprobe with saline, and appropriate activation and deactivation of the probe. No additional safety equipment other than that regularly used in the bronchoscopy suite is required for cryotherapy.

Anesthesia Considerations

When performed with flexible bronchoscopy, this procedure can be performed successfully under both general

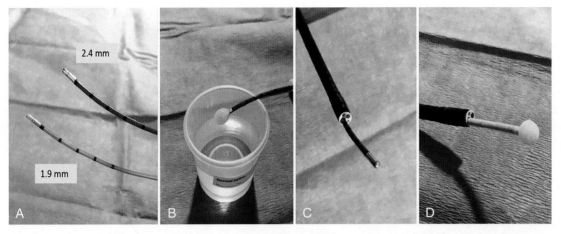

Fig. 9.7 Two commonly used flexible cryoprobes, 1.9 mm and 2.4 mm in diameter (A). Cryoprobe activation tested by making a saline ice ball before procedure (B). Cryoprobe inserted through working channel of flexible bronchoscope without freezing (C) and with freezing (D).

anesthesia and moderate sedation.[28] No studies comparing anesthesia techniques for cryotherapy ablation have been reported yet. Higher sedation requirements to avoid coughing and prevent airway injury during the procedure give an advantage to the use of general anesthesia; however, patients with significant comorbidities can be at additional risk with deeper anesthesia. The decision to use general anesthesia would be dictated by patient's condition, type of lesion, institutional availability, and provider preference.[27]

Advantages of Cryotherapy Over Other Ablative Modalities

1. The use of cryotherapy using a flexible bronchoscope provides easier access to upper lobe lesions and distal lesions, which is otherwise difficult to attain with rigid bronchoscopy.[13,30]
2. Less damage to cartilaginous structures is seen with cryotherapy due to their lesser water content.[13]
3. No safety equipment (e.g., goggles) is needed for cryoablation unlike when using laser therapy.[26]
4. There is no risk of airway fires or electric accidents during the procedure.[27]
5. Cryotherapy can be performed in patients requiring oxygenation at high supplemental oxygen levels, unlike thermal therapies.[30]
6. Cryotherapy equipment is less expensive than laser equipment used for debulking and ablation.[13]

Disadvantages of Cryotherapy

1. The effect of cryoablation is delayed and not immediate, sometimes necessitating repeat procedures.
2. Cryoablation is not the procedure of choice for high-grade emergent airway obstructions due to its delayed results.

PROCEDURAL TECHNIQUES

Variations in the technique of performing endobronchial cryoablation and cryoextraction are evident in literature around anesthesia, airway device, selection of equipment, freeze-thaw times, and so on. [23,26,27] Below is the outline of the most commonly applied technique.

1. A 2.4-mm or 1.9-mm flexible cryoprobe is advanced through the flexible fiberoptic bronchoscope inside the airways until the metallic tip is completely exposed. Rigid bronchoscopy is not needed to use the flexible cryoprobe; however, use of rigid and semi-rigid cryoprobes, which are used less commonly, requires rigid bronchoscopy.
2. The cryoprobe tip is brought in direct contact with the endobronchial target site and activated using the foot pedal.
3. Activation of the cryoprobe leads to formation and expansion of an ice ball in the target tissue until an adequate area is covered and adheres to the tip of the probe.

4. Following attachment of the cryoprobe tip to the desired area, alternate cycles of freezing and thawing the tissue for approximately 30 s each are applied (Fig. 9.8). Any overlying necrotic tissue should first be removed using cryoextraction for most benefit from the following delayed cryotherapy. Each new area should be located 5 mm apart from the last application, creating some overlap of treated area to ensure full coverage.

5. If a cryoprobe is being used to extract foreign bodies, mucus plugs, or blood clots (Figs. 9.9–9.11), then, once the desired adherence is achieved to the target tissue/object, the cryoprobe and bronchoscope are removed en bloc from the airway quickly. The probe is then thawed in saline at bedside to detach the adherent sample. An assistant should hold the endotracheal tube securely during scope removal to avoid inadvertent extubation.

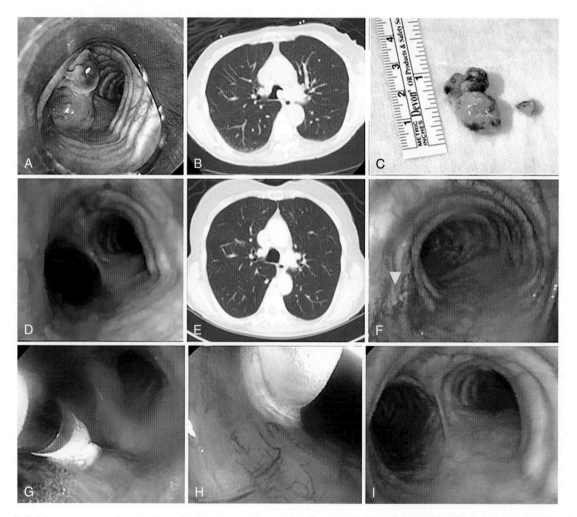

Fig. 9.8 Management of typical carcinoid tumor managed with cryotherapy. Preintervention imaging showing left mainstem tumor (A, B). Tumor extracted with combination therapy of cautery snare and cryoextraction during rigid bronchoscopy (C). Posttumor extraction, day 1 intervention (D). Postoperative CT of chest (E). Treatment of base of tumor attachment at the uptake of left mainstem with cryotherapy, freeze, and thaw technique (F–H). Local tumor control maintained with periodic cryotherapy, 3 months postintervention (I).

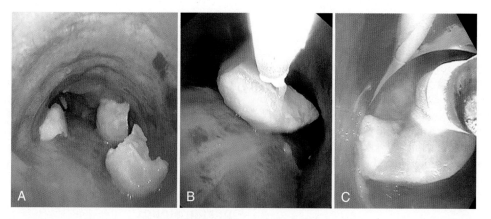

Fig. 9.9 Foreign body extraction (macadamia nuts) using cryofreezing and immediate extraction (A, B, C).

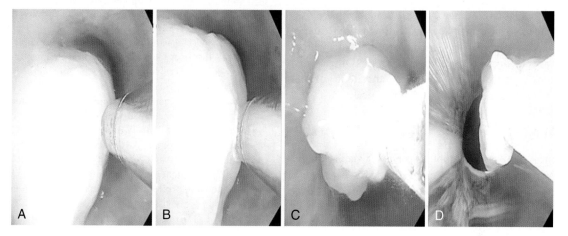

Fig. 9.10 Mucus plug extraction using cryotherapy (A–D). (From Van Holden MD, University of Maryland Medical Center.)

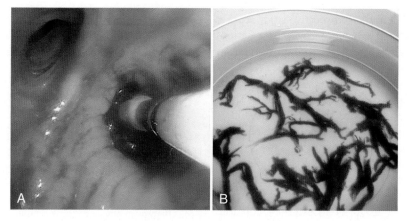

Fig. 9.11 Blood clot extraction using cryotherapy for immediate relief (A). Large organized blood clots cryoextracted in the form of airway clots extracted (B).

6. The bronchoscopist should take caution to ensure that the cryoprobe moves freely before the abrupt removal and does not attach to healthy tissue or the airway wall during removal to avoid inadvertent airway injury and/or bleeding.
7. If the cryoprobe does stick to an unintended area in the bronchus or endotracheal tube, it should be deactivated until the ice thaws and probe is spontaneously released from the tissue.[28]
8. Repeat bronchoscopy may be considered in 2–4 weeks to complete debridement of the sloughed tissue after the initial cryoablation.

COMPLICATIONS

Endobronchial cryotherapy is not associated with the risk of airway fire. However, following treatment, there can be associated airway edema and mucus accumulation, which can cause postoperative respiratory distress.[26] Other complications reported include ulceration and injury of the airway, bleeding, perforation, and, rarely, death.[26]

EVIDENCE

Evidence supports the application of cryoablation in improving intrinsic tumors and restoring the patency of airways. In a trial of 521 patients with malignant tracheobronchial tumors who underwent cryosurgery over 9 years, the investigators saw significant improvement in cough, dyspnea, hemoptysis, and quality of life.[13,26] In a study reported by Mathur and colleagues, cryoablation was able to altogether remove intrinsic tumors in 18/20 (90%) patients and led to symptom improvement in 75% of patients.[13] Another prospective study reports success rates of 77% in relieving airway obstruction. This improvement also correlates with improvement in symptoms as seen in other studies also.[13,31,32]

Cryoablation can also be applied in conjunction with other ablative therapies to achieve desired results. There is now accumulating evidence through small studies that chemotherapeutic agents may accumulate better in cryoablated tumors, leading to a better response to treatment.[33,34] Vergnon and colleagues reported a higher local tumor control (65% as compared to 35%) in patients with unresectable non–small cell lung cancer (NSCLC) who received cryotherapy prior to external radiation. This was also related to better survival as compared to radiation alone[35] (median 397 days vs. 144 days).

▉ SUMMARY

Cryotherapy is a useful, safe, and less expensive option of the currently available alternatives for endobronchial tumor debulking, ablation, clot or mucus retrieval, and foreign body aspiration. Its application depends on the urgency for recanalization, location and type of lesion, type of airway obstruction, and available expertise and equipment. Combining of tumor debulking and ablative techniques may have an additive advantage in expert hands to achieve best possible outcomes.

REFERENCES

1. Hayata Y, Kato H, Konaka C, et al. Fiberoptic bronchoscopic laser photoradiation for tumor localization in lung cancer. *Chest.* 1982;82(1):10–14.
2. Chaddha U, Hogarth DK, Murgu S. Bronchoscopic ablative therapies for malignant central airway obstruction and peripheral lung tumors. *Ann Am Thorac Soc.* 2019;16(10):1220–1229.
3. Kwiatkowski S, Knap B, Przystupski D, et al. Photodynamic therapy: mechanisms, photosensitizers and combinations. *Biomed Pharmacother.* 2018;106:1098–1107.
4. Dougherty TJ, Gomer CJ, Henderson BW, et al. Photodynamic therapy. *J Natl Cancer Inst.* 1998;90(12):889–905.
5. Gomer CJ, Dougherty TJ. Determination of [3H]- and [14C]hematoporphyrin derivative distribution in malignant and normal tissue. *Cancer Res.* 1979;39(1):146–151.
6. Moghissi K, Dixon K. Is bronchoscopic photodynamic therapy a therapeutic option in lung cancer? *Eur Respir J.* 2003;22(3):535–541.
7. Mahmood K, Wahidi MM. Ablative therapies for central airway obstruction. *Semin Respir Crit Care Med.* 2014;35(6):681–692.
8. Lee P, Kupeli E, Mehta AC. Therapeutic bronchoscopy in lung cancer. Laser therapy, electrocautery, brachytherapy, stents, and photodynamic therapy. *Clin Chest Med.* 2002;23(1):241–256.
9. McCaughan Jr JS, Williams TE. Photodynamic therapy for endobronchial malignant disease: a prospective fourteen-year study. *J Thorac Cardiovasc Surg.* 1997;114(6):940–946. discussion 946–947.
10. Kato H, Usuda J, Okunaka T, et al. Basic and clinical research on photodynamic therapy at Tokyo Medical University Hospital. *Lasers Surg Med.* 2006;38(5):371–375.
11. Moghissi K, Dixon K, Stringer M, Freeman T, Thorpe A, Brown S. The place of bronchoscopic photodynamic therapy in advanced unresectable lung cancer: experience of 100 cases. *Eur J Cardiothorac Surg.* 1999; 15(1):1–6.

12. Usuda J, Inoue T, Tsuchida T, et al. Clinical trial of photodynamic therapy for peripheral-type lung cancers using a new laser device in a pilot study. *Photodiagnosis Photodyn Ther.* 2020;30:101698.

13. Mathur PN, Wolf KM, Busk MF, Briete WM, Datzman M. Fiberoptic bronchoscopic cryotherapy in the management of tracheobronchial obstruction. *Chest.* 1996;110(3):718–723.

14. Arnott J. *On the Treatment of Cancer, by the Regulated Application of an Anaesthetic Temperature.* London: Churchill J; 1851.

15. Cooper IS, Lee AS. Cryostatic congelation: a system for producing a limited, controlled region of cooling or freezing of biologic tissues. *J Nerv Ment Dis.* 1961;133(3):259–263.

16. Gage AA, Koepf S, Wehrle D, Emmings F. Cryotherapy for cancer of the lip and oral cavity. *Cancer.* 1965;18(12):1646–1651.

17. Roebuck J, Murrell T, Miller E. The Joule-Thomson effect in carbon dioxide. *J Am Chem Soc.* 1942;64(2):400–411.

18. Roebuck J, Osterberg H. The Joule-Thomson effect in nitrogen. *Phys Rev.* 1935;48(5):450.

19. Niu L, Xu K, Mu F Cryosurgery for lung cancer. J Thorac Dis. 2012;4(4):408–419. https://doi:10.3978/j.issn.2072-1439.2012.07.13.

20. Xu KC, Niu LZ, He WB, Guo ZQ, Hu YZ, Zuo JS. Percutaneous cryoablation in combination with ethanol injection for unresectable hepatocellular carcinoma. *World J Gastroenterol.* 2003;9(12):2686.

21. Mouraviev V, Polascik TJ. Update on cryotherapy for prostate cancer in 2006. *Curr Opin Urol.* 2006;16(3):152–156.

22. Ernst A, Silvestri GA, Johnstone D. Interventional pulmonary procedures: guidelines from the American College of Chest Physicians. *Chest.* 2003;123(5):1693–1694.

23. Bolliger CT, Mathur PN, Beamis JF, et al. ERS/ATS statement on interventional pulmonology. European Respiratory Society/American Thoracic Society. *Eur Respir J.* 2002;19(2):356–373.

24. Mazur P. The role of intracellular freezing in the death of cells cooled at supraoptimal rates. *Cryobiology.* 1977;14(3):251–272.

25. Sunna R. Cryotherapy and cryodebridement. In: Ernst A, Herth FJF, eds. *Principles and Practice of Interventional Pulmonology*: Springer; 2013:343–350.

26. Shepherd RW, Radchenko C. Bronchoscopic ablation techniques in the management of lung cancer. *Ann Transl Med.* 2019;7(15):362.

27. DiBardino DM, Lanfranco AR, Haas AR. Bronchoscopic cryotherapy. Clinical applications of the cryoprobe, cryospray, and cryoadhesion. *Ann Am Thorac Soc.* 2016;13(8):1405–1415.

28. Hetzel M, Hetzel J, Schumann C, Marx N, Babiak A. Cryorecanalization: a new approach for the immediate management of acute airway obstruction. *J Thorac Cardiovasc Surg.* 2004;127(5):1427–1431.

29. Lentz RJ, Argento AC, Colby TV, Rickman OB, Maldonado F. Transbronchial cryobiopsy for diffuse parenchymal lung disease: a state-of-the-art review of procedural techniques, current evidence, and future challenges. *J Thorac Dis.* 2017;9(7):2186.

30. Dumon JF, Reboud E, Garbe L, Aucomte F, Meric B. Treatment of tracheobronchial lesions by laser photoresection. *Chest.* 1982;81(3):278–284.

31. Walsh D, Maiwand M, Nath A, Lockwood P, Lloyd M, Saab M. Bronchoscopic cryotherapy for advanced bronchial carcinoma. *Thorax.* 1990;45(7):509–513.

32. Maiwand M, Asimakopoulos G. Cryosurgery for lung cancer: clinical results and technical aspects. *Technol Cancer Res Treat.* 2004;3(2):143–150.

33. Homasson JP, Pecking A, Roden S, Angebault M, Bonniot JP. Tumor fixation of bleomycin labeled with 57 cobalt before and after cryotherapy of bronchial carcinoma. *Cryobiology.* 1992;29(5):543–548.

34. Ikekawa S, Ishihara K, Tanaka S, Ikeda S. Basic studies of cryochemotherapy in a murine tumor system. *Cryobiology.* 1985;22(5):477–483.

35. Vergnon JM, Schmitt T, Alamartine E, Barthelemy JC, Fournel P, Emonot A. Initial combined cryotherapy and irradiation for unresectable non-small cell lung cancer: preliminary results. *Chest.* 1992;102(5):1436–1440.

10

Stent Placement

A. Christine Argento and Sean B. Smith

INTRODUCTION

An airway stent is a hollow prosthesis that maintains airway patency and provides structural support. Stent deployment is an integral skill for an interventional pulmonologist. The indications and selection of airway stents will typically dictate the deployment technique used. Therefore the interventional pulmonologist must be familiar with a variety of techniques depending on the pathology that warrants stenting. In this chapter we will discuss stent types, indication, and placement.

HISTORY

The word "stent" is named after Charles Stent, a British dentist who created dental splints in the 19th century. The first stents were surgically placed by Trendelenburg and Bond to treat airway strictures and endoscopic placement was first performed by Brunings and Albrecht in 1915.[1] In 1965, a silicone stent with a tracheal stomal limb was invented by Montgomery, called the T-tube,[2] for treatment of subglottic stenosis. The first strictly endoluminal airway silicone stent was developed and described by Jean-François Dumon.[3] The silicone stent is what gave interventional pulmonology momentum, as this allowed central airway obstruction to be managed by pulmonologists with training in rigid bronchoscopy.[4] Since then there has also been the emergence of metallic stents.

TYPES OF STENTS

An ideal stent would (a) be easy to place and remove, (b) be resistant to migration, (c) not form granulation tissue, (d) not become obstructed with secretions, (e) be able to conform well to the patient's airway, (f) be customizable, (g) have sufficient radial force to maintain airway patency, and (h) be inexpensive. Unfortunately, this ideal stent does not (yet) exist.

Two main categories of stents exist: metallic and silicone. Both types of stents are used to manage central airway obstruction. A variety of stents are available for each main category (Fig. 10.1) and each stent has small nuances that will help you choose one over the other. A basic overview of the comparison of metallic versus silicone stents is shown in Table 10.1. One hybrid stent of special note is the dynamic stent, which is a bifurcated silicone stent that is constructed with anterior metal struts in the tracheal limb and only silicone at the posterior to simulate the tracheal rings and membranous trachea (Fig. 10.1H). This stent is placed with direct laryngoscopy and a pair of specialized rigid forceps. Finally, there are also hourglass stents that are made to resist migration when used to treat a stenotic airway and stent migration is a concern (Fig. 10.1G).

INDICATIONS FOR AIRWAY STENTING

Airway stents are placed when a patient develops respiratory symptoms and has imaging findings consistent with focal airway obstruction[1, 5] (Table 10.2). The amount of obstruction should be able to explain the patient's symptoms. Typically a 50% reduction in airway diameter is required for symptoms to arise. Generally a tracheal diameter of 8 mm or less is required before the patient will experience dyspnea on exertion, and a tracheal diameter of less than 5 mm will result in shortness of breath at rest.[4] Importantly, airways distal to

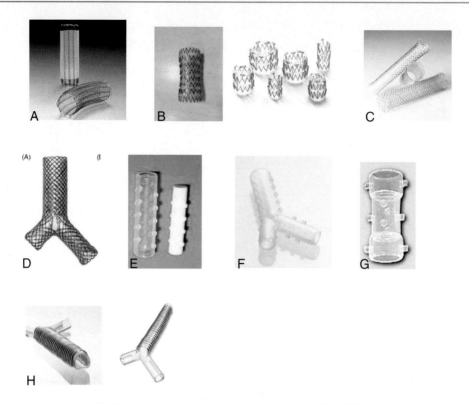

Fig. 10.1 Variety of stent types. (A) Ultraflex partially covered and uncovered. (B) AERO and AEROmini. (C) Bonastent. (D) Covered bifurcation/Y-stent. (E) Dumon silicone stents (radiolucent and radio-opaque). (F) Silicone bifurcation/Y-stent. (G) Hourglass stent. (H) Dynamic Y-stent.

the area of stent placement need to be patent for stent placement to be effective; this can sometimes be determined with imaging but often must be assessed during bronchoscopy. Airway stents can be particularly useful in patients with lung cancer, of which 30% present with airway obstruction and 35% will die from asphyxia, hemoptysis, or postobstructive pneumonia.[6] In a large, multicenter registry of 1115 procedures on 947 patients undergoing therapeutic bronchoscopy for central airway obstruction, one-third of patients underwent airway stenting that was associated with improvement in likelihood of achieving airway patency. Interestingly, patients with higher baseline dyspnea (Borg score) and nonlobar obstruction experienced greater improvements in dyspnea and health-related quality of life. Additionally, patients with higher American Society of Anesthesiology (ASA) score and lower functional status also had greater improvements in health-related quality of life.[7] Of note, the United States Food and Drug Administration of the United States issued a black box warning on the use of uncovered metallic stents in the trachea to treat benign tracheal obstruction in 2005.[8] The current standard of care is to treat benign tracheal obstruction with silicone stents or fully covered metallic stents. Fortin and colleagues reviewed the records of 30 patients who had third-generation fully covered metallic stents placed in the central airway for benign airway stenosis and found that 50% had to be removed for complications at a mean of 77 ± 96.6 days, the rest were removed at 122 ± 113.2 days without complication. The clinical success rate of stent treatment was 40.7% and no stent-related mortalities were reported.[9]

Stenting of more distal airways can be considered on a case-by-case basis to drain retained secretions, improve atelectasis, and assist with dyspnea, though this is technically more challenging and outcomes are less consistent, due for the most part to mucus clearance issues.[10]

TABLE 10.1   Comparison of Metallic and Silicone Stents

	Metal (Covered or Uncovered)	Silicone
Insertion with flexible scope	Yes	No
Insertion with rigid scope	Yes	Yes
Granulation tissue formation	Yes	Yes (ends)
Tumor ingrowth	Yes (uncovered)	No
Migration	Rarely	Yes
Fracture	Yes	Very rarely
Infection	Yes	Rarely
Airway perforation	Rarely	Very rarely
Mucus plugging	Rarely	Yes
Modifiable	No	Yes
Able to reposition	Immediately—yes Later—no	Yes
Ease of insertion	Easy	Requires rigid bronchoscopy expertise
Conforms to tortuous airway	Yes	No
Internal-to-external diameter ratio	High	Low
Radial strength/force	Medium	High
Mucociliary clearance	Uncovered—yes Covered—no	No
Cost	More	Less

TABLE 10.2   Indications for Metallic and Silicone Stents

Indication	Metallic	Silicone
Tracheal tumor	Yes	Yes
Bronchial tumor in central airways	Yes	Yes
Small airway with tumor	Yes	No
Malacia/EDAC	Sometimes	Yes
Tracheoesophageal fistula	No	Yes
Anastomotic dehiscence	Yes	Rarely
Extrinsic compression	Yes	Yes
Benign tracheal stenosis[a]	No	Yes

[a]This can include idiopathic, inhalational injury, posttracheostomy, postintubation, and autoimmune conditions (ex sarcoid, granulomatosis with polyangiitis, or systemic lupus erythematosus).
EDAC, Excessive dynamic airway collapse.

PREPROCEDURAL PLANNING

Patients' histories, physical examination, and computed tomography (CT) imaging should be carefully reviewed to confirm the need for airway stenting and to plan the procedure. Patients best suited for airway stenting are usually symptomatic with possible impending respiratory compromise, and so a team approach should be designed. Patients are best served in centers wherein there can be collaboration between multidisciplinary team members, including interventional pulmonologists, anesthesiologists, critical care physicians, and thoracic surgeons or otolaryngologists. Although some patients may be unstable for transport to other medical centers, it is essential to recognize that there can be risks of deploying airway stents without the proper equipment, team members, and facilities to care for the patient.[11]

It is important to recognize and plan for extrinsic, intrinsic, and complex stenoses. Tissue debulking may be necessary before stents can be deployed for intrinsic and complex stenoses, and so the proper equipment and expertise must be made available prior to the procedure, for example, rigid bronchoscopy, cryotherapy, argon plasma coagulation, electrocautery, or laser therapy.

The lung parenchyma distal to the stenosis should be carefully assessed. Airway stenting is most effective when the lung distal to the stenosis is viable. Stents placed in airways proximal to solid tissue masses may alleviate the stenosis and open the airway but not facilitate ventilation and therefore provide little clinical benefit. Likewise, CT imaging can help assess the vasculature in relation to airway stenosis, and if there is significant obstruction of distal lung perfusion, then stenting to improve ventilation may not yield clinical benefit. Therefore CT chest imaging with IV contrast can be extremely helpful for selection of patients most likely to benefit from stenting.

We recommend general anesthesia for stent deployment in order to facilitate airway management and adequate oxygenation and ventilation during the procedure. For distal tracheal or bronchial stenosis, the placement of an endotracheal tube may be routine, but for more proximal tracheal stenosis, endotracheal tube placement may be more difficult or impossible. Rigid bronchoscopy may therefore be necessary immediately upon the induction of anesthesia in order to secure the proximal trachea and follow with ablation or dilation of the stenosis before stenting. Rigid bronchoscopes also provide the interventional pulmonologist with more options for deployment of either silicone or metallic stents. Often the flexible scope is used through the rigid bronchoscope to assist with debulking or stent deployment. If a routine endotracheal tube is used, however, we recommend using at least an 8.0-size tube to facilitate ventilation around a therapeutic flexible bronchoscope.

DEPLOYING METALLIC STENTS

Metallic stents can be uncovered, partially covered, or completely covered by silicone or polyurethane. Although they used to be made of stainless steel, now these stents are made of nitinol, a nickel-titanium alloy that is elastic and has shape memory so will return to original form after being folded and loaded onto a catheter for deployment. No one stent is perfectly suited to all airway pathologies, and interventional pulmonologists should learn the benefits and limitations of each type. In general, metallic stents should be considered for malignant airways disease, when the provider wants to maximize internal-to-external diameter, if the airway is irregular, and when an uncovered portion may be desired to maintain patency of an adjacent airway. Uncovered metallic stents are used on occasion for benign disease, specifically for anastomotic dehiscence following lung transplantation.[12] All metallic stents share their ability to be easily folded into a low-profile deployment system. This means that they can be passed through a rigid bronchoscope or an endotracheal tube, and some can even pass through the working channel of a flexible bronchoscope, thus can be deployed without the use of rigid bronchoscopy. The most commonly used metallic stents today are the Ultraflex

(Boston Scientific, Marlborough, MA, USA) (Fig. 10.2), AERO and AEROmini (Merit Endotek, South Jordan, UT, USA) (Fig. 10.3), and the Bonastent (Thoracent, Huntington, NY, USA) (Fig. 10.4). Ultraflex stents are either uncovered or partially covered and are held onto the delivery catheter using a silk thread that you unwind by pulling on the string and releasing a series of crochet knots (Fig. 10.2). They have both proximal and distal release options. The AERO, AEROmini, and Bonastent are all metallic, fully covered with silicone or polyurethane, and use an external clear deployment catheter to compress the stent that is subsequently unsheathed for deployment (Figs. 10.3 and 10.4).

After the airway has been secured, flexible or rigid bronchoscopy is performed to inspect the stenosis and perform any necessary measure for dilation or ablation. Once the diameter of the airway lumen has been maximized, the provider should make measurements of the length and diameter of residual stenosis in order to select the appropriate stent size. Measurement of length can be done by passing the scope to the distal end of the stenosis, placing a finger on the scope to use as a marker, and then retracting to the proximal end of the stenosis. The distance from the distal to proximal end can then be measured using a ruler. If there are adjacent airway orifices, providers should consider the risks of occluding the orifice with any covered portion of a metallic stent. The diameter of the airway lumen can sometimes be estimated by visual inspection in relation to the scope, but balloon dilation can be useful to measure by inflating a balloon to the diameter required to occlude the lumen briefly. Finally, some companies offer sizing balloons to measure the airway luminal diameter more accurately (Fig. 10.5). As a general rule, diameter of the stent should be sized 2 mm greater than the airway diameter in order for the stent to exert radial force to the airway wall. We encourage two or three assessments of measurements to ensure accuracy. While taking measurements for placement, one can also place external radio-opaque devices (e.g., paperclips) on the patient's chest wall under fluoroscopy guidance to correspond to the proximal and distal ends of the stenosis as marked by the scope. This provides an external fluoroscopic assessment of the length of the stenosis for when the stent is deployed if not deploying with direct bronchoscopic visualization.

Once the stent type and size have been selected, a guidewire (typically 0.035 inch diameter) is placed

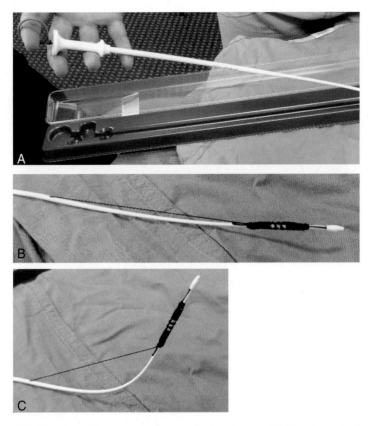

Fig. 10.2 Ultraflex stent. (A) Handle with ring to release crochet knots. (B) Stent on deployment catheter, distal release. (C) Stent on deployment catheter, proximal release.

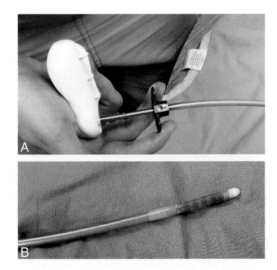

Fig. 10.3 AERO and AEROmini. (A) Handle and (B) stent on deployment catheter.

through the bronchoscope under visual and/or fluoroscopic guidance. The wire is passed through the stenosis to the distal airway, and again an assessment of the external metallic markers corresponding to the proximal and distal ends of the stenosis is made. If a flexible bronchoscope is being used, the scope is then removed using the Seldinger technique, keeping gentle forward pressure on the wire in order to leave the wire in place across the stenosis. Live fluoroscopy is useful to maintain the wire in the desired location. With the flexible scope removed and the wire exiting via the endotracheal tube or rigid scope, the stent deployment device can be positioned over the wire. It is important to assess the endotracheal tube or rigid bronchoscope size and ventilator connectors to ensure that the deployment device can fit smoothly over the wire, through the tube or scope and into the airway. The deployment device is then advanced over the wire and across the stenosis,

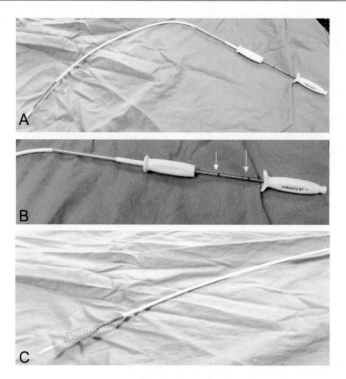

Fig. 10.4 Bonastent. (A) Full stent, (B) handle demonstrating indicators for when the stent starts to deploy *(white arrow)* and is 70% deployed *(yellow arrow)*, this is the point beyond which the stent can no longer be retrieved for repositioning, and (C) stent in mid-deployment.

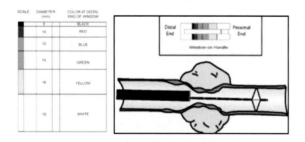

Fig. 10.5 Example of a sizing balloon (Aerosizer by Merit Endotek).

using direct visualization with an ultrathin or pediatric scope with or without live fluoroscopy to ensure that the stent will land in the desired location. When the stent is deployed, there tends to be some backward tension and movement of the stent, and so keeping the stent slightly distal to the desired location is advised.

Deployment devices differ by brand of metallic stent. The principle involves the unsheathing of the folded stent with either retraction of a cord or removal of a covering sheath. As the stent is uncovered, use direct visualization with a bronchoscope or live fluoroscopy and gentle forward pressure on the deployment device to keep the stent from migrating during deployment. Some brands with a retractable sheath allow for readvancing the sheath back over the stent up to a certain point during deployment if the stent location needs adjustment. During deployment, the metallic stent will expand to its manufactured diameter depending on its interaction with and the compliance of the airway wall. It is useful to remember that although metallic, the radial force of a metallic stent is less than that of a silicone stent, and so extrinsic pressure from the airway wall may limit full expansion. Once fully uncovered, the deployment device will be disengaged from the stent and must be removed from the airway. We often continue direct visualization with a scope or live fluoroscopy guidance to ensure that the deployment device disengages fully and does not unintentionally catch or retract the stent.

In cases where the deployment device is small enough, it can be deployed via the working channel of a flexible therapeutic bronchoscope (Bonastents 8 mm or 10 mm diameter). Rigid bronchoscopy, however, can also be used to deploy a metallic stent. The rigid scope serves as the endotracheal tube for ventilation and can be large enough in diameter to accommodate a deployment device. Depending on the sizes, a flexible or rigid optic device may also pass through the scope to provide real-time endoscopic guidance during deployment. This may help the bronchoscopist get an assessment of how the stent interacts and fits within the proximal end of the stenosis.[13] We would still encourage concomitant live fluoroscopy to help assess the distal end that is unlikely to be well visualized endoscopically.

After deployment, either flexible or rigid bronchoscopy should be used to perform a thorough assessment of the stent within the stenosis. Adjacent airway orifices should be examined in order to determine how, if at all, there has been any obstruction than may limit ventilation or mucus drainage. Metallic stents can be adjusted once deployed. Some brands have strings woven within the proximal and/or distal ends that can facilitate grasping with a flexible or rigid forceps. The forceps can then be used to pull the stent proximally across the stenosis for better positioning. We recommend not applying significant force on any single metallic strut without the help of a string, as the struts may fracture. Finally, balloon dilation may be used to improve the deployment of a stent that is not completely unfolded or may be compressed by extrinsic force of the airway wall. Please access Video 10.1 (Tracheobronchial Esophageal Fistula) online to watch deployment of a covered metallic stent for tracheobronchial esophageal fistula.

If a metallic stent needs to be removed, this can be accomplished by either flexible or rigid bronchoscopy. If the stent was just deployed, or if granulation tissue has not encroached upon the stent, then a simple pulling maneuver with flexible forceps may disengage the stent from the airway wall. If there has been encroachment by granulation tissue or tumor, however, then ablative therapies or rigid bronchoscopy may be needed to carefully disengage the stent from the airway wall. Once mobilized, the metallic stent can be pulled out of the airway via the endotracheal tube, rigid scope, or even the native airway through the vocal cords, though using moderate sedation for stent removal is not advised given the possible difficulties that could be encountered and potential damage to the vocal cords.

DEPLOYING SILICONE STENTS

As with metallic stents, there is no perfect stent for a specific airway obstruction. Silicone stents can be used in either benign or malignant disease, apply more radial force to extrinsic compression of the airway wall, and can generally remain in airways for longer periods of time with less granulation tissue formation. Silicone stents, however, are more prone to migration and are more likely to impair mucus clearance. All silicone stents require deployment with a rigid bronchoscope, and so the expertise with rigid techniques and equipment is absolutely necessary for the bronchoscopist, team, and facility planning to deploy a silicone stent.

The procedures described earlier regarding bronchoscopic examination and planning before stent deployment apply similarly to silicone stents. Unlike metallic stents, however, silicone stents are not routinely placed over guidewires, but rather folded and deployed through the barrel of a rigid bronchoscope. This requires the rigid scope to be large enough to accommodate the folded silicone stent but also small enough to pass through the airway stenosis. Therefore diligent examination of the stenosis and manipulation of the scope through the stenosis should be performed prior to selecting and loading a stent.

The silicone stent should be prepared for deployment. There are a wide variety of shapes and designs for silicone stents. Some are simple tube stents, while others have external studs to help minimize migration, and some are Y-shaped with three limbs in order to fit at a carina. Simple tube stents are symmetric, but silicone stents with special features require the provider to be very thoughtful when folding so as to ensure proper positioning of features within the airway after deployment. Some providers will use sandpaper or abrasive devices to shave or smooth down sharp edges on the ends of silicone stents in hopes of minimizing granulation tissue for long-term deployment. Also, the length can be customized using scissors or a scalpel and "windows" can be created using a rongeur (Fig. 10.6) to allow for ventilation and mucus clearance from airways that would otherwise have been occluded by the stent. This technique of window customization is most often used

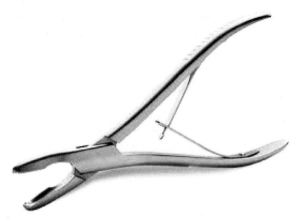

Fig. 10.6 Rongeur used to create a window in a silicone stent, most commonly used for the right upper lobe orifice.

for the right upper lobe orifice. Customization of these stents can lead to successful stenting of difficult lesions with a good short-term safety profile.[14]

Depending on the brand of rigid bronchoscope, there are loading devices that assist in the folding and insertion of a silicone stent into a rigid introducer. The introducer is a hollow tube that can accommodate the folded stent within its own lumen, and then the introducer can be fit through the barrel of the rigid scope for stent deployment. The loading device helps keep the stent in folded position so that it can be pushed into the introducer (Figs. 10.7 and 10.8). Ample lubrication is helpful to slide the folded stent into the loader and introducer. Finally, a matched-size plunger will be placed through the back of the introducer (Fig. 10.9). The plunger is a rigid rod that will abut the proximal end of the stent within the introducer. The bronchoscopist will not be able to see the interaction of the plunger and the stent through the introducer, and so careful handling is required in order to ensure that the stent is not pushed out of the introducer. In general, the length of the stent should correspond to the length between the plunger and introducer handles when properly positioned (Fig. 10.7G).

When ready for deployment, the rigid bronchoscope should be placed through the airway stenosis and positioned near its distal end. The rigid optic and suction catheters will need to be removed, and depending on the rigid scope brand and ventilation strategy used (conventional vs. jet), adjustments to the caps or ventilation tubing may be required so that nothing is obstructing the barrel of the rigid scope proximally. Although brief, there will be a pause in effective ventilation during deployment, and so the anesthesia team should be prepared. The introducer, already loaded with the folded stent and plunger, can then be placed through the back end of the rigid scope. The introducer should be matched to the size of the barrel, thus allowing both for smooth passage of the introducer through the barrel as well as for correct positioning of the end of the introducer at the end of the barrel of the rigid bronchoscope.

Some introducers allow for a rigid optic to be placed through the plunger or introducer, but in most cases the next steps of deployment will be blind. Silicone stents are not readily visible fluoroscopically, unless using a radio-opaque version, and so we do not find that fluoroscopy is useful during deployment. As the introducer is maneuvered through the barrel of the rigid scope, the bronchoscopist must keep the barrel in a steady position. Unknowingly advancing or retracting the scope before deployment will lead to malposition of the stent after deployment. With one hand steadying the barrel of the rigid scope, the bronchoscopist can use their other hand to push the plunger through the introducer, thus pushing the folded stent out of the introducer and into the airway. As the plunger is moved forward, we suggest gentle retraction of the barrel of the rigid scope so that the distal end of the stent remains in alignment, just beyond the distal edge of the stenosis. Simply deploying the plunger and stent without retracting the barrel can lead to the stent being pushed out far distal to the stenosis. After the plunger has been fully advanced through the introducer and the stent deployed, the introducer and plunger are removed so that the optic and suction catheters can be replaced.

As with the deployment of metallic stents, there should be careful bronchoscopic inspection of a newly deployed silicone stent. Rigid manipulation is often required to achieve proper positioning and complete unfolding. The radial force and configuration memory of silicone stent will often cause it to open spontaneously from its folded configuration, but rigid forceps can be needed to pull, push, or twist a silicone stent into the desired position. Twisting of a silicone stent will cause it to fold into itself and reduce external diameter, and this maneuver can be useful to help slide a stent through the airway or stenosis. The rigid forceps, the barrel of the rigid scope, or an expansion balloon are all tools that can be used to help unfold and properly deploy silicone stents.

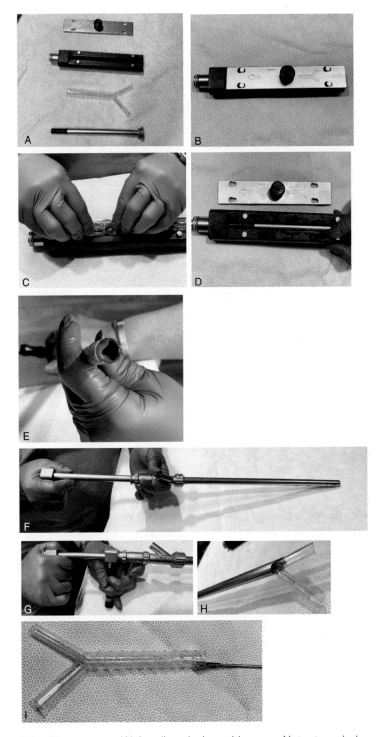

Fig. 10.7 Silicone Y-stent loading system. (A) Loading device with cover, Y-stent, and plunger. (B) Loading device closed with cover. (C) Loading the Y-stent into the loading device. (D) Loading device once the stent has been put into the introducer. (E) Y-stent loaded into the introducer. (F) Positioning the introducer through the rigid bronchoscope. (G) The introducer and plunger ready for stent deployment through a rigid bronchoscope. (H) Y-stent as it deploys. (I) Rigid forceps that can be used to grasp and manipulate the stent to adjust into appropriate position within the airway.

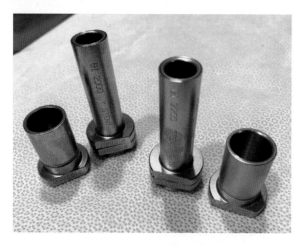

Fig. 10.8 Tubular silicone stent loaders.

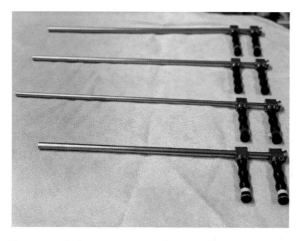

Fig. 10.9 Different-sized rigid stent introducer and plunger sets.

If a silicone stent needs to be removed because of malpositioning after deployment, or for any other reasons thereafter, rigid bronchoscopy will be required. The twisting maneuver with rigid forceps can help fold the stent such that it can be pulled within the barrel of a rigid scope. Once the stent has mobilized from the airway and engaged within the barrel, the stent can either be pulled through the barrel entirely if small enough or the stent (firmly grasped by forceps) and scope can be removed en bloc from the airway. This latter maneuver requires extubation with the rigid scope, and so the bronchoscopist and anesthesiologist must communicate and plan for airway management after rigid extubation.

POSTPROCEDURAL CARE

After deployment of an airway stent, the bronchoscopic and anesthesiologist must make a careful assessment of the patient's physiology and airway. Many patients will have been intubated just for the procedure, but others may have required intubation for respiratory failure because of the stenosis itself prior to bronchoscopy. If the stenosis has been fully dilated and protected with the stent, extubation in the operating room may be possible even for those patients with preexisting respiratory failure provided their oxygenation, ventilation, hemodynamics, and mental status allow. Awakening from anesthesia following rigid bronchoscopy is a unique situation often done with the placement of a new endotracheal tube or laryngeal mask airway (LMA) to assist with ventilation and oxygenation as the patient awakens. While LMA placement would not interact with airway stents, a new endotracheal tube may come into contact with a high- or mid-tracheal stent. Telescoping an endotracheal tube within a stent is possible, but final extubation is then best facilitated with a flexible bronchoscope to assure that the stent remains in position after retraction of the tube. Once extubated and transferred to anesthesia recovery areas, patients should be observed before the final decision regarding disposition.

Airway stents are artificial devices that will inherently affect patients' normal mucus clearance and bronchial hygiene. Silicone stents are especially prone to impair clearance and cause mucostasis, which can lead to disastrous obstructions of stents that are sometimes critical to maintain central airway patency. Indefinite bronchial hygiene is therefore required to maintain stent patency, and we recommend combination nebulized therapy of bronchodilator agents (e.g., albuterol) along with mucolytic agents (e.g., hypertonic saline or N-acetyl-cysteine) for all silicone stents. Surveillance bronchoscopy following stent placement is not standardized, and some institutions follow a particular schedule of intervals to perform it, whereas others perform bronchoscopy based on patient's reported symptoms. In all cases, patients with airway stents require close follow-up with the inserting team. Finally, a stent card should be provided to the patient to carry with them detailing the type, position, and size of stent as well as the physician's contact information in case the patient requires intubation.

COMPLICATIONS

Complications of airway stenting are frequent but not typically severe. With metallic stents, granulation tissue formation can occur from 4% to 25% of the time at the ends of the stent and can be treated with thermal therapies (cryotherapy, laser, or argon plasma coagulation). Mucus impaction, tumor ingrowth, and infection occur 5%–15% of the time. Stent fracture is variable and will depend on the indication for stent placement as well as the stent location.[15] For silicone stents, migration is most common at 9.5%, granulation tissue formation occurs ~7.9% of the time, and obstruction from secretions occurs 36% of the time.

When there is significant tumor ingrowth or obstruction from mucus, this can be life-threatening and the stent should be removed. Although removal is fairly straightforward with silicone stents (though does require rigid bronchoscopy) or fully covered metallic stents, uncovered metallic stent removal can prove to be challenging and cause complications, particularly if the stent has been in position for longer than 3 months. In one study, Lunn and colleagues describe their experience with removal of 30 metallic stents and reported the following complications: retained stent pieces (7/30), mucosal tear with bleeding (4/30), reobstruction requiring silicone stent placement (14/30), need for postoperative mechanical ventilation (6/30), and tension pneumothorax (1/30).[16] By contrast, a study by Noppen and colleagues described removal of 49 fully covered metallic stents without major complications. All patients were extubated postoperatively, and follow-up was unremarkable.[17] Most reports demonstrate some difficulty with metallic stent removal and expertise should be available to manage these complications should metallic stent retrieval be attempted.

■ SUMMARY

Airway stents are an important aspect of therapeutic bronchoscopy and improve success at achieving and maintaining airway patency in patients with either benign or malignant central airway obstruction. Stent selection and method of placement will vary depending on indication and location of obstruction as well as local expertise.

REFERENCES

1. Lee P, Kupeli E, Mehta AC. Airway stents. *Clin Chest Med*. 2010;31:141–150.
2. Montgomery WW. T-tube tracheal stent. *Arch Otolaryngol*. 1965;82:320–321.
3. Dumon JF. A dedicated tracheobronchial stent. *Chest*. 1990;97:328–332.
4. Ernst A, Herth F. *Principles and Practice of Interventional Pulmonology*. New York: Springer; 2013.
5. Guibert N, Saka H, Dutau H. Airway stenting: technological advancements and its role in interventional pulmonology. *Respirology*. 2020;25:953–962.
6. Cavaliere S, Venuta F, Foccoli P, Toninelli C, La Face B. Endoscopic treatment of malignant airway obstructions in 2,008 patients. *Chest*. 1996;110:1536–1542.
7. Ost DE, Ernst A, Grosu HB, et al. Therapeutic bronchoscopy for malignant central airway obstruction: success rates and impact on dyspnea and quality of life. *Chest*. 2015;147:1282–1298.
8. Food and Drug Administration. FDA Public Health Notification: Complications From Metallic Tracheal Stents in Patients With Benign AIRWAY Disorders. 2005.
9. Fortin M, Lacasse Y, Elharrar X, et al. Safety and efficacy of a fully covered self-expandable metallic stent in benign airway stenosis. *Respiration*. 2017;93:430–435.
10. Argento AC, Puchalski JT. Distal airway stenting: how far is too far? *J Bronchology Interv Pulmonol*. 2015;22:e15–e16.
11. Flannery A, Daneshvar C, Dutau H, Breen D. The art of rigid bronchoscopy and airway stenting. *Clin Chest Med*. 2018;39:149–167.
12. Mughal MM, Gildea TR, Murthy S, Pettersson G, DeCamp M, Mehta AC. Short-term deployment of self-expanding metallic stents facilitates healing of bronchial dehiscence. *Am J Respir Crit Care Med*. 2005;172:768–771.
13. Herth F, Becker HD, LoCicero 3rd J, Thurer R, Ernst A. Successful bronchoscopic placement of tracheobronchial stents without fluoroscopy. *Chest*. 2001;119:1910–1912.
14. Breen DP, Dutau H. On-site customization of silicone stents: towards optimal palliation of complex airway conditions. *Respiration*. 2009;77:447–453.
15. Saad CP, Murthy S, Krizmanich G, Mehta AC. Self-expandable metallic airway stents and flexible bronchoscopy: long-term outcomes analysis. *Chest*. 2003;124:1993–1999.
16. Lunn W, Feller-Kopman D, Wahidi M, Ashiku S, Thurer R, Ernst A. Endoscopic removal of metallic airway stents. *Chest*. 2005;127:2106–2112.
17. Noppen M, Stratakos G, D'Haese J, Meysman M, Vinken W. Removal of covered self-expandable metallic airway stents in benign disorders: indications, technique, and outcomes. *Chest*. 2005;127:482–487.

11

The Endoscopic Application of Medication to the Airway

Megan Acho, Roy Semaan and Lonny Yarmus

INTRODUCTION

Since its discovery in 1876, bronchoscopy has served a fundamental role in the diagnosis and management of pulmonary disease.[1] Over the past few decades, the therapeutic capabilities of bronchoscopy have evolved dramatically. Indeed, technologies such as laser therapy, argon plasma coagulation, cryotherapy, brachytherapy, and endobronchial stenting have revolutionized the management of malignant and nonmalignant central airway disease, ushering in a new age of interventional pulmonology. More recently, there has been increased interest in the direct application of medications to the airways utilizing a bronchoscopic approach. This chapter discusses the endoscopic application of medication to a variety of malignant and nonmalignant thoracic diseases.

MALIGNANT THORACIC DISEASE

Transbronchial Needle Injections

Despite widespread anti-tobacco campaigns and lung cancer screening initiatives, lung cancer remains the leading cause of cancer death in the United States with a projected mortality of over 147,000 deaths in 2019 alone.[2] The majority of lung cancers are non–small cell lung cancer (NSCLC), many of which are advanced at the time of initial presentation.[3] Given the significant morbidity and mortality associated with lung cancer, early diagnosis is of paramount importance. In the late 1970s, Ko-Pen Wang developed flexible transbronchial needle aspiration (TBNA)[1] through a fiberoptic bronchoscope, allowing for endoscopic tissue sampling with

possible rapid on-site evaluation (ROSE) of histopathologic specimens. The use of TBNA for the diagnosis and staging of lung cancer significantly increased after the introduction of endobronchial ultrasonography (EBUS).[4] EBUS allows for direct visualization of the lesion being biopsied, not only increasing the diagnostic yield of the procedure[5] but also rendering the procedure safer by allowing operators to visualize advancement and retraction of the needle in real time. Today EBUS-guided TBNA has become an integral component in the diagnosis of thoracic malignancy and mediastinal lymph node staging, providing a minimally invasive alternative to mediastinoscopy and video-assisted thoracoscopic surgery as a means by which to diagnose and stage lung cancer.[3,6-8] EBUS-TBNA has also previously been shown to reduce the time to diagnosis of lung cancer, allowing for earlier initiation of therapy,[9] as well as expedited care coordination between patients, oncologists, pulmonologists, and surgeons.

Given the impressive diagnostic capabilities of TBNA, especially in conjunction with EBUS, there has been growing interest in the role of transbronchial needle injections (TBNI) as a therapeutic modality. This is particularly relevant to lung cancer. Treatment of NSCLC is based on cancer staging, with advanced stages (II–IV) typically requiring radiation and/or chemotherapeutic agents. Among patients diagnosed with lung cancer, approximately 20%–30% will develop some degree of malignant airway obstruction.[10] These obstructive lesions can be associated with progressively worsening dyspnea, resulting in a diminished quality of life. Malignant airway obstructions may also give way to such complications as hemoptysis, postobstructive pneumonia, and, in severe cases, respiratory failure. In these situations, rapid, safe, and effective recanalization of the airway is imperative.

In contrast to intravenous therapies, TBNI allows for localized delivery of (oftentimes cytotoxic) medications into these lesions, not only potentially minimizing the systemic toxicities associated with these agents but also increasing the intratumoral concentrations of the drugs. In the 1980s, TBNI (without EBUS) was used to deliver ethanol into endobronchial tumors with the goal of alleviating central airway obstruction and minimizing tumoral bleeding.[11] Fujisawa et al. injected 0.5–3 mL of 99.5% ethanol into the tumors of 13 patients with tracheobronchial tumors invading the central airway to potentiate tissue necrosis, allowing pieces of the necrotic tumor to be debrided with forceps in order to improve airway patency.[12] Sawa et al. performed a similar intervention, injecting 4.5 mL (on average) of 99% ethanol into the endobronchial lesions of eight patients utilizing an endoscopic video information system to assess for leakage of ethanol beyond the tumor margins.[13]

In addition to ethanol, chemotherapeutic agents have also been directly injected into intra- and extraluminal tumors endoscopically. When chemotherapy is administered via TBNI, the procedure is termed *endobronchial intratumoral chemotherapy* (EITC).[14] One of the first descriptions of EITC came from Celikoglu et al. in Turkey.[15] This study was designed to evaluate EITC as a potential palliative intervention for individuals with lung cancer (primarily squamous cell carcinoma) that was not amenable to surgery. Ninety-three patients with inoperable cancers and evidence of more than 50% exophytic obstruction of at least one major airway were enrolled. Of these patients, 68 carried a diagnosis of previously untreated bronchogenic carcinoma (with plans to initiate systemic chemotherapy and radiation following treatment with intratumoral injections), whereas 25 had a history of cancer that had recurred despite prior treatment with chemotherapy and/or radiation. Utilizing a flexible bronchoscope and 23-gauge (G) flexible needle (Olympus Corp, Tokyo, Japan), the authors injected 1–3 mL each of 50 mg/mL 5-fluorouracil, 1 mg/mL mitomycin, 5 mg/mL methotrexate, 10 mg/mL bleomycin, and 2 mg/mL mitoxantrone into different sites on the tumor. Injections took place over the course of one to six sessions. Following the treatment, the authors noted a reduction in tumor size and improvement in airway obstruction in 81 patients, 39 of whom experienced a more than 50% relative increase in the luminal diameter of their airways. The authors did report postprocedural fevers in a small percentage of the patients, though no significant adverse events were noted.

A follow-up study was performed by Celikoglu using 5-fluorouracil monotherapy intratumorally for the palliative management of severe airway obstruction.[16] The authors again studied patients with severe obstruction of at least one major airway. Among the 65 patients enrolled, the mean degree of luminal patency pretreatment was 22%; 56 patients experienced anatomic improvement of their airway obstruction with an average luminal patency of 58.5% following flexible bronchoscopic injection of 0.5–1 g of 50 mg/mL 5-fluorouracil with a 23-G TBNA needle. Again, no significant side effects were noted.

In addition to 5-fluorouracil, there are data to support the use of other chemotherapeutic agents. Additional studies have been done demonstrating the safety and efficacy of intratumoral injections of paclitaxel,[17] carboplatin,[18] and cisplatin,[19–21] with many recent studies utilizing the latter. Drugs are selected based on their pharmacologic profile with regard to both safety and biometabolism. From a safety standpoint, chemotherapeutic agents selected for EITC must be directly cytotoxic but should not induce necrosis in the healthy tissues that are adjacent to the malignant lesions. Additionally, in terms of metabolism, the drugs must not require systemic metabolism in order to be effective.[16] Though the optimal dose of cisplatin remains unclear, computational modeling studies have shown that lower cumulative doses may be achieved by performing multiple small, spaced injections of cisplatin as opposed to a larger bolus injection into the tumor center.[22] More research must be done to determine which chemotherapeutic agents and dosages are most appropriate, as well as the optimal number of injections and their location. Additionally, more longitudinal follow-up data of patients who have undergone TBNI must also be conducted in order to determine the appropriate duration of therapy and the long-term implications of this therapeutic intervention.

EBUS-Guided TBNI

More recently, EBUS has been employed to help bolster the safety of EITC. Khan et al. described the first use of EBUS-guided TBNI in 2014,[21] in which the authors utilized EBUS-guided TBNI to inject cisplatin into an endobronchial lesion in a patient with previously treated, recurrent squamous cell carcinoma (Fig. 11.1).

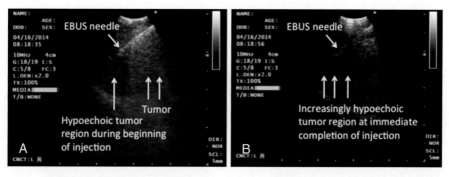

Fig. 11.1 Cisplatin injection into an endobronchial lesion via EBUS-TBNI. (From Khan F, Anker CJ, Garrison G, Kinsey CM. Endobronchial ultrasound-guided transbronchial needle injection for local control of recurrent non-small cell lung cancer. *Ann Am Thorac Soc.* 2015;12:101–104.)

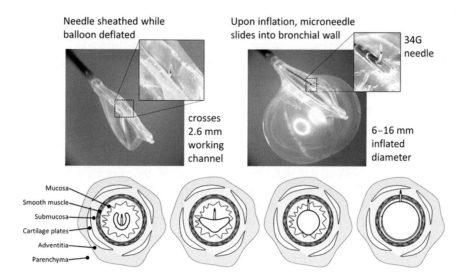

Fig. 11.2 Blowfish catheter with the balloon deflated and inflated. (From Yarmus L, Mallow C, Akulian J, et al. Prospective multicentered safety and feasibility pilot for endobronchial intratumoral chemotherapy. *Chest.* 2019;156:562–570.)

They noted that EBUS allows not only for direct visualization of drug injection into the tumor but also for the use of Doppler ultrasonography, which minimizes the risk that the needle could be inserted into a highly vascularized region.

Endobronchial Balloon Drug Delivery Catheter

TBNI used in conjunction with a flexible or rigid bronchoscope can lead to logistical difficulties for injection into lesions located perpendicular to the airway wall. Classic TBNI into airway walls may also lead to deep penetration of medication with the risk of airway dehiscence. A novel endobronchial balloon drug delivery catheter (Blowfish Catheter, Mercator MedSystems, Inc., CA, USA) was recently developed that is able to be passed down a flexible bronchoscope. Once deployed through the working channel of a bronchoscope, the distal balloon is inflated and extrudes a 34-G microneedle perpendicular to the catheter (Fig. 11.2). Medications can then be injected through this needle into the tumor and bronchial wall directly into the submucosa and bronchial adventitia, but not past the cartilaginous layer. Porcine studies showed that the Blowfish catheter was

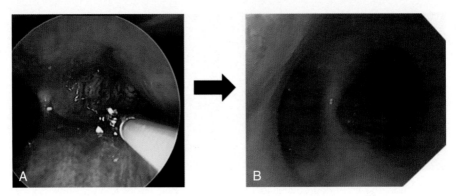

Fig. 11.3 (A) 100% occlusion of the right mainstem bronchus by a malignant airway obstruction. (B) Patent right mainstem bronchus 6 weeks after paclitaxel injection. (From Yarmus L, Mallow C, Akulian J, et al. Prospective multi-centered safety and feasibility pilot for endobronchial intratumoral chemotherapy. *Chest.* 2019;156:562-570.)

able to circumferentially inject medication into 60% of the airway wall per injection.[23] This catheter was studied in a multicenter human safety and feasibility pilot looking at the efficacy of injections of a cumulative dose of 1.5 mg of paclitaxel in 19 patients with NSCLC and malignant central airway obstruction (Fig. 11.3).[17] All patients underwent rigid bronchoscopy with recanalization of their airways with successful injection of paclitaxel using the Blowfish microinjection catheter. This required an average of 3.4 injections per patient. The authors noted significantly less airway stenosis following the intervention and reported no significant adverse events. None of the patients enrolled in the study required further interventions in the 6-week follow-up period. No patients required airway stenting.

Gene Therapy

There are very early and preliminary studies of tumor suppressor gene therapy delivered via TBNI.[11,24] The most common genetic anomaly associated with lung cancer is a mutation in the *p53* tumor suppressor gene.[25,26] In the 1990s, Roth et al. used TBNI to administer wild-type copies of *p53* via a retroviral vector into the endobronchial lesions of four patients with recurrent NSCLC.[27] The authors reported regression of the tumor mass in three patients on subsequent bronchoscopic examinations, with follow-up biopsies revealing no viable tumor (though patients did experience progression of disease elsewhere). More recently multiple studies have been performed using recombinant adenoviral vectors. Weill et al. administered adenoviral-mediated

p53 gene (*Adp53*) through TBNI to 12 patients with endobronchial NSCLC associated with a known *p53* mutation; they noted significant improvement in airway obstruction in half of the patients.[28] The authors reported minimal toxicity associated with the therapy. It is important to note that in this cohort 5 of the 12 patients received *Adp53* alone, whereas 7 received *Adp53* in conjunction with cisplatin; of these subgroups, only one of the patients who received *Adp53* alone experienced significant improvement in endobronchial obstruction, whereas 5 of the 7 in the *Adp53*/cisplatin group experienced improvement. An additional study looked at the coadministration of *Adp53* and cisplatin in 24 patients with NSCLC; 17 patients had disappearance of their endobronchial lesions posttreatment for at least 4 weeks based on imaging and/or physical examination, whereas 2 patients demonstrated partial response.[29]

Beyond cisplatin, other therapies have been administered alongside *p53*. Schuler et al. studied the concurrent administration of intratumoral injections of adenovirus-mediated wild-type *p53* genes with either carboplatin/paclitaxel or cisplatin/vinorelbine.[30] Ultimately the authors did not detect a difference in response rates between those who received chemotherapy and *p53* versus those who received chemotherapy alone. They did note, however, that local tumor regression appeared to be more significant among those who received cisplatin/vinorelbine and *p53* relative to those who received carboplatin/paclitaxel and *p53*.

The impact of tumor suppressor gene injections has also been considered in the setting of radiation therapy. Swisher et al. studied patients with nonmeta-static NSCLC who were ineligible for chemotherapy or surgical intervention.[31] Patients were given intratumoral injections of *Adp53* in the setting of also receiving radiation therapy (at 60 Gy) over 6 weeks. After several months, the biopsies of 12 of 19 patients revealed no viable tumor.

All of these studies are fairly preliminary and lack the sample size to either prove or disprove efficacy of various agents delivered bronchoscopically. As such, the data should be viewed as exploratory, the main emphasis here being that bronchoscopy as a platform for delivery of drugs and other therapeutic agents is starting to be explored. In this context, it is important for the interventional bronchoscopist to understand the available data, the limitations of these data, and the procedural aspects of bronchoscopic drug delivery in case it is needed.

NONMALIGNANT THORACIC DISEASE

Postintubation or Tracheostomy Laryngotracheal Stenosis

In addition to lung cancer, there are a variety of nonmalignant airway-centric pathologies that may benefit from endobronchially administered medications. One such disorder, benign laryngotracheal stenosis, is most commonly seen in patients who have previously required endotracheal intubation and/or tracheostomy for a prolonged period of time (typically greater than 7–10 days[32]). Other risk factors for developing laryngotracheal stenosis include a history of difficult or emergency intubation, placement of an oversized endotracheal tube, or excessively high cuff pressures.[33] Symptoms of laryngotracheal stenosis may take weeks to months after extubation or decannulation to manifest. Patients will often complain of subacute, progressive dyspnea, as well as wheezing that is refractory to treatment with bronchodilators.[34] Laryngotracheal stenoses can be subdivided into simple versus complex stenoses. Simple lesions are defined as those impacting a short region (less than 1 cm long) of the airway without evidence of tracheomalacia. In contrast, complex lesions are those involving extensive areas (greater than 1 cm in length) of stenosis and/or cartilaginous involvement and tracheomalacia. Simple stenoses are typically amenable to a bronchoscopic intervention, usually consisting of radial incision (e.g., with an electrocautery knife) followed by balloon dilation. Complex stenoses may require multiple, repeated interventions including deployment of airway stents, argon plasma coagulation, cryotherapy, balloon dilation, or eventually surgical resection.[35]

Recently, the use of mitomycin C in the management of benign laryngotracheal stenosis has been gaining popularity. Mitomycin C is an antineoplastic agent that derives from *Streptomyces caespitosus*. It has historically been used in the treatment of a variety of cancers, including breast cancer, colorectal cancer, gastric cancer, and NSCLC,[36] and its use as an antiproliferative agent in the treatment of diseases like glaucoma is well established in the ophthalmology literature.[37] Dalar et al. reported on the use of topical 0.2 mg/mL mitomycin C in a limited number of patients with simple and complex tracheal stenoses (Fig. 11.4). The authors noted that mitomycin appeared to delay time to consecutive stent dilations in patients with complex stenoses and decreased the need for repeated dilations in patients with simple stenoses.[35] Though there are not yet any randomized controlled trials studying the impact of mitomycin C on this condition, Perepelitsyn and Shapshay performed a retrospective cohort study comparing the efficacy of carbon dioxide laser incisions combined with bronchoscopic dilatation alone versus steroid injections versus topical application of mitomycin C. They reported symptomatic improvement in the group that received topical mitomycin C.[38] There are also some data to suggest that two applications of mitomycin C, spaced approximately 1 month apart, can help to postpone (but not prevent) episodes of restenosis.[39] Additional research must be done to further explore these results and determine the optimal dosing frequency of topical mitomycin C in these patients.

Granulomatosis With Polyangiitis

Granulomatosis with polyangiitis (GPA, formerly Wegener's granulomatosis) is a form of small-vessel, antineutrophil cytoplasmic antibodies (ANCA)-associated vasculitis. According to the American College of Rheumatology, there are four criteria used to diagnosis the disease:
1. Abnormal urinary sediment
2. Abnormal chest imaging findings
3. The presence of oral ulcers or nasal discharge
4. The presence of granulomas on biopsy.[40]

From a pulmonary standpoint, GPA can have a wide variety of manifestations, including (potentially

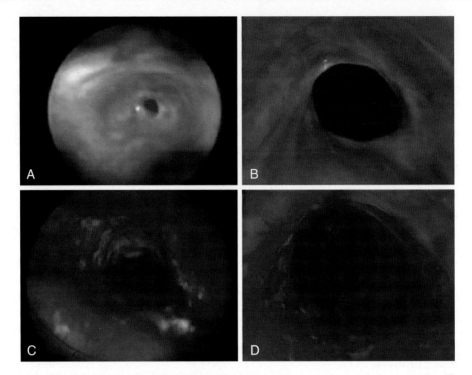

Fig. 11.4 Postintubation tracheal stenosis (A) and magnified (B), before bronchoscopic intervention. The same trachea visualized again (C) and magnified (D) following three treatments with topical mitomycin. (From Dalar L, Karasulu L, Abul Y, et al. Bronchoscopic treatment in the management of benign tracheal stenosis: choices for simple and complex tracheal stenosis. *Ann Thorac Surg.* 2016;101:1310–1317.)

cavitary) lung nodules, ground-glass opacities in the setting of alveolar hemorrhage, airway stenoses, and mucosal ulcerations.[41] The disease is typically managed with systemic immunosuppressive therapy and avoidance of airway manipulation, as this can lead to worsening inflammation and further stenosis in the future. However, central airway involvement can be the primary derangement in a small proportion of patients and may progress even with appropriate systemic therapy; this situation may necessitate endoscopic intervention.

Upper respiratory tract involvement is relatively common in GPA, particularly involving the subglottic region of the trachea.[42] Indeed, 16% of patients with active disease develop subglottic stenosis, which can be life-threatening.[43] Multiple studies have suggested a role for endoscopic glucocorticoid injections, performed in conjunction with bronchoscopic dilation.[42–45] Additionally, prior research has demonstrated that patients may develop subglottic stenosis while receiving

systemic immunosuppression, suggesting that immunosuppressive therapy may not always be sufficient to prevent/manage this complication.[46] Hoffman et al. performed intralesional long-acting corticosteroid injections and dilatations in 21 patients with GPA complicated by subglottic stenosis.[42] In this study, 40 mg/mL of methylprednisolone acetate was injected into the submucosa of the stenotic region using a 20-G laryngeal needle in a four-quadrant distribution. They noted that patients with no prior airway scarring required an average of 2.4 procedures approximately 12 months apart in order to maintain patency of the subglottic region. In contrast, patients with evidence of airway scarring (from prior procedures) required an average of 4.1 procedures approximately 7 months apart in order to maintain regional patency. Based on their findings, the authors suggest that steroid injections and dilatation are a reasonable therapeutic modality for patients with subglottic stenosis and GPA not responsive to systemic therapy.

Sarcoidosis

Sarcoidosis is a multisystem disease characterized by the presence of noncaseating granulomas. Though presentations of sarcoidosis can vary significantly based on the affected organ systems, the respiratory system is impacted in more than 90% of cases.[47] Pulmonary manifestations of sarcoidosis include bilateral hilar adenopathy, pulmonary micronodules, ground-glass opacities, and, in advanced disease, fibrosis. Airway involvement of the disease is typically indicative of the presence of endobronchial mucosal granulomas, causing scarring and stenosis.[48] The resulting narrowing of the airway can be detected radiographically and bronchoscopically and often leads to symptoms of dyspnea and wheezing. On imaging, extensive involvement of the small airways can result in evidence of air-trapping on expiratory films.[49]

Corticosteroids are among the most commonly used therapies for active sarcoidosis.[50] When endobronchial airway involvement occurs in sarcoidosis, intraluminal injections of corticosteroids (including dexamethasone[51] and triamcinolone[11]) may be of benefit, although data on efficacy are limited. Butler et al. performed a retrospective chart review of 10 patients with laryngeal involvement from sarcoidosis. Among these patients, six had sarcoidosis that was limited to the larynx, whereas four had other systemic manifestations; two patients had symptoms that were so severe that they required emergency tracheostomy. All had received high doses of systemic corticosteroids prior to intervention. Patients underwent multiple steroid injections into the base of each lesion, using 40–120 mg of 40 mg/mL methylprednisolone acetate, as well as laser photoreduction using a carbon dioxide laser. They completed anywhere from one to four sessions.[52] The authors reported significant improvement in the patients' Medical Research Council (MRC) dyspnea scales[53] following treatment, as well as a significant reduction in systemic steroid usage.

There may also be a role for topical mitomycin C in the management of sarcoidosis of the airway. In a case report describing a woman with endobronchial involvement of her sarcoidosis who had failed systemic steroid therapy, balloon dilation, and the application of topical 0.4 mg/mL mitomycin C resulted in transient improvement in the patient's symptoms.[54] More research must be done on the potential role of mitomycin C in the management of sarcoidosis involving the airways.

Idiopathic Laryngotracheal Stenosis

Idiopathic laryngotracheal stenosis is a rare inflammatory disorder that almost exclusively affects women, typically those who are pre- and perimenopausal. Patients generally present with exertional dyspnea, wheezing, and, occasionally, a change in the quality of their voice. As its name suggests, *idiopathic* laryngotracheal stenosis is a diagnosis of exclusion. As such, it is incumbent on the provider to rule out infectious, traumatic, and rheumatologic processes in order to make the diagnosis.[55] Recently, derangements in estrogen and progesterone, as may be seen at the time of menopause, have been studied as possible contributors to the pathogenesis of this disorder.[56]

Idiopathic laryngotracheal stenosis is characterized by stenosis within the upper airway, often impacting the subglottic region.[57] Histopathologically there is evidence of fibrous inflammation in the lamina propria of the subglottis and proximal trachea.[58] Traditionally this disorder has been managed surgically, with laryngotracheal or tracheal resection and reconstruction. Outcomes with this surgical approach have been favorable.[59] One study described 73 patients who underwent operative intervention for idiopathic laryngotracheal stenosis; of this group, 19 patients described no difficulties in breathing or vocal quality postoperatively, 47 reported some difficulty projecting loudly after surgery, 5 reported some ongoing dyspnea or stridor, and 1 needed ongoing management with dilations.[60]

Despite the efficacy of surgery, there has been increasing interest in the role of bronchoscopy for the management of this disorder, as extensive surgical resection may not be tolerated by a large subset of patients with this disease due to medical comorbidities. As with benign laryngotracheal stenoses, bronchoscopic interventions for idiopathic stenoses include balloon dilatation, laser as well as other thermal ablative therapies, stenting, and cryotherapy.[35] Shabani et al. attempted endoscopic balloon dilation and steroid injection in 37 patients with subglottic stenosis due to idiopathic laryngotracheal stenosis. Of the 37 patients, 13 received steroid injections (triamcinolone or dexamethasone) for all procedures, whereas 4 received no concurrent steroid injections. Though the results did not reach statistical significance, the authors noted that the patients who received steroid injections tended to require fewer dilations (on average, approximately 4 vs. 7) with a longer time between dilations (on average, approximately 556 days as opposed to 283 days) than those who did not receive the steroid injections.[58] Given the small sample size, more research must be done to determine the utility of concurrent steroid injections, as well as the optimal timing of these treatments.

Recurrent Respiratory Papillomatosis

Recurrent respiratory papillomatosis (RRP) is a benign disorder characterized by the development of numerous papillomatous, exophytic lesions throughout the respiratory tract. Very rarely there may also be parenchymal involvement of RRP, characterized by the presence of solid or cavitary pulmonary nodules.[61] The disease is attributed to infection with human papillomavirus (HPV), most commonly subtypes 6 and 11, which together account for more than 90% of cases of RRP. There is general consensus that HPV 11 represents the more virulent strain, as patients afflicted with RRP due to HPV 11 typically are those who require more aggressive airway interventions (including tracheostomy) and have a higher risk of malignant transformation.[62] RRP may affect children, who frequently contract HPV at the time of birth through vaginal delivery, though there is evidence that some children become infected through placental transmission of the virus.[63] Adults may also contract HPV and develop RRP following orogenital sexual contact.[64]

The traditional approach to management of RRP has focused on surgical debulking of the papillomas, typically using laser therapy, in order to restore airway patency. Still, given the recurring nature of the disease, frequent surgeries may be required, placing (oftentimes pediatric) patients at risk for laryngotracheal stenosis and scarring, burns, and fistulae formation.[65] As a result, there has been increased focus on adjuvant therapies intended to minimize the need for repeated operative interventions. The use of intralesional cidofovir has been evaluated as a potential intervention to minimize the need for invasive procedures in this population.[66–69] Cidofovir is an antiviral medication that inhibits viral DNA polymerases.[70] Much of the data describing use of cidofovir come from case reports, with varying descriptions of the efficacy of the drug. Wierzbicka et al. noted complete remission in 18 of 32 patients with recurring papillomatous disease who underwent intralesional cidofovir injections (ranging from a total of one to seven injections, using 2–33 mL in total of 5 mg/mL

cidofovir); importantly, the authors reported that one patient developed gastrointestinal symptoms following the procedure, whereas two more developed a transient transaminitis.[66] Naiman et al. performed monthly intralesional injections of 5 mg/mL cidofovir in 26 patients (including adults and children). Repeat endoscopies were performed at 3 months to assess for ongoing disease burden and, if present, cidofovir injections were repeated at the time on the persisting papillomas. The authors reported complete remission in eight patients (of whom 2 had undergone 1 injection, 2 had 2 injections, and 4 had an average of 4.2 injections). Seventeen patients had mild disease at the end of the therapeutic trial. The authors did not note any significant adverse events.[71]

There are limited data at present describing the long-term efficacy of cidofovir injections for the management of RRP. Milczuk followed four children with RRP who had each undergone six treatments, 6–8 weeks apart, consisting of surgical papilloma excision and intralesional injections of cidofovir. One year after completing treatment, one patient continued to experience remission of his disease, whereas two patients had recurrence of symptoms (which began to recur during the initial treatment protocol). The fourth patient did not respond to cidofovir injections.[72] Tanna et al. followed 13 adults who had previously experienced disease remission after an average of six cidofovir injections, reporting that 6 did not require subsequent interventions, whereas 7 required further treatment of their RRP after an average of 1 year.[73] Additional research must be done in order to determine the long-term efficacy of intralesional cidofovir injections.

Lung Transplant–Associated Bronchial Stenosis

Despite improvements in surgical techniques over the past several decades, airway complications remain a relatively common complication of lung transplantation, with approximately 15% of lung transplant recipients affected.[74,75] Airway complications may have tremendous implications on a patient's quality of life, oftentimes provoking cough, progressive dyspnea, and/or recurrent infections. These complications frequently require multiple posttransplantation interventions depending on the underlying etiology of the complication. There are a wide variety of airway complications, including anastomotic necrosis and dehiscence, anastomotic infections, fistulas (bronchopleural, bronchovascular, or broncho-mediastinal), and, most commonly, bronchial stenosis.[74] Bronchial stenoses may occur at or distal to the anastomotic site and can develop months to years following transplant. According to a review by Yousem et al., histopathologic studies of bronchial cartilage in posttransplant recipients demonstrate ossification, calcification, and fibrovascular ingrowth, presumably due (at least in part) to inflammation and decreased bronchial perfusion following transplantation.[76]

The bronchoscopic management of posttransplant bronchial stenosis encompasses a variety of interventions aimed at dilating the airway. Historically, rigid bronchoscopy with bougie dilation was the standard treatment modality, though flexible bronchoscopy with balloon dilation has become increasingly prevalent in recent years.[77] Other interventions include airway stenting, cryotherapy, electrocautery, laser therapy, and endobronchial brachytherapy. There are also data to support the bronchoscopic application of topical agents, most notably mitomycin C, to regions affected by bronchial stenosis. Erard et al. published the first case report describing the local application of mitomycin C in recurring bronchial stenosis in 2001 (Fig. 11.5). They describe a patient with a history of cystic fibrosis and multidrug-resistant *Burkholderia cepacia* who underwent bilateral lung transplantation complicated by recurrent bronchial stenosis despite treatment with argon laser electrocoagulation and multiple attempts at dilatation and stenting. At postoperative week 42, the authors applied a cotton swab soaked in a solution of 2 mg/mL of mitomycin C to granulation tissue in the patient's stenosed right upper lobe bronchus and bronchus intermedius for 2 min. They reported improvement in the patient's FEV_1 (forced expiratory volume in the first second) that persisted for several months, though they did note that the patient developed a recurring stricture in the bronchus intermedius, which was treated again with topical mitomycin C with good efficacy.[78]

A recent retrospective cohort study from Duke University evaluated posttransplant patients with bronchial stenosis in whom mitomycin C was injected submucosally into the stenotic airway. The study included 11 patients who had undergone lung transplantation complicated by airway stenosis that recurred despite balloon dilatation and/or airway stent placement. The patients underwent bronchoscopy with balloon bronchoplasty, after which 5 mL of 0.4 mg/mL solution of mitomycin C was administered through a submucosal injection with a 21-G needle. In order to determine the impact of the mitomycin C injection, the authors

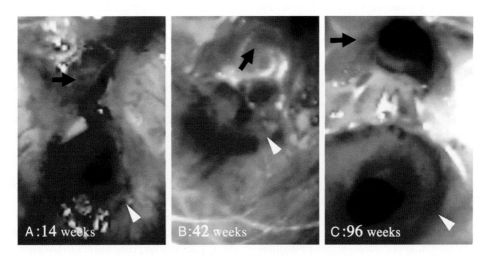

Fig. 11.5 Bronchial stenosis in a lung transplantation patient. (A) Stenosis of the right upper lobar bronchus and bronchus intermedius 14 weeks posttransplantation; (B) 42 weeks posttransplantation, following stent placement in the right upper lobe bronchus; (C) 96 weeks posttransplantation, following topical mitomycin C application. (From Erard AC, Monnier P, Spiliopoulos A, Nicod L. Mitomycin C for control of recurrent bronchial stenosis: a case report. *Chest.* 2001;120:2103–2105.)

compared the number of airway dilations performed in the months prior to intervention and in the months following this therapy. They reported that a median of three dilations was performed per patient in the 6 months that preceded intervention, in contrast to two dilations in the following 6 months. The authors also described nonsignificant improvements in the patients' FEV_1 values and forced vital capacities (FVCs) and noted that the injections were well tolerated.[79]

ENDOSCOPIC APPLICATION OF MEDICATIONS AND CHOICE OF TECHNIQUE

The endoscopic application of medications can be performed using four general techniques:
1. Topical application
2. Injection under direct visualization
3. Injection under ultrasound visualization
4. Circumferential injection using an endobronchial balloon catheter.

The topical application of medications is generally the least invasive of these techniques and is less likely to cause deep penetration; as a result, there are typically fewer complications associated with this technique. Topical application of medications may be performed by soaking the pledget in the desired medication, grasping the pledget with rigid forceps, and, finally, placing the soaked pledget on the central airway lesion. The time needed to apply the pledget varies from 30 seconds up to several minutes, depending on the indication. The amount of medication absorbed into the mucosa will vary depending on the concentration of the solution in which the pledget is soaked, the duration of time for which the pledget is held against the mucosa, and the number of applications. It should be noted that this technique can also be accomplished by grasping the pledget with flexible forceps through a bronchoscope, though this typically leads to less forceful apposition of the pledget to the airway and, as such, lower concentrations of medication absorption.

In contrast to topical applications, medications may also be injected endoscopically. The endoscopic injection of agents can be performed under direct visualization through a TBNA needle or using ultrasound guidance through an EBUS-TBNA needle. Direct injection with a standard TBNA needle can be performed easily using a flexible bronchoscope and should be considered in patients who have lesions that extend into the lumen of a central airway and/or completely obstruct the airway. In contrast, EBUS-TBNA is preferred for mediastinal masses that are not visible in central airways. Still, both of these treatment modalities remain experimental, as the most effective volumes, concentrations, and types of medications are still unknown.

Finally, medications may also be administered using the flexible endobronchial balloon (Blowfish) catheter, described earlier in this chapter. This device consists of a double lumen catheter that is passed down a flexible bronchoscope with the balloon deflated and the needle sheathed. One lumen inflates an endobronchial balloon at the tip of the catheter, which then extrudes a 34-G needle perpendicularly. This needle is then inserted into the submucosa. Once the balloon is fully inflated, the drug is delivered down the second lumen via the needle. Generally, four injections are completed in a circumferential manner. Contrast dye can be mixed with the drug being injected in an effort to monitor the extent of extravasation of the drug into the submucosa, though this is not completely necessary.

SUMMARY

This chapter provides a brief overview of the ways in which a variety of pulmonary pathologies may be managed through the endoscopic administration of medications. All of these therapeutic options have yet to be validated through large, randomized controlled trials, and, as such, the level of evidence behind these interventions is limited. The efficacy of the bronchoscopic delivery of medications to the airway varies not only by disease, but also by the medication delivered. The proper dosing and delivery schedule of each medication need to be determined and validated. Similarly, the method of drug delivery (e.g., injection with direct visualization using classic TBNA needles, EBUS-assisted TBNI, or bronchial balloon drug delivery catheters) is likely to impact outcomes. Despite these limitations, the available data do suggest that the use of bronchoscopy as a drug delivery platform for select airway diseases may be worthwhile. Additional research is required to determine the appropriate indications for the bronchoscopic administration of medication, as well as the optimal drug dosing, delivery method, and frequency of administration.

REFERENCES

1. Panchabhai TS, Mehta AC. Historical perspectives of bronchoscopy. Connecting the dots. *Ann Am Thorac Soc.* 2015;12:631–641.
2. Siegel RL, Miller KD, Jemal A. Cancer statistics, 2019. *CA Cancer J Clin.* 2019;69:7–34.
3. Reck M, Heigener DF, Mok T, Soria JC, Rabe KF. Management of non-small-cell lung cancer: recent developments. *Lancet.* 2013;382:709–719.
4. Hurter T, Hanrath P. Endobronchial sonography: feasibility and preliminary results. *Thorax.* 1992;47:565–567.
5. Herth F, Becker HD, Ernst A. Conventional vs endobronchial ultrasound-guided transbronchial needle aspiration: a randomized trial. *Chest.* 2004;125:322–325.
6. Gomez M, Silvestri GA. Endobronchial ultrasound for the diagnosis and staging of lung cancer. *Proc Am Thorac Soc.* 2009;6:180–186.
7. Andolfi M, Potenza R, Capozzi R, Liparulo V, Puma F, Yasufuku K. The role of bronchoscopy in the diagnosis of early lung cancer: a review. *J Thorac Dis.* 2016;8: 3329–3337.
8. Krasnik M, Vilmann P, Larsen SS, Jacobsen GK. Preliminary experience with a new method of endoscopic transbronchial real time ultrasound guided biopsy for diagnosis of mediastinal and hilar lesions. *Thorax.* 2003;58:1083–1086.
9. Navani N, Nankivell M, Lawrence DR, et al. Lung cancer diagnosis and staging with endobronchial ultrasound-guided transbronchial needle aspiration compared with conventional approaches: an open-label, pragmatic, randomised controlled trial. *Lancet Respir Med.* 2015;3:282–289.
10. Ernst A, Feller-Kopman D, Becker HD, Mehta AC. Central airway obstruction. *Am J Respir Crit Care Med.* 2004;169:1278–1297.
11. Seymour CW, Krimsky WS, Sager J, et al. Transbronchial needle injection: a systematic review of a new diagnostic and therapeutic paradigm. *Respiration.* 2006;73:78–89.
12. Fujisawa T, Hongo H, Yamaguchi Y, et al. Intratumoral ethanol injection for malignant tracheobronchial lesions: a new bronchofiberscopic procedure. *Endoscopy.* 1986;18:188–191.
13. Sawa T, Ikoma T, Yoshida T, et al. [Intratumoral ethanol injection therapy using endoscopic video information system]. *Gan To Kagaku Ryoho.* 1999;26:1865–1868.
14. Celikoglu F, Celikoglu SI, Goldberg EP. Bronchoscopic intratumoral chemotherapy of lung cancer. *Lung Cancer.* 2008;61:1–12.
15. Celikoglu SI, Karayel T, Demirci S, Celikoglu F, Cagatay T. Direct injection of anti-cancer drugs into endobronchial tumours for palliation of major airway obstruction. *Postgrad Med J.* 1997;73:159–162.
16. Celikoglu F, Celikoglu SI. Intratumoural chemotherapy with 5-fluorouracil for palliation of bronchial cancer in patients with severe airway obstruction. *J Pharm Pharmacol.* 2003;55:1441–1448.
17. Yarmus L, Mallow C, Akulian J, et al. Prospective multicentered safety and feasibility pilot for endobronchial intratumoral chemotherapy. *Chest.* 2019;156:562–570.
18. Liu M, Ma P, Lu Z. [Local chemotherapy by fibrobronchoscopy for advanced bronchogenic carcinoma]. *Zhonghua Jie He He Hu Xi Za Zhi.* 2000;23:550–551.
19. Mehta HJ, Begnaud A, Penley AM, et al. Treatment of isolated mediastinal and hilar recurrence of lung cancer with bronchoscopic endobronchial ultrasound guided intratumoral injection of chemotherapy with cisplatin. *Lung Cancer.* 2015;90:542–547.
20. Celikoglu SI, Celikoglu F, Goldberg EP. Endobronchial intratumoral chemotherapy (EITC) followed by surgery in early non-small cell lung cancer with polypoid growth causing erroneous impression of advanced disease. *Lung Cancer.* 2006;54:339–346.
21. Khan F, Anker CJ, Garrison G, Kinsey CM. Endobronchial ultrasound-guided transbronchial needle injection for local control of recurrent non-small cell lung cancer. *Ann Am Thorac Soc.* 2015;12:101–104.
22. Mori V, Roy GS, Bates JHT, Kinsey CM. Cisplatin pharmacodynamics following endobronchial ultrasound-guided transbronchial needle injection into lung tumors. *Sci Rep.* 2019;9:6819.
23. Tsukada H, Seward KP, Rafeq S, Kocher O, Ernst A. Experimental pilot study of a novel endobronchial drug delivery catheter. *J Bronchology Interv Pulmonol.* 2015;22:312–318.
24. Harris K, Puchalski J, Sterman D. Recent advances in bronchoscopic treatment of peripheral lung cancers. *Chest.* 2017;151:674–685.
25. Lubin R, Zalcman G, Bouchet L, et al. Serum p53 antibodies as early markers of lung cancer. *Nat Med.* 1995;1:701–702.
26. Iggo R, Gatter K, Bartek J, Lane D, Harris AL. Increased expression of mutant forms of p53 oncogene in primary lung cancer. *Lancet.* 1990;335:675–679.
27. Roth JA, Nguyen D, Lawrence DD, et al. Retrovirus-mediated wild-type p53 gene transfer to tumors of patients with lung cancer. *Nat Med.* 1996;2:985–991.
28. Weill D, Mack M, Roth J, et al. Adenoviral-mediated p53 gene transfer to non-small cell lung cancer through endobronchial injection. *Chest.* 2000;118:966–970.
29. Nemunaitis J, Swisher SG, Timmons T, et al. Adenovirus-mediated p53 gene transfer in sequence with cisplatin to tumors of patients with non-small-cell lung cancer. *J Clin Oncol.* 2000;18:609–622.
30. Schuler M, Herrmann R, De Greve JL, et al. Adenovirus-mediated wild-type p53 gene transfer in patients

receiving chemotherapy for advanced non-small-cell lung cancer: results of a multicenter phase II study. *J Clin Oncol.* 2001;19:1750–1758.

31. Swisher SG, Roth JA, Komaki R, et al. Induction of p53-regulated genes and tumor regression in lung cancer patients after intratumoral delivery of adenoviral p53 (INGN 201) and radiation therapy. *Clin Cancer Res.* 2003;9:93–101.

32. Whited RE. A prospective study of laryngotracheal sequelae in long-term intubation. *Laryngoscope.* 1984;94:367–377.

33. Tadie JM, Behm E, Lecuyer L, et al. Post-intubation laryngeal injuries and extubation failure: a fiberoptic endoscopic study. *Intensive Care Med.* 2010;36:991–998.

34. Spittle N, McCluskey A. Lesson of the week: tracheal stenosis after intubation. *BMJ.* 2000;321:1000–1002.

35. Dalar L, Karasulu L, Abul Y, et al. Bronchoscopic treatment in the management of benign tracheal stenosis: choices for simple and complex tracheal stenosis. *Ann Thorac Surg.* 2016;101:1310–1317.

36. Verweij J, Pinedo HM. Mitomycin C: mechanism of action, usefulness and limitations. *Anticancer Drugs.* 1990;1:5–13.

37. Cheng JW, Cai JP, Li Y, Wei RL. Intraoperative mitomycin C for nonpenetrating glaucoma surgery: a systematic review and meta-analysis. *J Glaucoma.* 2011;20:322–326.

38. Perepelitsyn I, Shapshay SM. Endoscopic treatment of laryngeal and tracheal stenosis-has mitomycin C improved the outcome? *Otolaryngol Head Neck Surg.* 2004;131:16–20.

39. Smith ME, Elstad M. Mitomycin C and the endoscopic treatment of laryngotracheal stenosis: are two applications better than one? *Laryngoscope.* 2009;119:272–283.

40. Leavitt RY, Fauci AS, Bloch DA, et al. The American College of Rheumatology 1990 criteria for the classification of Wegener's granulomatosis. *Arthritis Rheum.* 1990;33:1101–1107.

41. Ananthakrishnan L, Sharma N, Kanne JP. Wegener's granulomatosis in the chest: high-resolution CT findings. *AJR Am J Roentgenol.* 2009;192:676–682.

42. Hoffman GS, Thomas-Golbanov CK, Chan J, Akst LM, Eliachar I. Treatment of subglottic stenosis, due to Wegener's granulomatosis, with intralesional corticosteroids and dilation. *J Rheumatol.* 2003;30:1017–1021.

43. Stappaerts I, Van Laer C, Deschepper K, Van de Heyning P, Vermeire P. Endoscopic management of severe subglottic stenosis in Wegener's granulomatosis. *Clin Rheumatol.* 2000;19:315–317.

44. Girard C, Charles P, Terrier B, et al. Tracheobronchial stenoses in granulomatosis with polyangiitis (Wegener's): a report on 26 cases. *Medicine (Baltimore).* 2015;94:e1088.

45. Nouraei SA, Obholzer R, Ind PW, et al. Results of endoscopic surgery and intralesional steroid therapy for airway compromise due to tracheobronchial Wegener's granulomatosis. *Thorax.* 2008;63:49–52.

46. Langford CA, Sneller MC, Hallahan CW, et al. Clinical features and therapeutic management of subglottic stenosis in patients with Wegener's granulomatosis. *Arthritis Rheum.* 1996;39:1754–1760.

47. Polychronopoulos VS, Prakash UBS. Airway involvement in sarcoidosis. *Chest.* 2009;136:1371–1380.

48. Westcott JL, Noehren TH. Bronchial stenosis in chronic sarcoidosis. *Chest.* 1973;63:893–897.

49. Nunes H, Uzunhan Y, Gille T, Lamberto C, Valeyre D, Brillet PY. Imaging of sarcoidosis of the airways and lung parenchyma and correlation with lung function. *Eur Respir J.* 2012;40:750–765.

50. Judson MA. An approach to the treatment of pulmonary sarcoidosis with corticosteroids: the six phases of treatment. *Chest.* 1999;115:1158–1165.

51. Judson MA, Uflacker R. Treatment of a solitary pulmonary sarcoidosis mass by CT-guided direct intralesional injection of corticosteroid. *Chest.* 2001;120:316–317.

52. Butler CR, Nouraei SA, Mace AD, Khalil S, Sandhu SK, Sandhu GS. Endoscopic airway management of laryngeal sarcoidosis. *Arch Otolaryngol Head Neck Surg.* 2010;136:251–255.

53. Bestall JC, Paul EA, Garrod R, Garnham R, Jones PW, Wedzicha JA. Usefulness of the Medical Research Council (MRC) dyspnoea scale as a measure of disability in patients with chronic obstructive pulmonary disease. *Thorax.* 1999;54:581–586.

54. Teo F, Anantham D, Feller-Kopman D, Ernst A. Bronchoscopic management of sarcoidosis related bronchial stenosis with adjunctive topical mitomycin C. *Ann Thorac Surg.* 2010;89:2005–2007.

55. Costantino CL, Mathisen DJ. Idiopathic laryngotracheal stenosis. *J Thorac Dis.* 2016;8:S204–S209.

56. Fiz I, Bittar Z, Piazza C, et al. Hormone receptors analysis in idiopathic progressive subglottic stenosis. *Laryngoscope.* 2018;128:E72–E77.

57. Grillo HC, Mark EJ, Mathisen DJ, Wain JC. Idiopathic laryngotracheal stenosis and its management. *Ann Thorac Surg.* 1993;56:80–87.

58. Shabani S, Hoffman MR, Brand WT, Dailey SH. Endoscopic Management of idiopathic subglottic stenosis. *Ann Otol Rhinol Laryngol.* 2017;126:96–102.

59. Taylor SC, Clayburgh DR, Rosenbaum JT, Schindler JS. Clinical manifestations and treatment of idiopathic and Wegener granulomatosis-associated subglottic stenosis. *JAMA Otolaryngol Head Neck Surg.* 2013;139:76–81.

60. Grillo HC, Mathisen DJ, Ashiku SK, Wright CD, Wain JC. Successful treatment of idiopathic laryngotracheal

stenosis by resection and primary anastomosis. *Ann Otol Rhinol Laryngol.* 2003;112:798–800.

61. Marchiori E, Araujo Neto C, Meirelles GS, et al. Laryngotracheobronchial papillomatosis: findings on computed tomography scans of the chest. *J Bras Pneumol.* 2008;34:1084–1089.

62. Donne AJ, Hampson L, Homer JJ, Hampson IN. The role of HPV type in recurrent respiratory papillomatosis. *Int J Pediatr Otorhinolaryngol.* 2010;74:7–14.

63. Rombaldi RL, Serafini EP, Mandelli J, Zimmermann E, Losquiavo KP. Transplacental transmission of human papillomavirus. *Virol J.* 2008;5:106.

64. Fortes HR, von Ranke FM, Escuissato DL, et al. Recurrent respiratory papillomatosis: a state-of-the-art review. *Respir Med.* 2017;126:116–121.

65. Carifi M, Napolitano D, Morandi M, Dall'Olio D. Recurrent respiratory papillomatosis: current and future perspectives. *Ther Clin Risk Manag.* 2015;11:731–738.

66. Wierzbicka M, Jackowska J, Bartochowska A, Jozefiak A, Szyfter W, Kedzia W. Effectiveness of cidofovir intralesional treatment in recurrent respiratory papillomatosis. *Eur Arch Otorhinolaryngol.* 2011;268:1305–1311.

67. Dikkers FG. Treatment of recurrent respiratory papillomatosis with microsurgery in combination with intralesional cidofovir–a prospective study. *Eur Arch Otorhinolaryngol.* 2006;263:440–443.

68. Lee AS, Rosen CA. Efficacy of cidofovir injection for the treatment of recurrent respiratory papillomatosis. *J Voice.* 2004;18:551–556.

69. Shehab N, Sweet BV, Hogikyan ND. Cidofovir for the treatment of recurrent respiratory papillomatosis: a review of the literature. *Pharmacotherapy.* 2005;25:977–989.

70. Cundy KC. Clinical pharmacokinetics of the antiviral nucleotide analogues cidofovir and adefovir. *Clin Pharmacokinet.* 1999;36:127–143.

71. Naiman AN, Ceruse P, Coulombeau B, Froehlich P. Intralesional cidofovir and surgical excision for laryngeal papillomatosis. *Laryngoscope.* 2003;113:2174–2181.

72. Milczuk HA. Intralesional cidofovir for the treatment of severe juvenile recurrent respiratory papillomatosis: long-term results in 4 children. *Otolaryngol Head Neck Surg.* 2003;128:788–794.

73. Tanna N, Sidell D, Joshi AS, Bielamowicz SA. Adult intralesional cidofovir therapy for laryngeal papilloma: a 10-year perspective. *Arch Otolaryngol Head Neck Surg.* 2008;134:497–500.

74. Frye L, Machuzak M. Airway complications after lung transplantation. *Clin Chest Med.* 2017;38:693–706.

75. Oberg CL, Holden VK, Channick CL. Benign central airway obstruction. *Semin Respir Crit Care Med.* 2018;39:731–746.

76. Yousem SA, Dauber JH, Griffith BP. Bronchial cartilage alterations in lung transplantation. *Chest.* 1990;98:1121–1124.

77. Chhajed PN, Malouf MA, Tamm M, Spratt P, Glanville AR. Interventional bronchoscopy for the management of airway complications following lung transplantation. *Chest.* 2001;120:1894–1899.

78. Erard AC, Monnier P, Spiliopoulos A, Nicod L. Mitomycin C for control of recurrent bronchial stenosis: a case report. *Chest.* 2001;120:2103–2105.

79. Davidson KR, Elmasri M, Wahidi MM, Shofer SL, Cheng GZ, Mahmood K. Management of lung transplant bronchial stenosis with mitomycin C. *J Bronchology Interv Pulmonol.* 2019;26:124–128.

12

Bronchial Thermoplasty

Waqas Aslam, Ajay Sheshadri and Carla R. Lamb

INTRODUCTION

Asthma affects over 300 million people throughout the world, with a high burden of morbidity and mortality.[1] According to World Health Organization (WHO) estimates, approximately 250, 000 people die prematurely each year from asthma.[2] Approximately 5%–10% of patients with asthma are categorized as severe with failure of symptom control despite maximal inhaler therapy.[3] The definition of severe asthma sometimes varies, but is generally characterized by recurrent exacerbations or ongoing symptoms despite maximal treatment.[4] Frequent emergency room visits, unscheduled clinic visits, hospitalizations, missed school or work, and a reduced quality of life impact patients with severe asthma. About 1000 people die each day from asthma.[5] Asthma is among the top 20 causes of years of life lived with disability.[5] The significant global impact on health care costs and resource utilization is ongoing and exceeds 56 billion dollars annually in the United States alone.[5] Asthma is a disease hallmarked by inflammation and hyperresponsiveness of the peripheral airways. When asthma is left unchecked, airway remodeling leads to increased airway smooth muscle (ASM) mass, mucus metaplasia, and airway wall fibrosis. The cornerstone of asthma therapy is a combination of both short- and long-acting beta-2 receptor adrenergic agonists, corticosteroids, leukotriene antagonists, and sometimes monoclonal antibody therapy.[6] Chronic medical management of asthma focuses on bronchodilation and the reduction of airway inflammation, but the reversal of airway remodeling remains a challenge. Bronchial thermoplasty (BT) is a therapy that can reverse the effects of smooth muscle hypertrophy and other mucosal changes through the application of controlled thermal energy directly to airway walls. The approval of BT by the Food and Drug Administration (FDA) on April 27, 2010 has set a new paradigm in the treatment for moderate to severe persistent asthma.

SCIENTIFIC BASIS FOR BRONCHIAL THERMOPLASTY

The direct application of controlled thermal energy of 65°C to the airway wall using a thermal energy probe deployed during bronchoscopy reduces ASM mass.[7–12] Early studies in canines showed that the reduction in ASM mass could result in decreased bronchial constriction in response to various intrinsic and extrinsic inflammatory mediators.[13] Reduction in ASM mass, type 1 collagen deposition, and reticular basement membrane thickness have been confirmed by biopsy in humans.[14] BT causes a reduction in nerve fibers innervating the epithelium and ASM.[12,15] BT changes epithelial cell phenotype leading to reduced mucin production and goblet cell hyperplasia, perhaps driven by decreased interleukin (IL)-13 expression.[16] BT may also alter several other genes involved in pathogenesis of asthma and exert immunomodulatory actions by altering T-cell subpopulations in the airway.[17,18] BT increases luminal airway volume and reduces gas trapping in small airways.[19–22] These changes may not always be evident by spirometry or impedance oscillometry, but changes in ventilation can be quantified using advanced imaging techniques, such as hyperpolarized ³He magnetic resonance imaging (MRI).[23,24] However, the benefit of increased airway caliber in the absence of improvements in pulmonary function is not entirely clear. In summary, BT induces many changes in the airways, including reduction in ASM mass and nerve fibers, beneficial changes in the airway epithelium, and improves ventilation, potentially by increasing airway caliber.

CLINICAL EVIDENCE FROM HUMAN STUDIES

Miller and colleagues[25] performed the first prospective feasibility study of BT in humans. BT was performed in eight patients preoperatively up to 3 weeks prior to the planned lung resection for suspected or proven lung cancer. Treatment was limited to the segmental bronchi planned to be removed. There were no adverse effects related to the procedure. There was no bronchoscopic evidence of scarring in the airways, and histologic examination confirmed a reduction in ASM in the treated airways and immediate peribronchial area.

Cox and colleagues[26] performed the first nonrandomized feasibility study of BT in 16 patients with stable asthma and demonstrated a significant increase in methacholine PC20 and mean symptom-free days.

The Asthma Intervention Research (AIR) trial was the first randomized controlled trial enrolling 112 patients and compared BT plus standard-of-care therapy (inhaled corticosteroids [ICS] and long-acting beta agonists [LABA]) with standard-of-care therapy (ICS and LABA) alone in patients with moderate to severe persistent asthma.[27] The trial demonstrated a significant decrease in the rate of mild exacerbations (not severe exacerbations) and an increase in morning peak expiratory flow rate among patients receiving BT compared to the control group.[27] Long-term follow-up of BT patients revealed a stable rate of respiratory adverse events, without increase in emergency visits or hospitalizations for respiratory symptoms and stable lung function over 5 years.[28]

The Research in Severe Asthma (RISA) trial was a randomized multicenter trial enrolling 34 patients with severe asthma.[29] The patients were randomized to receive either BT or continue high-dose ICS and LABA.[29] The trial showed a significant increase in prebronchodilator forced expiratory volume in the first second of expiration (FEV_1) and improvement in asthma control and quality of life in BT group compared to the control group.[29] Long-term follow-up for 5 years revealed stable respiratory adverse events and decrease in hospitalizations and emergency department visits for respiratory symptoms.[30]

The AIR2 trial was the first double-blind, sham-controlled randomized control trial of BT comparing the effectiveness and safety of BT versus a sham procedure in patients with severe asthma.[31] A total of 288 patients were randomized to either BT or sham control.[31] Primary outcome was the difference in asthma quality-of-life questionnaire (AQLQ) scores from baseline to average of 6, 9, and 12 months (integrated AQLQ).[31] The improvement in integrated AQLQ score from baseline was superior in the BT group compared to the sham group.[31] More BT patients (6% more) were hospitalized in the treatment period.[31] BT patients experienced fewer exacerbations, emergency room visits, and days missed from work or school compared to the sham group.[31] Five-year follow-up of BT-treated patients from AIR2 trial demonstrated 5-year durability of benefits of BT.[32] BT-treated patients had fewer severe exacerbations and emergency visits on 5-year follow-up (average 5-year reduction of 44% in severe exacerbations and 78% for emergency visits) compared to those observed in the 12 months prior to their BT.[32]

The Post-FDA Approval Clinical Trial Evaluating Bronchial Thermoplasty in Severe Persistent Asthma (PAS2) is a prospective, observational, multicenter study designed to confirm the safety and efficacy of BT in clinical practice.[33] The primary endpoint is the proportion of subjects experiencing severe exacerbations during the subsequent 12-month period for years 2, 3, 4, and 5 compared with the first 12-month period after BT.[33] PAS2 data show that BT is safe and associated with lower rates of severe asthma exacerbations, emergency visits, and hospitalization at 3 years after BT (45%, 55%, and 40% decrease, respectively) compared to the 12 months before BT.[33]

Burn and colleagues[34] analyzed the efficacy and safety of BT in the UK and found mean improvement in AQLQ score at 12 months and a significant reduction in hospital admissions at 24 months follow-up without any deterioration in FEV_1, consistent with other clinical trials.

PREPROCEDURE MANAGEMENT OVERVIEW AND PATIENT SELECTION

Patient selection remains a key component to successful outcomes as described in the literature. A multidisciplinary approach in the setting of an asthma center with nurse practitioner, clinical pharmacist, and physician allows for a complete assessment of the patient, socioeconomic support, awareness about asthma, technique and compliance with inhaler usage, environmental exposures, tobacco history, and evaluation of other underlying diseases that may directly impact asthma care, such as rhinitis or sinusitis, atopy, immunodeficiency, gastroesophageal reflux, and obesity. Patients should be evaluated for other diseases that can mimic asthma, such as cardiac disease, vocal cord dysfunction, structural tracheal diseases, connective tissue diseases, or vasculitis syndromes. A thorough clinical assessment to identify factors to improve the patient's asthma symptoms is necessary to more accurately rate the severity of the disease while screening for the potential role for BT in moderate to severe persistent asthma (Fig. 12.1).

Practically speaking, many clinicians continue to adhere to the inclusion and exclusion criteria reported in the prior clinical trials. The series of clinical trials have developed specific selection criteria as well as general considerations for patient selection for bronchial thermoplasty (Boxes 12.1 and 12.2).[33,35–37] Future studies and outcome reports will be needed to determine if a broader range of patients will benefit from BT, such as those with severely impaired lung function.

PATIENT PREPARATION

- Patients are prescribed prophylactic prednisone 50 mg per day 3 days before the procedure, the day of the procedure, and the day after the procedure to reduce periprocedural inflammation.
- Procedural consent is completed after discussing all risks and benefits of BT and bronchoscopy along with the specifics of sedation, analgesia, and anesthesia (if needed).
- Majority of patients can undergo BT with moderate sedation: midazolam and fentanyl along with topical lidocaine. General anesthesia is safe and feasible as well.[38] F_{IO_2} less than 40% is recommended to avoid the possibility of airway ignition.[36]
- Albuterol nebulization prior to the bronchoscopy is mandatory.
- Oral codeine 30–60 mg may be prescribed 1 h prior to the procedure to further eliminate the cough reflex. This is ordered in patients who undergo the procedure under moderate sedation and is not ordered if the procedure is performed under general anesthesia.
- Topical anesthesia regimen applied to the airway may include nebulized 1% lidocaine.
- Glycopyrrolate can be administered intravenously with a very rapid onset of action to reduce airway secretions, if deemed necessary.

IMMEDIATE PREPROCEDURE ASSESSMENT

The day of the procedure the clinician should assure that the patient is at baseline before proceeding and the patient should undergo spirometry demonstrating an FEV_1 within 10% of their established baseline.

The procedure should be postponed and rescheduled if:
- Patient did not take the prescribed preprocedure prednisone
- SpO_2 <90% on room air
- Asthma symptoms have increased in the preceding 48 h with escalation of rescue bronchodilator use more than four puffs/day
- Active respiratory infection
- Active sinusitis
- Less than 14 days from completion of oral steroid therapy due to asthma exacerbation
- Any other contraindication.
  The procedure should be terminated if:
- Airways become excessively edematous
- Extensive bronchoconstriction
- Significant mucus in the airways
- Inability to access the airways due to patient's anatomy
- Excessive coughing or secretions that obscure visibility of the airways.

BRONCHIAL THERMOPLASTY EQUIPMENT

The Alair Bronchial Thermoplasty System (Boston Scientific, Natick, MA, USA) consists of a catheter and a radiofrequency (RF) controller (Figs. 12.2 and 12.3). The patient is initially grounded to the device with a standard gel electrode and connected to the controller. Each single-use catheter passes through the working channel of the bronchoscope and contains an expandable electrode array at one end and a deployment handle at the other end. Ideally, a 2-mm minimum working channel bronchoscope is required. The electrode array, once expanded, makes contact with the airway wall at four points and is then activated by a foot pedal. Each activation delivers RF electrical energy to heat the airways to a temperature of 65°C. The preset controller delivers a set intensity and duration of energy to the ASM without impacting other airway structures. Energy will not be

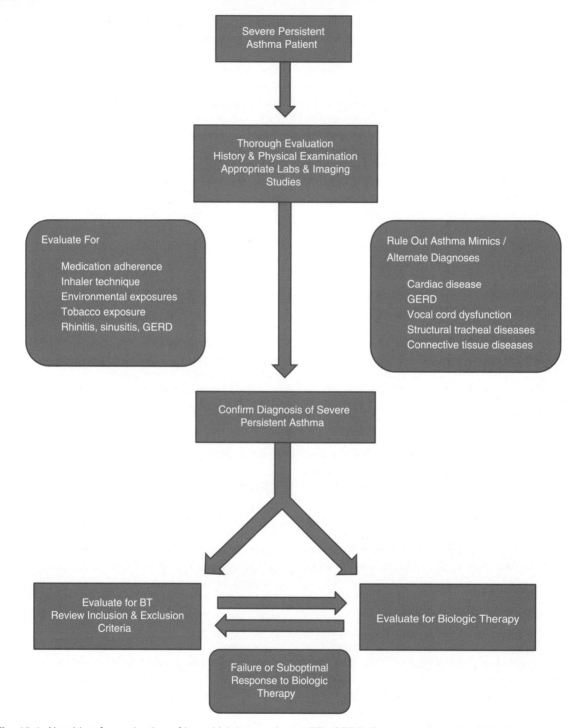

Fig. 12.1 Algorithm for evaluation of bronchial thermoplasty (*BT*). *GERD*, Gastroesophageal reflux disease.

BOX 12.1 Inclusion Criteria for Bronchial Thermoplasty

- Adult age 18 to 65 years
- Diagnosis of asthma and taking regular maintenance medication to include inhaled corticosteroid (ICS) at a dosage >1000 μg beclomethasone daily or equivalent and long-acting beta-2 agonist (LABA) at a dosage ≥100 μg daily of salmeterol or equivalent
- In addition to ICS and LABA, the patient may be on leukotriene antagonists, anti-IgE, other biologic therapies, or oral corticosteroids at a dosage of up to 10 mg daily or 20 mg every other day
- Stability of asthma symptoms on maintenance medications
- No current respiratory tract infection or severe asthma exacerbation within 4 weeks preceding a scheduled bronchial thermoplasty (BT)
- No unstable or untreated comorbid condition that would increase the risk of bronchoscopy
- Prebronchodilator forced expiratory volume in the first second of expiration (FEV$_1$) ≥60% predicted
- Postbronchodilator FEV$_1$ ≥65% predicted
- FEV$_1$ within 10% of the individual's best value
- Patient had at least 2 days of asthma symptoms in the last 4 weeks
- Nonsmoker for 1 year or more and less than a 10-pack-year tobacco history
- Able to undergo an outpatient bronchoscopy
- No contraindications to medications required to perform bronchoscopy (lidocaine, opiates, benzodiazepines)

BOX 12.2 Exclusion Criteria for Bronchial Thermoplasty

- Participation in another clinical trial within 6 weeks of baseline period of study enrollment
- Patient requires rescue medication over the last week of a 4-week medication stable period, exceeding average of eight puffs per day of short-acting bronchodilator, or four puffs per day of long-acting rescue bronchodilator, or two nebulizer treatments per day
- Postbronchodilator FEV$_1$ <65%
- History of life-threatening asthma: past intubations for asthma, ICU admission for asthma in the past 2 years
- Three or more hospitalizations for asthma exacerbation in the prior year
- Four or more infections of the lower respiratory tract requiring antibiotics in the past year
- Four or more pulses of systemic corticosteroids for asthma symptoms in the past year
- Known sensitivity to medications required to perform bronchoscopy
- Concomitant respiratory diseases such as tracheal stenosis, tracheobronchomalacia, emphysema, cystic fibrosis, bronchiectasis, vocal cord dysfunction, mechanical upper airway obstruction, Churg-Strauss syndrome, and allergic bronchopulmonary aspergillosis
- Segmental atelectasis, lobar consolidation, significant or unstable pulmonary infiltrate, or pneumothorax confirmed on chest radiograph
- Significant cardiovascular disease, including myocardial infarction, angina, cardiac dysfunction, cardiac dysrhythmia, conduction defect, cardiomyopathy, or stroke
- Known aortic aneurysm
- Comorbid illness: cancer, renal failure, liver disease, or cerebral vascular disease
- Uncontrolled hypertension; systolic pressure >200 mmHg or diastolic pressure >100 mmHg
- Implanted electrical stimulation device such as pacemaker, cardiac defibrillator, deep nerve, or brain stimulator
- Coagulopathy; international normalized ratio (INR) >1.5
- Inability to discontinue anticoagulants or antiplatelets prior to the procedure
- Known bleeding disorder
- Prior treatment with bronchial thermoplasty
- Age <18 years
- Pregnancy

delivered unless each equipment connection is secured and appropriate airway wall contact is made with the probe. An audio and visual feedback is emitted from the controller to alert the clinician if the catheter is not in contact with the airway wall and needs repositioning. The number of successful actuations is also recorded and displayed on the front panel of the controller.

BRONCHIAL THERMOPLASTY PROCEDURE OVERVIEW

BT procedures involve sequential bronchoscopic treatment of the peripheral airways over three consecutive bronchoscopic sessions, each occurring at 3-week intervals. The sequence of treatments is as follows: (1) right lower lobe, (2) left lower lobe, and (3) both upper lobes. The right middle lobe is not treated due to its hypothetical susceptibility to transient obstruction, atelectasis, and right middle lobe syndrome. However, Eisenmann and colleagues[39] performed BT in the right

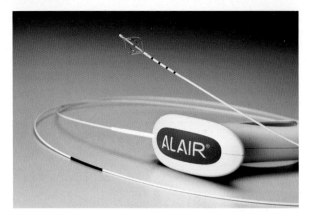

Fig. 12.2 Alair electrode array disposable catheter. (With permission from Boston Scientific, Natick, MA, USA.)

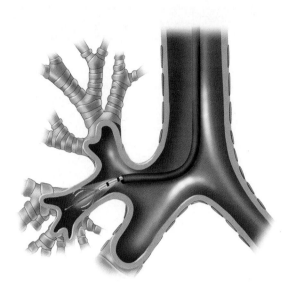

Fig. 12.4 Illustration of bronchial thermoplasty treatment with electrode array deployed in the peripheral airway. (With permission from Boston Scientific, Natick, MA, USA.)

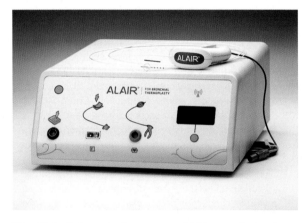

Fig. 12.3 Alair controller system. (With permission from Boston Scientific, Natick, MA, USA.)

activations delivered during BT correlates with the clinical response to treatment as well as the transient deterioration in lung function (FEV_1) after BT.[40,41] A thinner bronchoscope (outer diameter 4.2 mm) may increase the delivery of RF activations to the bronchial tree.[42]

POSTPROCEDURE ASSESSMENT AND FOLLOW-UP

After completion of each BT treatment, the patients undergo observation as is standard for moderate sedation. Increased respiratory symptoms are common immediately following bronchoscopy. In addition, patients remain under observation until they have achieved a postbronchodilator FEV_1 within 80% of the preprocedure value and are feeling well without any evidence of procedural complication. Postprocedural plan and instructions should be verified in detail with patients prior to discharge. Post-BT symptoms often present in a delayed fashion and should be treated as needed with the addition of corticosteroids, increased rescue bronchodilators, and antibiotics when clinically indicated. The patient should be assessed by phone call

middle lobe safely without any complications, suggesting these concerns may be overstated. All treatments utilizing the thermal probe are done under methodic visualization of the peripheral airways distal to the mainstem bronchi, ranging from 3 to 10 mm, utilizing the 2-mm working channel flexible bronchoscope in a contiguous and nonoverlapping fashion from distal to proximal airway. Expanding the electrode array allows contact along four points of the peripheral airway wall at 12, 3, 6, and 9 o'clock position followed by activating the energy source with the foot pedal (Figs. 12.4 and 12.5). The typical procedure time varies from 30 to 45 min, with an average 40 to 65 actuations per treatment session. Recent studies have shown that the number of RF

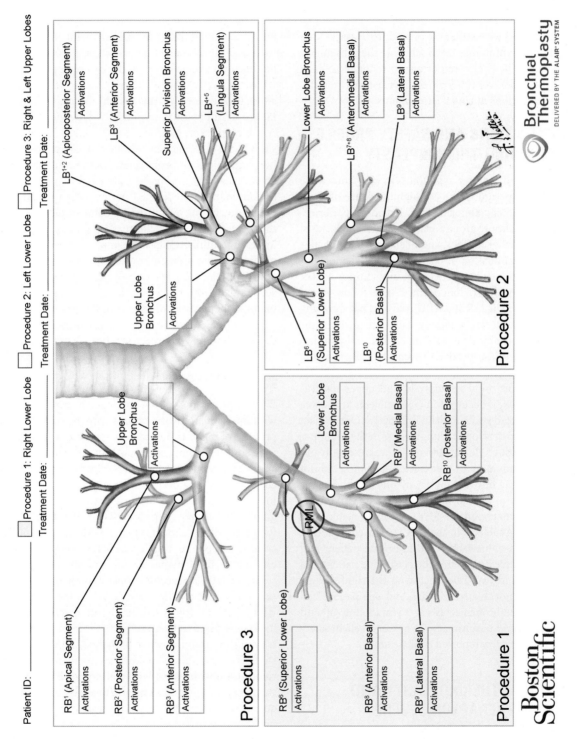

Fig. 12.5 Anatomic map of all lobar subsegments for recording treated areas of each sequential bronchial thermoplasty treatment. (With permission from Boston Scientific, Natick, MA, USA.)

1, 2, and 7 days postprocedure. An office visit should be scheduled 2 to 3 weeks after the procedure to assess lung function and symptoms and to schedule the subsequent BT treatment. It is also important to reiterate to each patient that they continue all of their asthma maintenance medications during BT treatments.

COMPLICATIONS AND SAFETY PROFILE OF BRONCHIAL THERMOPLASTY

BT can worsen asthma symptoms in the immediate posttreatment period. There is a high incidence of acute transient radiologic abnormalities, including peribronchial consolidations, ground-glass opacities, atelectasis, partial bronchial occlusions, and dilatations shortly after BT due to inflammation or edema. All these abnormalities resolve spontaneously without any clinical consequences.[43–45] However, long-term 5-year follow-up of patients enrolled in AIR and AIR2 trials did not show any case of pneumothorax, respiratory failure requiring intubation and mechanical ventilation, cardiac arrhythmias, or death.[28,32] Respiratory adverse events typical of asthma (including dyspnea, cough, wheeze, and nasal congestion), chest discomfort, mild hemoptysis, and upper respiratory tract infection occurred in ≥3% subjects at a stable rate from year 2 to year 5 in the BT group.[28,32] One subject in the BT group developed a lung abscess in the left upper lobe at 14 months.[28] He underwent surgical resection and histologic examination of the resected specimen did not show any airway obstruction or any other contributory abnormality from BT causing lung abscess.[28] Lung function and prebronchodilator FEV_1 remained stable over 5 years.[32] Three subjects in the AIR2 trial were found to have increased or new bronchiectasis; one patient had worsening of preexisting bronchiectasis, one patient had bronchiectasis in two lobes including the right middle lobe that was not treated with BT, and one patient had newly identified bronchiectasis at 3 years follow-up and remained stable.[32] In summary, BT has an excellent safety profile with very few reported complications.

BRONCHIAL THERMOPLASTY AND BIOLOGIC THERAPY IN SEVERE UNCONTROLLED ASTHMA

The Global Initiative for Asthma (GINA) 2019 guidelines recommend consideration of BT and biologic therapies (omalizumab, mepolizumab, reslizumab, benralizumab, dupilumab) for patients with severe uncontrolled asthma, despite maximal standard therapy. There has been no trial comparing BT and biologic therapies. BT is an effective therapy in nonallergic asthma and an alternative or add-on therapy in allergic asthma with failure or suboptimal response to biologic therapies.[46] An indirect comparison of BT versus omalizumab showed no difference in relative risk of asthma-related hospitalizations and emergency room visits between BT and omalizumab groups.[47] Relative risk of severe exacerbations in the immediate BT perioperative period favors omalizumab, but overall BT is comparable to biologic therapy.[47] Seeley and colleagues[48] reported a significant increase in mini-AQLQ score and a decrease in asthma medication requirement, including omalizumab 1 year after BT treatment. The cost of performing BT may be substantially lower than the long-term treatment with biologic therapy.[49–51] Modifications to the standard BT schedule may allow for even more efficient treatment delivery, but these approaches require validation.

■ SUMMARY

BT is a promising option for management of patients with moderate to severe asthma with an excellent safety profile. All patients should be assessed at a center experienced in managing severe asthma. BT should be considered for adult patients with moderate to severe poorly controlled asthma despite optimal medical therapy and may be cost effective in such situations. GINA 2019 guidelines have recommended BT as a treatment option for adult asthma patients at step 5. The success of BT is contingent upon thorough patient screening, optimizing existing medical management, and successful patient selection. BT is a procedure that requires skill and expertise in flexible bronchoscopy as well as the technique of BT application. The procedure should first be performed in a supervised setting with standardized procedural training and training of the bronchoscopy suite support staff. The procedure should be performed by an experienced bronchoscopist with training in BT. Physicians with expertise and training in advanced bronchoscopy and interventional pulmonology practicing in high-volume centers are best suited for performing BT due to the relatively higher risk associated with this specific patient population. Postprocedural care and subsequent follow-up further ensure safe and favorable BT outcomes.

REFERENCES

1. Global Initiative for Asthma (GINA). Global strategy for asthma management and prevention, 2019. Available from http://www.ginasthma.org.
2. World Health Organization. Global surveillance, prevention and control of chronic respiratory diseases: a comprehensive approach. https://apps.who.int/iris/handle/10665/43776; 2007.
3. Moore WC, Bleecker ER, Curran-Everett D, et al. Characterization of the severe asthma phenotype by the National Heart, Lung, and Blood Institute's Severe Asthma Research Program. *J Allergy Clin Immunol.* 2007;119:405–413.
4. Chung KF, Wenzel SE, Brozek JL, et al. International ERS/ATS guidelines on definition, evaluation and treatment of severe asthma. *Eur Respir J.* 2014;43:343–373.
5. The Global Asthma Report 2018. Auckland, New Zealand: Global Asthma Network, 2018.
6. Wahidi M, Kraft M. Bronchial thermoplasty for severe asthma. *Am J Respir Crit Care Med.* 2012;185:709–714.
7. Gordon IO, Husain AN, Charbeneau J, Krishnan JA, Hogarth DK. Endobronchial biopsy: a guide for asthma therapy selection in the era of bronchial thermoplasty. *J Asthma.* 2013;50(6):634–641.
8. Pretolani M, Dombret MC, Thabut G, et al. Reduction of airway smooth muscle mass by bronchial thermoplasty in patients with severe asthma. *Am J Respir Crit Care Med.* 2014;190(12):1452–1454.
9. d'Hooghe JNS, Goorsenberg AWM, Ten Hacken NHT, et al. Airway smooth muscle reduction after bronchial thermoplasty in severe asthma correlates with FEV$_1$ TASMA Research Group. *Clin Exp Allergy.* 2019;49(4):541–544.
10. Pretolani M, Bergqvist A, Thabut G, et al. Effectiveness of bronchial thermoplasty in patients with severe refractory asthma: clinical and histopathologic correlations. *J Allergy Clin Immunol.* 2017;139(4):1176–1185.
11. Chakir J, Haj-Salem I, Gras D, et al. Effects of bronchial thermoplasty on airway smooth muscle and collagen deposition in asthma. *Ann Am Thorac Soc.* 2015;12(11):1612–1618.
12. Ichikawa T, Panariti A, Audusseau S, et al. Effect of bronchial thermoplasty on structural changes and inflammatory mediators in the airways of subjects with severe asthma. *Respir Med.* 2019;150:165–172.
13. Danek CJ, Lombard CM, Dungworth DL, et al. Reduction in airway hyperresponsiveness to methacholine by the application of RF energy in dogs. *J Appl Physiol (1985).* 2004;97(5):1946–1953.
14. Salem IH, Boulet LP, Biardel S, et al. Long-term effects of bronchial thermoplasty on airway smooth muscle and reticular basement membrane thickness in severe asthma. *Ann Am Thorac Soc.* 2016;13(8):1426–1428.
15. Facciolongo N, Di Stefano A, Pietrini V, et al. Nerve ablation after bronchial thermoplasty and sustained improvement in severe asthma. *BMC Pulm Med.* 2018;18(1):29.
16. Haj Salem I, Gras D, Joubert P, et al. Persistent reduction of mucin production after bronchial thermoplasty in severe asthma. *Am J Respir Crit Care Med.* 2019;199(4):536–538.
17. Liao SY, Linderholm AL, Yoneda KY, Kenyon NJ, Harper RW. Airway transcriptomic profiling after bronchial thermoplasty. *ERJ Open Res.* 2019;5(1):00123–02018.
18. Marc Malovrh M, Rozman A, Škrgat S, et al. Bronchial thermoplasty induces immunomodulation with a significant increase in pulmonary CD4$^+$25$^+$ regulatory T cells. *Ann Allergy Asthma Immunol.* 2017;119(3):289–290.
19. Langton D, Sloan G, Banks C, Bennetts K, Plummer V, Thien F. Bronchial thermoplasty increases airway volume measured by functional respiratory imaging. *Respir Res.* 2019;20(1):157.
20. Langton D, Ing A, Bennetts K, et al. Bronchial thermoplasty reduces gas trapping in severe asthma. *BMC Pulm Med.* 2018;18(1):155.
21. Konietzke P, Weinheimer O, Wielpütz MO, et al. Quantitative CT detects changes in airway dimensions and air-trapping after bronchial thermoplasty for severe asthma. *Eur J Radiol.* 2018;107:33–38.
22. Zanon M, Strieder DL, Rubin AS, et al. Use of MDCT to assess the results of bronchial thermoplasty. *AJR Am J Roentgenol.* 2017;209(4):752–756.
23. Langton D, Ing A, Sha J, et al. Measuring the effects of bronchial thermoplasty using oscillometry. *Respirology.* 2019;24(5):431–436.
24. Thomen RP, Sheshadri A, Quirk JD, et al. Regional ventilation changes in severe asthma after bronchial thermoplasty with (3)He MR imaging and CT. *Radiology.* 2015;274(1):250–259.
25. Miller JD, Cox G, Vincic L, Lombard CM, Loomas BE, Danek CJ. A prospective feasibility study of bronchial thermoplasty in the human airway. *Chest.* 2005;127(6):1999–2006.
26. Cox G, Miller JD, McWilliams A, Fitzgerald JM, Lam S. Bronchial thermoplasty for asthma. *Am J Respir Crit Care Med.* 2006;173(9):965–969.
27. Cox G, Thomson NC, Rubin AS, et al. Asthma control during the year after bronchial thermoplasty AIR Trial Study Group. *N Engl J Med.* 2007;356(13):1327–1337.
28. Thomson NC, Rubin AS, Niven RM, et al. Long-term (5 year) safety of bronchial thermoplasty: Asthma Intervention Research (AIR) trial AIR Trial Study Group. *BMC Pulm Med.* 2011;11:8.
29. Pavord ID, Cox G, Thomson NC, et al. Safety and efficacy of bronchial thermoplasty in symptomatic, severe asthma RISA Trial Study Group. *Am J Respir Crit Care Med.* 2007;176(12):1185–1191.

30. Pavord ID, Thomson NC, Niven RM, et al. Safety of bronchial thermoplasty in patients with severe refractory asthma Research in Severe Asthma Trial Study Group. *Ann Allergy Asthma Immunol.* 2013;111(5):402–407.

31. Castro M, Rubin AS, Laviolette M, et al. AIR2 Trial Study Group. Effectiveness and safety of bronchial thermoplasty in the treatment of severe asthma: a multicenter, randomized, double-blind, sham-controlled clinical trial. *Am J Respir Crit Care Med.* 2010;181(2):116–124.

32. Wechsler ME, Laviolette M, Rubin AS, et al. Asthma Intervention Research 2 Trial Study Group. Bronchial thermoplasty: long-term safety and effectiveness in patients with severe persistent asthma. *J Allergy Clin Immunol.* 2013;132(6):1295–1302.

33. Chupp G, Laviolette M, Cohn L, et al. Other members of the PAS2 Study Group. Long-term outcomes of bronchial thermoplasty in subjects with severe asthma: a comparison of 3-year follow-up results from two prospective multicentre studies. *Eur Respir J.* 2017;50(2):1700017.

34. Burn J, Sims AJ, Patrick H, Heaney LG, Niven RM. Efficacy and safety of bronchial thermoplasty in clinical practice: a prospective, longitudinal, cohort study using evidence from the UK Severe Asthma Registry. *BMJ Open.* 2019;9(6):e026742.

35. Mayse MI, Laviolette M, Rubin A, et al. Clinical pearls for bronchial thermoplasty. *J Bronchol.* 2007;14:115–123.

36. Bonta PI, Chanez P, Annema JT, Shah PL, Niven R. Bronchial thermoplasty in severe asthma: best practice recommendations from an expert panel. *Respiration.* 2018;95(5):289–300.

37. Niven R, Aubier M, Bonta P, Puente-Maestu L, Facciolongo N, Ryan D. European consensus meeting/statement on bronchial thermoplasty. Who? Where? How? *Respir Med.* 1502019161–164.

38. Aizawa M, Ishihara S, Yokoyama T, Katayama K. Feasibility and safety of general anesthesia for bronchial thermoplasty: a description of early 10 treatments. *J Anesth.* 2018;32(3):443–446.

39. Eisenmann S, Schütte W, Funke F, Oezkan F, Islam S, Darwiche K. Bronchial thermoplasty including the middle lobe bronchus significantly improves lung function and quality of life in patients suffering from severe asthma. *Lung.* 2019;197(4):493–499.

40. Langton D, Sha J, Ing A, Fielding D, Thien F, Plummer V. Bronchial thermoplasty: activations predict response. *Respir Res.* 2017;18(1):134.

41. Langton D, Wang W, Thien F, Plummer V. The acute effects of bronchial thermoplasty on FEV_1. *Respir Med.* 2018;137:147–151.

42. Langton D, Gaffney N, Wang WC, Thien F, Plummer V. Utility of a thin bronchoscope in facilitating bronchial thermoplasty. *J Asthma Allergy.* 2018;11:261–266.

43. Goorsenberg AWM, d'Hooghe JNS, de Bruin DM, van den Berk IAH, Annema JT, Bonta PI. Bronchial thermoplasty-induced acute airway effects assessed with optical coherence tomography in severe asthma. *Respiration.* 2018;96(6):564–570.

44. d'Hooghe JNS, van den Berk IAH, Annema JT, Bonta PI. Acute radiological abnormalities after bronchial thermoplasty: a prospective cohort trial. *Respiration.* 2017;94(3):258–262.

45. Debray MP, Dombret MC, Pretolani M, et al. Early computed tomography modifications following bronchial thermoplasty in patients with severe asthma. *Eur Respir J.* 2017;49(3):1601565.

46. Minami D, Kayatani H, Sato K, et al. Clinical characteristics of severe refractory asthma associated with the effectiveness of bronchial thermoplasty. *Acta Med Okayama.* 2019;73(2):155–160.

47. Niven RM, Simmonds MR, Cangelosi MJ, Tilden DP, Cottrell S, Shargill NS. Indirect comparison of bronchial thermoplasty versus omalizumab for uncontrolled severe asthma. *J Asthma.* 2018;55(4):443–451.

48. Seeley EJ, Alshelli I, Canfield J, Lum M, Krishna G. The impact of bronchial thermoplasty on asthma-related quality of life and controller medication use. *Respiration.* 2019;98(2):165–170.

49. Zafari Z, Sadatsafavi M, Marra CA, Chen W, FitzGerald JM. Cost-effectiveness of bronchial thermoplasty, omalizumab, and standard therapy for moderate-to-severe allergic asthma. *PLoS One.* 2016;11(1):e0146003.

50. Cangelosi MJ, Ortendahl JD, Meckley LM, et al. Cost-effectiveness of bronchial thermoplasty in commercially-insured patients with poorly controlled, severe, persistent asthma. *Expert Rev Pharmacoecon Outcomes Res.* 2015;15(2):357–364.

51. Zein JG, Menegay MC, Singer ME, et al. Cost effectiveness of bronchial thermoplasty in patients with severe uncontrolled asthma. *J Asthma.* 2016;53(2):194–200.

13

Bronchoscopic Lung Volume Reduction

Jason Beattie and Adnan Majid

INTRODUCTION

Chronic obstructive pulmonary disease (COPD) causes considerable morbidity, mortality, and health care expenditure both in the United States and globally. For COPD patients with burdensome symptoms despite standard medical therapy, historically, few treatment options have been available. In the last 20 years, a variety of bronchoscopic interventions have expanded therapeutic options for emphysema patients with hyperinflation. Several techniques are now recognized by the Global Initiative for Chronic Obstructive Lung Disease (GOLD), and two devices have gained FDA approval.[1] With increasing treatment options for patients with emphysema, practical knowledge of available technologies, proper patient evaluation and selection, and preparedness for procedures and for procedure-related complications will be integral to optimized care for these vulnerable patients.[1]

DEFINITION

Bronchoscopic lung volume reduction (BLVR) interventions are performed with a standard bronchoscope for the treatment of emphysema. The goal of these treatment methods is to deflate or promote physical changes of the severely emphysematous lung in order to improve respiratory mechanics and physiology. BLVR treatments were developed as alternatives to lung volume reduction surgery (LVRS). They include one-way valves, coils, thermal vapor ablation, and biological lung volume reduction. Stents placed for airway bypass were developed in the past; however, they failed in clinical trials and their use has been abandoned. Of the aforementioned interventions, one-way valves are currently the most widely accepted and recommended devices, whereas the others remain largely investigational. As of 2020, one-way valves are the only BLVR intervention approved in the United States; other treatments have approval in other countries.

PREPROCEDURAL PREPARATION

Patient Selection and Initial Patient Evaluation

Appropriate patients for BLVR include patients with advanced emphysema and hyperinflation who have significant dyspnea despite standard-of-care noninvasive management strategies, including smoking cessation, maintenance medications such as inhaled bronchodilators and corticosteroids, and pulmonary rehabilitation. Evaluation of BLVR candidates is ideally made by a multidisciplinary team, with consideration of surgical interventions including lung transplantation, LVRS, and bullectomy when appropriate.[2] Emerging evidence may also assist in proper patient profiling; the relative benefit of surgical versus BLVR is currently under investigation.

Upon initial work up for BLVR, a general medical and pulmonary evaluation should be performed, including basic laboratory analysis, blood gas, electrocardiogram (ECG), echocardiogram, and pulmonary function tests including spirometry, lung volumes, diffusion capacity for carbon monoxide (DLCO), and 6-min walk test (6MWT). Pulmonary function tests should reveal severe obstruction (forced expiratory volume in 1 s, FEV_1, of 15%–45%), hyperinflation (total lung capacity, TLC $\geq$100%), and air trapping with residual volume (RV) $\geq$150%. 6MWT should demonstrate diminished exercise capacity (100–500 m).

Patients should lack significant comorbidities that may compromise short-term survival and performance status. Severe hypercapnia ($Paco_2$ >55 mmHg) or hypoxia (Pao_2 <45 mmHg) (measured on room air), severely decreased D_{LCO} (<20%), and pulmonary hypertension (right ventricular systolic pressure [RVSP] $\geq$50) are generally contraindications as well. If echocardiogram demonstrates concern for pulmonary hypertension, further evaluation with right heart catheterization may be needed.[3]

A noncontrast, thin-cut computed tomography (CT) chest ($\leq$1.5-mm slice thickness) is also part of the initial evaluation.[4] The CT is useful to examine the extent and distribution of emphysema and the radiographic integrity of lobar fissures. The CT also functions to screen patients for other potential contraindications including severe bronchiectasis, concerning pulmonary nodules and masses, and interstitial lung disease. The amount of emphysema in individual lung lobes can be assessed by quantifying the proportion of lung voxels below an attenuation threshold such as −910 or −950 (this correlates with emphysema pathologically), which is accomplished by evaluating the chest CT via specialized software programs. This emphysema severity information is used for targeting sites for treatment and for quantifying the distribution of the disease (heterogeneous vs. homogeneous). Additionally, perfusion scintigraphy can be used to quantify relative perfusion. This can facilitate target lobe selection in patients with homogeneous and heterogeneous disease where there are two potential target lobes for treatment.[5] It is important to avoid targeting lobes with high perfusion (compared to other lobes), as this can lead to imbalances in perfusion/ventilation matching and subsequent respiratory failure.

For one-way valve placement, subgroup analysis from initial multicenter studies demonstrated that clinical benefit with placement of these devices is dependent on lack of collateral ventilation (CV) due to intact fissures.[6,7] Quantification of fissure integrity can be accomplished by analyzing the patient's high-resolution computed tomography (HRCT) chest with dedicated software. Fissure completeness less than 80% is considered incomplete and not amenable to one-way valve placement. A fissure integrity of $\geq$95% is considered complete and amenable to endobronchial valve (EBV) therapy.[8] Fissure integrity of 80%–94% can be further assessed with a proprietary balloon occlusion-based system (Chartis) during bronchoscopy to evaluate for CV.[9] The balloon is typically inserted via the bronchoscope and inflated in the target

lobe. The tip of the catheter distal to the balloon remains open and can measure the flow returning from the obstructed target lobe. If CV exists, then air flow from the obstructed lobe will continue. If CV is absent, then air flow from the obstructed lobe will gradually decrease until it ceases. In contrast to one-way valves, lack of CV is not a prerequisite for other BLVR techniques.

Equipment and Procedural Techniques
One-Way Valves

One-way valve devices cause target lung region collapse by preventing air entry during inspiration while allowing air to exit during exhalation. The valves are placed within all the segments of the most emphysematous lobe target in order to elicit a lobar atelectasis. There are two commercially available valves, both of which received US Food and Drug Administration (FDA) approval: an EBV (Zephyr, Pulmonx Corporation, Redwood City, CA, USA) and an intrabronchial valve (IBV) (Spiration Valve System [SVS], Spiration Inc./Olympus Respiratory America, Redmond, WA, USA). Both valve devices can be placed under general anesthesia or moderate sedation.

Zephyr Endobronchial Valve

Recent landmark trials that studied the Zephyr EBV used the Chartis Pulmonary Assessment System (Pulmonx Corporation) for bronchoscopic evaluation for the presence or absence of CV as part of the inclusion/exclusion criteria.[10-13] The Chartis system uses a single-use balloon catheter with a central channel that can measure pressure and flow during balloon occlusion of a lung segment in order to quantify CV. Chartis assessment is generally performed during the same procedure as EBV placement, as part of final evaluation of eligibility for valve placement. Targets for treatment can also be modified based on Chartis evaluation: if the right upper lobe (RUL) is the primary target, but CV is found at the RUL, the integrity of the major fissure can then be assessed by placing the Chartis balloon in the right lower lobe (RLL). If there is no CV at the RLL, there is the option of treating both the RUL and right middle lobe (RML).

The Zephyr valve is a silicone, "duckbill"-shaped valve device mounted within a self-expanding nitinol silicone covered stent-like retainer structure (Fig. 13.1). The valve comes in four sizes: 4.0, 4.0 low-profile (LP), 5.5, and 5.5 LP. The 4.0-size valves can be deployed for airways between 4 and 7 mm, whereas the 5.5 valve can be deployed for airways between 5.5 and 8.5 mm. The LP valve has a shorter

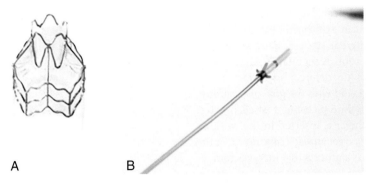

Fig. 13.1 Zephyr endobronchial valve. (A) Valve device. (B) Sizing catheter. (Courtesy Pulmonx. © 2019 Pulmonx Corporation or its affiliates. All rights reserved.)

proximal to distal length, allowing placement in shorter bronchial segments. Zephyr valve delivery catheters have delivery gauges for selecting proper valve size. The valves are intended for segmental and/or subsegmental airway placement with no defined limit to the number of valves placed within a lobe. The propeller-like sizing catheters should verify that the target airway is appropriate for the selected valve size (Fig. 13.1). There are also depth markers for choosing between LP and standard-length valves. Once a valve size is selected, the endobronchial loader system is used to load the valve into the delivery catheter. Within the bronchoscope (either in a central airway or outside the patient), the delivery catheter is advanced until the tip of the catheter can be viewed with the bronchoscope camera. The bronchoscope is then navigated to the target airway orifice and the delivery catheter is advanced into the airway until the diameter gauge is flush with the airway orifice. Valve deployment is initiated by partially advancing the actuator of the delivery catheter handle; as the valve begins deployment, the position of the distal end should be verified as against the carina distal to the valve target, after which the actuator can be advanced to complete valve deployment. The main body of the stent-like retainer portion of the valve should fully interface with the target airway and should not protrude outside of the airway orifice. If the valve is malpositioned and/or concluded to be the wrong size, it can be removed using rat tooth forceps with grasping of the retainer portion of the valve device and subsequent removal en bloc.

Spiration Valve System

The Spiration valve system is composed of a nitinol frame and polyurethane membrane with an umbrella

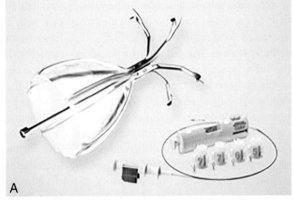

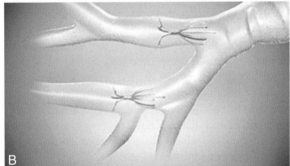

Fig. 13.2 Spiration valve system. (A) Valve device, loading device, and deployment catheter. (B) Illustration of valves deployment in airways. (Courtesy Olympus America. © 2019 Olympus America Corportation or its affiliates. All rights reserved.)

shape with anchors that hold it in place through superficial airway wall penetration (Fig. 13.2). The struts of the umbrella expand and contract with the respiratory cycle so that the airway is occluded during inspiration, whereas air and mucus can exit during expiration. The valves come in four different sizes: 5, 6, 7, and 9 mm. The valves are placed in lobar, segmental, and/or sub-segmental airways with no defined limitation to the number of valves placed, and with the goal of occluding the entire target lobe. Before placement of each valve, a calibrated balloon catheter is inserted in the working channel for sizing of the target airway (calibration of the balloon catheter system is a process that involves removing air from the catheter system with saline, precise saline volume measurement with a dedicated syringe, and sizing of the saline-filled balloon; this process takes approximately 5 min and is best done before the procedure begins).[14]

Once the valve size is chosen, the valve is then loaded from a cartridge into the deployment catheter with a dedicated loading device (Fig. 13.2). The deployment catheter is then inserted into the working channel with the bronchoscope within a central airway until the tip of the catheter and the tip of the removal rod and the yellow valve line are visible. The catheter tip should be retracted as needed to eliminate any gap between the stabilization wire and the tip of the removal rod. Once the bronchoscope is in position with the catheter within the target airway, the yellow valve line on the catheter should be aligned with the ostium of the target bronchial branch when deploying valve sizes 5, 6, and 7. On the other hand, when deploying the 9-mm valve size, it is recommended to align the yellow line 1 mm proximal to the ostium to correct for the fact that these valves can advance distally 1–2 mm over time following deployment. If valve removal is desired due to improper sizing or positioning, the valve can easily be removed with standard forceps. The center nitinol hub is a rod with a knob at the end that facilitates grasping the valve with forceps; once the valve is grasped, the bronchoscope and forceps can be withdrawn en bloc.

Coils

Endobronchial coil placement is a BLVR technique that targets one lobe of both lungs (each lung is treated in an individual procedure with the contralateral side treated 4–8 weeks after the initial procedure). These devices are nitinol wire with shape memory that are delivered into subsegmental airways in a straight conformation but transition into a predetermined angled shape after deployment (Fig. 13.3). This change in shape allows

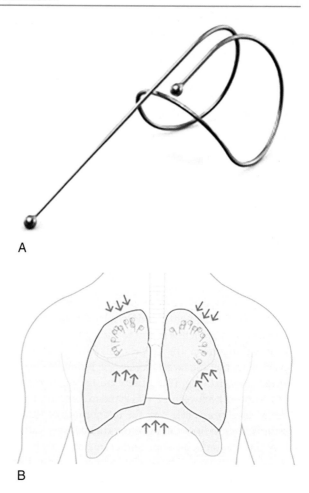

Fig. 13.3 PneumRx endobronchial coils. (A) Endobronchial coil. (B) Illustration of endobronchial coils deployed in the chest. (Image provided courtesy of Boston Scientific. © 2022 Boston Scientific Corporation or its affiliates. All rights reserved.)

the coils to apply traction on the airways, which leads to compression of the emphysematous lung tissue in the target lobe (Fig. 13.3). Rather than atelectasis, the desired effect to the target lung territory is compression and improved elastic recoil. Given the physical compression mechanism, unlike one-way valves, coils do not rely on lack of CV for efficacy of lung volume reduction. Coils are generally thought of as permanent implants, though bronchoscopic removal, including late removal, has been reported.[15] They can be placed under general anesthesia (preferred) or moderate sedation, under fluoroscopic guidance.[16,17]

The coils are available in three different lengths (100, 125, and 150 mm). The coil delivery system consists of a guidewire, catheter, cartridge, and forceps that are inserted via the working channel of a standard bronchoscope. The guidewire guides the catheter to the target airway and is used for selecting the length of the coil. The cartridge is used to straighten and load the coil into the delivery catheter. The forceps are used to grasp the proximal end of the coil to deliver the coil through the catheter. The catheter and forceps can also be used to reposition the coil if needed. Once the bronchoscope is in position within a distal airway of the targeted treatment lobe, the catheter position is verified with fluoroscopy. The coils are deployed under fluoroscopic guidance ensuring there is a safe distance from the pleura. The coils are placed with an algorithm that facilitates anatomically dispersed placement; 8–12 coils are generally placed in the upper lobes and 10–14 in the lower lobes.

Thermal Vapor Ablation

Thermal vapor ablation uses heated water vapor to cause scarring of lung tissue as a lung volume reduction technique. This irreversible treatment modality was developed with the potential advantage of targeting severely emphysematous segments within a lobe rather than obligatory treatment of entire lobes as in one-way valves and coils. At present, published trials involving this technique have only been performed in patients with upper-lobe, heterogeneous emphysema.[18,19] The equipment includes a catheter-based system with a multi-use vapor generator and a single-use catheter for proximal balloon occlusion of the targeted segment and delivery of the vapor distally over 3–10 s with a target dose of 8.5 calories per gram of lung tissue (Fig. 13.4).

Biological Lung Volume Reduction

Biological lung volume reduction is another irreversible BLVR treatment modality that can be applied at individual segments. The technique involves administering a synthetic polymer as a foam sealant to block airways and CV, leading to collapse of lung tissue. The sealant is prepared using an aqueous polymer solution and cross-linker in a 20-mL syringe with polymerization occurring over 3 min. The resulting 5 mL solution is mixed with 15 mL of air within the syringe to yield a 20-mL foam sealant. The bronchoscope is wedged within a targeted airway segment, and then a single-lumen catheter is advanced into the targeted segment. This sealant is then

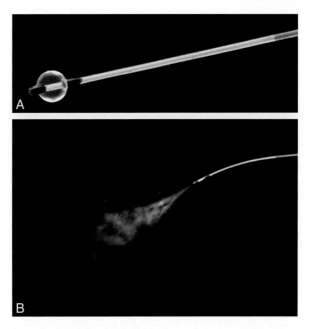

Fig. 13.4 Bronchoscopic thermal vapor ablation. (A) Catheter system with balloon occlusion. (B) Catheter with vapor deployment. (Courtesy Uptake Medical. © 2019 Uptake Medical Corporation or its affiliates. All rights reserved.)

delivered over 10–20 s via the catheter. The scope is then left wedged in the segment for 1 min post instillation, after which the next segment can be targeted.[20]

Notable Complications of BLVR Procedures

- Pneumothorax (most notable with one-way valve placement)
- Exacerbation of chronic obstructive pulmonary disease (COPD)
- Respiratory failure
- Hemoptysis
- Pneumonia
- Post treatment acute inflammatory response (lung sealant and vapor ablation)
- Device malposition or migration (one-way valves).

Management and Mitigation of Treatment-Specific Complications

Pneumothorax is the most frequent complication with one-way valve placement and has been associated with notable morbidity. Rupture of blebs or bullae or shearing of emphysematous lung tissue in the setting of volume shifts that occur in the ipsilateral adjacent nontarget lobe during atelectasis of the target lobe following valve placement is thought to be the principal mechanism for clinically important pneumothorax.[21] A chest x-ray should be obtained within 1 h of valve placement to evaluate for pneumothorax. In landmark clinical trials, most pneumothorax complications occurred within the first 3 days following valve placement and as such patients should generally be kept hospitalized following the procedure for at least 3 days for monitoring. Management of pneumothorax following one-way valve placement is centered around chest tube placement and observation of the patient until the air leak stops. Although most pneumothoraces resolve with chest tube placement within a few days, a small percentage develop a prolonged air leak. If the air leak persists for 7 days after valve placement, then one valve should be removed. If the air leak persists for 48 h following the removal of a single valve, then all valves should be removed. In very rare instances, surgical intervention may be required to repair an ongoing air leak despite removal of all valves. Expert algorithms for this management are available.

An acute inflammatory response following lung sealant instillation and vapor ablation is a syndrome that includes fever, dyspnea, cough, chest pain, and elevated inflammatory markers. Its description in pilot studies

has led to prophylactic peri procedure steroids, nonsteroidal antiinflammatory drugs (NSAIDs), and antibiotics in some clinical trials.[22]

EVIDENCE

For summaries of respiratory outcomes and complications of BLVR trials, see Tables 13.1 and 13.2.

Zephyr Endobronchial Valve

Randomized trial evidence for efficacy of EBVs has included patients with homogeneous and heterogeneous emphysema with valve implantations performed in upper and lower lobe targets and follow-up of up to 1 year. These trials have shown clinically meaningful improvements in lung function (including FEV_1 and RV), quality of life, 6MWT distance, and dyspnea scores. As mentioned earlier, the most common serious adverse event in these trials has been pneumothorax, occurring in 22% to 29.2% of patients. Of patients treated with valves in four recent landmark trials, death within 60 days of valve placements related to pneumothorax hospitalization or to respiratory failure occurred in 2.2% (6/276) of patients.

Long-term follow-up in small cohorts has demonstrated survival advantage in patients treated with EBVs with radiographically intact fissures in comparison to those without, and in patients with atelectasis

TABLE 13.1	**Respiratory Outcomes of BLVR Trials**								
Trial	Device	*n*	Emphysema Type	Treatment Location	FEV$_1$ (mL)	RV (mL)	6MWT (m)	SGRQ
IMPACT[12]	EBV	43	Homogeneous	Unilateral, UL/LL	120	−430	28	−7.6
TRANSFORM[11]	EBV	65	Heterogeneous	Unilateral, UL/LL	230	−670	79	−6.5
STELVIO[13]	EBV	40	All	Unilateral, UL/LL	147	−672	61	−11
LIBERATE[10]	EBV	128	Heterogeneous	Unilateral, UL/LL	106	−522	39	−7.1
REACH[26]	IBV	58	Heterogeneous	Unilateral, UL/LL	108	a	42	−12.8
EMPROVE[32]	IBV	113	Heterogeneous	Unilateral, UL/LL	101	−361	15	−8.5
REVOLENS[28]	Coils	50	All	Bilateral, UL/LL	80	−360	a	−10.6
RENEW[30]	Coils	158	All	Bilateral, UL/LL	50	−310	15	−8.9
STEP-UP[18]	Steam	44	Heterogeneous	Bilateral, UL	103	−303	31	−11.1

[a]Not statistically significant.

AECOPD, Acute exacerbation of COPD; *BLVR*, bronchoscopic lung volume reduction; *EBV*, endobronchial valve; *FEV$_1$*, forced expiratory volume in 1 s; *IBV*, intrabronchial valve; *RV*, residual volume; *SGRQ*, St. George's respiratory questionnaire; *UL/LL*, treatment applied to either upper lobe or lower lobe; *6MWT*, 6-min walk test.

Modified from Herth FJF, Slebos DJ, Criner GJ, Valipour A, Sciurba F, Shah PL. Endoscopic lung volume reduction: an expert panel recommendation - update 2019. *Respiration.* 2019;97(6):548-557.

TABLE 13.2   Complications in BLVR Trials (%)

Trial	Pneumothorax	AECOPD	Pneumonia/ Respiratory Infection	Hemoptysis
IMPACT[12]	25.6	34.9	7	×
TRANSFORM[11]	29.2	37	11	6.2
STELVIO[13]	17.6	11.8	5.9	2.9
LIBERATE[10]	29.7	19.5	4.7	8.6
REACH[26]	7.6	19.7	1.5	×
EMPROVE[32]	25.7	16.8	8.9	×
REVOLENS[28]	6	26	18	2
RENEW[30]	10.3	11.6	20	3.9
STEP-UP[18]	2	24	18	2

AECOPD, Acute exacerbation of chronic obstructive pulmonary disease; *BLVR*, bronchoscopic lung volume reduction; ×, not reported.
Modified from Herth FJF, Slebos DJ, Criner GJ, Valipour A, Sciurba F, Shah PL. Endoscopic lung volume reduction: an expert panel recommendation - update 2019. *Respiration*. 2019;97(6):548-557.

following valve placement in comparison to those without atelectasis. Furthermore, a single-center retrospective review of 449 patients treated with one-way valves demonstrated a 5-year survival benefit in patients with lobar atelectasis following valve placement, and did not detect decreased survival in patients who developed pneumothorax in comparison to those who did not. Long-term survival data from prospective randomized trials are yet to be demonstrated, however.[23–25]

Intrabronchial Valves: Spiration Valve System

Two randomized trials have evaluated treatment with the SVS. In the REACH study patients with heterogeneous emphysema and radiographically intact interlobar fissures (≥90%) were randomized to SVS versus standard of care.[26] The SVS-treated group showed clinically and statistically significant improvement in FEV_1 at 3 months (sustained at 6 months), as well as improvement in exercise capacity and quality of life. The most common adverse event was COPD exacerbation, occurring in 21% of patients. Pneumothorax rate was 7.6% in the treatment group with 60% of pneumothorax occurring within 30 days. In the EMPROVE trial, patients with heterogeneous emphysema treated with SVS showed statistically and clinically significant improvement in pulmonary function, dyspnea, and quality of life (but a borderline clinically significant

change in 6MWT) in comparison to controls. Adverse events occurred in 31% of the valve patients including 12.4% rate of pneumothorax; there was one death (0.9%) attributed to study treatment in a patient who developed pneumothorax.

Coils

Several studies have provided randomized controlled data for coils. Cumulative long-term data from these studies have shown benefit in terms of RV and dyspnea scores with modest clinical benefit in FEV_1 and 6MWT.[27–29] Common serious adverse events have included pneumonia (in up to 18%–20%) and pneumothorax (6%–12%). Although a recently published large randomized controlled trial (RENEW trial) failed to demonstrate significant clinical improvement in lung function and exercise capacity, a subgroup analysis demonstrated that patients with severe heterogeneous emphysema and hyperinflation (RV >200%) derived more significant benefit in RV reduction, improvement in FEV_1, quality of life, and exercise capacity.[30]

Thermal Vapor Ablation

Current randomized controlled data for thermal vapor ablation are available from the STEP-UP multicenter trial conducted on patients with upper lobe predominant heterogeneous severe emphysema.[31] Patients treated with this technique were managed with a selective sequential treatment of more diseased upper lobe segments. At 12 months this trial showed a clinically significant benefit in FEV_1, RV, and improved dyspnea scores in favor of the thermal ablation group. The most common serious adverse event in the treatment group was COPD exacerbation, occurring in 24% of patients. Trials in homogeneous and lower lobe disease have already begun, and the results are expected in the near future.

Biological Lung Volume Reduction

The efficacy of biological lung volume reduction has been evaluated in two pilot studies as well as one randomized multicenter trial. The ASPIRE trial randomized patients with upper lobe predominant severe emphysema to lung sealant treatment of the two most severe upper lobe segments in each lung.[22] Lung function, dyspnea, and quality of life improved significantly in the treatment arm relative to controls and persisted at 6-month follow-up. Although effective, there are some concerns about the safety of this technology since 44% of the patients in the treatment group experienced a severe adverse event requiring hospital admission (2.5-fold more than the control group) and 6% died.

SUMMARY

Emphysema remains an irreversible disease process with devastating morbidity, mortality, and limited effective treatments. BLVR with EBVs has shown to be a safe and effective option to treat patients with severe emphysema, hyperinflation, and minimal or no CV. Other BLVR techniques, although promising, continue to be experimental at the present time. As supportive data for these interventions grow, so will more tailored therapy to meet individual patient needs. For the bronchoscopist, delivering optimal care to patients with advanced emphysema will involve technical skills and proper experience with emerging technology, clinical expertise in careful patient selection, and a clinical program that offers proper patient support, monitoring, and follow-up.

REFERENCES

1. Singh D, Agusti A, Anzueto A, et al. Global strategy for the diagnosis, management, and prevention of chronic obstructive lung disease: the GOLD science committee report 2019. *Eur Respir J.* 2019;53(5):1900164.

2. Marchetti N, Criner GJ. Surgical approaches to treating emphysema: lung volume reduction surgery, bullectomy, and lung transplantation. *Semin Respir Crit Care Med.* 2015;36(4):592–608.

3. Herth FJF, Slebos DJ, Criner GJ, Valipour A, Sciurba F, Shah PL. Endoscopic lung volume reduction: an expert panel recommendation—update 2019. *Respiration.* 2019;97(6):548–557.

4. Labaki WW, Martinez CH, Martinez FJ, et al. The role of chest computed tomography in the evaluation and management of the patient with chronic obstructive pulmonary disease. *Am J Respir Crit Care Med.* 2017;196(11):1372–1379.

5. Argula RG, Strange C, Ramakrishnan V, Goldin J. Baseline regional perfusion impacts exercise response to endobronchial valve therapy in advanced pulmonary emphysema. *Chest.* 2013;144(5):1578–1586.

6. Sciurba FC, Ernst A, Herth FJ, et al. A randomized study of endobronchial valves for advanced emphysema. *N Engl J Med.* 2010;363(13):1233–1244.

7. Herth FJ, Noppen M, Valipour A, et al. Efficacy predictors of lung volume reduction with Zephyr valves in a European cohort. *Eur Respir J.* 2012;39(6):1334–1342.

8. Koster TD, van Rikxoort EM, Huebner RH, et al. Predicting lung volume reduction after endobronchial valve therapy is maximized using a combination of diagnostic tools. *Respiration.* 2016;92(3):150–157.

9. Herth FJ, Eberhardt R, Gompelmann D, et al. Radiological and clinical outcomes of using Chartis to plan endobronchial valve treatment. *Eur Respir J.* 2013;41(2):302–308.

10. Criner GJ, Sue R, Wright S, et al. A multicenter randomized controlled trial of Zephyr endobronchial valve treatment in heterogeneous emphysema (LIBERATE). *Am J Respir Crit Care Med.* 2018;198(9):1151–1164.

11. Kemp SV, Slebos DJ, Kirk A, et al. A multicenter randomized controlled trial of Zephyr endobronchial valve treatment in heterogeneous emphysema (TRANSFORM). *Am J Respir Crit Care Med.* 2017;196(12): 1535–1543.

12. Valipour A, Slebos DJ, Herth F, et al. Endobronchial valve therapy in patients with homogeneous emphysema. Results from the IMPACT study. *Am J Respir Crit Care Med.* 2016;194(9):1073–1082.

13. Klooster K, ten Hacken NH, Hartman JE, Kerstjens HA, van Rikxoort EM, Slebos DJ. Endobronchial valves for emphysema without interlobar collateral ventilation. *N Engl J Med.* 2015;373(24):2325–2335.

14. Olympus. Spiration Valve System. Available from: *Spiration*.com. Instructions for use.

15. Dutau H, Bourru D, Guinde J, Laroumagne S, Deslée G, Astoul P. Successful late removal of endobronchial coils. *Chest.* 2016;150(6):e143–e145.

16. Slebos DJ, Ten Hacken NH, Hetzel M, Herth FJF, Shah PL. Endobronchial coils for endoscopic lung volume reduction: best practice recommendations from an expert panel. *Respiration*. 2018;96(1):1–11.

17. Klooster K, Ten Hacken NH, Slebos DJ. The lung volume reduction coil for the treatment of emphysema: a new therapy in development. *Expert Rev Med Devices*. 2014;11(5):481–489.

18. Herth FJ, Valipour A, Shah PL, et al. Segmental volume reduction using thermal vapour ablation in patients with severe emphysema: 6-month results of the multicentre, parallel-group, open-label, randomised controlled STEP-UP trial. *Lancet Respir Med*. 2016;4(3):185–193.

19. Snell GI, Hopkins P, Westall G, Holsworth L, Carle A, Williams TJ. A feasibility and safety study of bronchoscopic thermal vapor ablation: a novel emphysema therapy. *Ann Thorac Surg*. 2009;88(6):1993–1998.

20. Herth FJ, Gompelmann D, Stanzel F, et al. Treatment of advanced emphysema with emphysematous lung sealant (AeriSeal®). *Respiration*. 2011;82(1):36–45.

21. Valipour A, Slebos DJ, de Oliveira HG, et al. Expert statement: pneumothorax associated with endoscopic valve therapy for emphysema–potential mechanisms, treatment algorithm, and case examples. *Respiration*. 2014;87(6):513–521.

22. Come CE, Kramer MR, Dransfield MT, et al. A randomised trial of lung sealant versus medical therapy for advanced emphysema. *Eur Respir J*. 2015;46(3):651–662.

23. Hopkinson NS, Kemp SV, Toma TP, et al. Atelectasis and survival after bronchoscopic lung volume reduction for COPD. *Eur Respir J*. 2011;37(6):1346–1351.

24. Venuta F, Anile M, Diso D, et al. Long-term follow-up after bronchoscopic lung volume reduction in patients with emphysema. *Eur Respir J*. 2012;39(5):1084–1089.

25. Gompelmann D, Benjamin N, Bischoff E, et al. Survival after endoscopic valve therapy in patients with severe emphysema. *Respiration*. 2019;97(2):145–152.

26. Li S, Wang G, Wang C, et al. The REACH trial: a randomized controlled trial assessing the safety and effectiveness of the Spiration(R) Valve System in the treatment of severe emphysema. *Respiration*. 2019;97(5):416–427.

27. Shah PL, Zoumot Z, Singh S, et al. Endobronchial coils for the treatment of severe emphysema with hyperinflation (RESET): a randomised controlled trial. *Lancet Respir Med*. 2013;1(3):233–240.

28. Deslée G, Mal H, Dutau H, et al. Lung volume reduction coil treatment vs usual care in patients with severe emphysema: the REVOLENS randomized clinical trial. *JAMA*. 2016;315(2):175–184.

29. Zoumot Z, Kemp SV, Singh S, et al. Endobronchial coils for severe emphysema are effective up to 12 months following treatment: medium term and cross-over results from a randomised controlled trial. *PLoS One*. 2015;10(4):e0122656.

30. Sciurba FC, Criner GJ, Strange C, et al. Effect of endobronchial coils vs usual care on exercise tolerance in patients with severe emphysema: the RENEW randomized clinical trial. *JAMA*. 2016;315(20):2178–2189.

31. Shah PL, Gompelmann D, Valipour A, et al. Thermal vapour ablation to reduce segmental volume in patients with severe emphysema: STEP-UP 12 month results. *Lancet Respir Med*. 2016;4(9):e44–e45.

32. Criner GJ, Delage A, Voelker K, et al. Improving lung function in severe heterogenous emphysema with the Spiration Valve System (EMPROVE). A multicenter, open-label randomized controlled clinical trial. *Am J Respir Crit Care Med*. 2019;200(11):1354–1362.

14

Multimodality Approach to Malignant Airway Obstruction

David E. Ost

INTRODUCTION

The goal of this chapter is to provide an effective, systematic, multimodality bronchoscopic approach to the problem of malignant airway obstruction that facilitates proper integration of all of the various technologies currently available. The approach outlined is multimodality and focuses on bronchoscopic interventions, but bronchoscopic interventions are just one component of the multidisciplinary care of the cancer patient, so we will also discuss how and when bronchoscopic interventions should be integrated with chemotherapy, radiation therapy, and surgery.

To do this we will first establish a clear classification system for the different types of malignant airway obstruction. Different types of malignant airway obstruction are best treated by different techniques. The focus is on the decision process of when to use a given technique and how to integrate multiple techniques into a unified approach. The details of how to do the actual techniques are provided in other chapters. We will then use this classification scheme to delineate the indications for therapeutic bronchoscopy for malignant airway obstruction, preprocedural management, intraprocedural management, and postprocedural management.

TYPES OF MALIGNANT CENTRAL AIRWAY OBSTRUCTION

Malignant central airway obstruction occurs frequently in patients with lung cancer and in patients with pulmonary metastases from other malignancies, including breast, colon, and renal cell cancer.[1] Central airway obstruction in this case refers to an obstruction in the trachea, mainstem bronchi, bronchus intermedius, or at the entrance of a lobar orifice. There are three main types of malignant airway obstruction: endobronchial, extrinsic compression, and a mixed pattern (Fig. 14.1). Endobronchial obstructing tumors are typically polypoid or fungating and are predominantly intraluminal with a relatively intact bronchial wall such that if the intraluminal component of the tumor is destroyed, the airway has sufficient structural integrity to remain open with a normal luminal diameter thereafter. Extrinsic compression by tumors can also lead to obstruction. In cases of extrinsic compression, the airway wall itself may be tumor free, but the mass effect of the tumor compresses the airway to such a degree that the airway is compromised. Of course, many lesions demonstrate a mixed pattern of disease, with some intraluminal tumor as well as some airway compression.

The type of intervention chosen depends on the type of malignant airway obstruction. Ablative techniques that destroy tissue are useful for malignant endobronchial obstruction. Ablative techniques include lasers, electrocautery, argon plasma coagulation (APC), photodynamic therapy, microdebriders, cryotherapy, and mechanical debridement. Stents are the primary modality for patients with malignant extrinsic compression leading to airway compromise. For patients with a mixed pattern of disease, multiple modalities are usually required. Typically the endobronchial component of the obstruction will first need to be ablated followed by stenting if required.

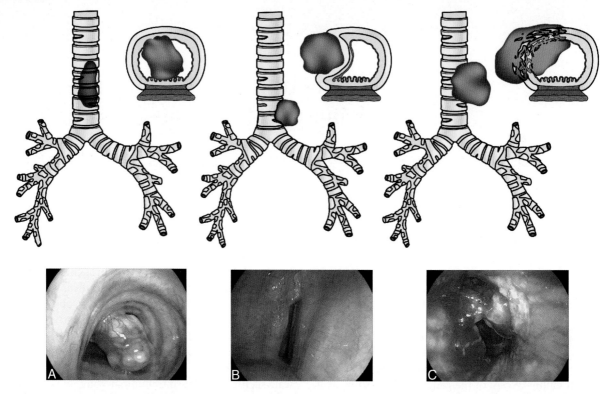

Fig. 14.1 Type of malignant central airway obstruction. (A) Endobronchial lesion, (B) extrinsic compression, (C) mixed disease. Each panel shows an overview of the airway as well as a cross-sectional view of the lesion as it would be seen at the time of bronchoscopy. Beneath the illustration is a prototypical example as seen during bronchoscopy. (A) Endobronchial obstruction—the tumor is located in the airway. If the tumor is removed, the airway walls have sufficient structural integrity that the airway will stay open. (B) Extrinsic obstruction—the tumor is located outside of the airway, but is pressing on the airway causing a stenosis. The airway wall is intact but not strong enough to stay open. Buttressing the wall with a stent will reestablish the airway lumen. You do not want to use an ablative tool (e.g., laser), since this will merely make a hole in the normal wall, making things worse. (C) Mixed pattern of endobronchial obstruction combined with extrinsic compression. First treat the endobronchial component with an ablative therapy, then, if necessary, stent.

INDICATIONS FOR BRONCHOSCOPY IN PATIENTS WITH MALIGNANT CENTRAL AIRWAY OBSTRUCTION

Indications for bronchoscopic intervention include relief of obstruction that is causing dyspnea, infection, or clinically significant bleeding. Although therapeutic bronchoscopy in this setting may indeed prolong life modestly for some patients (e.g., enable them to get off the ventilator), the majority of patients benefit from changes in quality of life rather than duration. When deciding whether to perform therapeutic bronchoscopy for malignant central airway obstruction it is important to consider:

- The probability of technical success, defined as the probability of being able to reestablish and maintain central airway patency at ≥50% of normal.
- How likely is it that the procedure, if technically successful, will also result in a clinically meaningful improvement in dyspnea and health-related quality of life (HRQOL)? A procedure that is technically successful (i.e., 100% reopening of a previously 70% obstructed left mainstem bronchus) may or may not result in a clinically significant improvement in dyspnea.
- The risk if the obstruction were to remain unrelieved versus the risks of the procedure. Both short-term and long-term risks need to be considered.

Technical Success

Clinically significant malignant central airway obstruction is typically defined as ≥50% obstruction of the cross-sectional area of the trachea, mainstem bronchi, bronchus intermedius, or a lobar orifice. Obstructions involving <50% of the cross-sectional area of the airways are less likely to cause symptoms and are likely to have little or no immediate physiologic impact. Bronchoscopic intervention is usually warranted for symptomatic lesions resulting in ≥50% obstruction, provided that there are patent airways with viable lung distal to the obstruction. If the airways distal to the obstruction are themselves occluded or the lung is nonviable, then relief of the central airway obstruction will not result in any meaningful improvement, so therapeutic bronchoscopy is not warranted. Of course, obstructing lesions can grow, so a 40% obstruction that is asymptomatic may progress to 80% obstruction with symptoms in the future. Therefore in select cases of asymptomatic central airway obstruction that are <50%, bronchoscopic intervention may be warranted if the probability of disease progression in the future is high.

Technical success of therapeutic bronchoscopy in this context is therefore defined anatomically. A technically successful bronchoscopy is one that relieves the targeted anatomic obstruction(s) such that central airway patency is >50% of normal upon completion of the procedure. It is a short-term outcome, since the airways may close back up in the future. Factors associated with a higher probability of technical success include endobronchial lesions (as opposed to extrinsic compression or mixed obstructions) and placement of airway stents. Factors associated with a lower probability of technical success include American Society of Anesthesia (ASA) score >3, renal failure, primary lung cancer (as opposed to other types of cancer), left mainstem disease, and tracheal-esophageal fistula.[2]

Impact on Dyspnea and HRQOL

It is important to remember that therapeutic bronchoscopy for malignant central airway obstruction is essentially a palliative intervention, since most patients have advanced disease that is incurable. So while relief of anatomic obstruction defines technical success, this is only a short-term tactical goal of bronchoscopic intervention. The true strategic goal is to decrease dyspnea, improve HRQOL, and improve quality-adjusted survival.[3] Not every patient with a technically successful procedure will have a meaningful improvement in dyspnea and quality-adjusted survival. Clinically significant improvement in dyspnea occurs in approximately 50% of patients undergoing therapeutic bronchoscopy, whereas clinically significant improvement in HRQOL occurs in 40%. Patients with more shortness of breath at baseline (as measured by the Borg score) are more likely to experience significant improvements in dyspnea and HRQOL.[2,3] Conversely, patients with lobar obstruction (as opposed to obstruction in the mainstem bronchi, bronchus intermedius, or trachea) are less likely to have a significant improvement in dyspnea or HRQOL. The magnitude of the improvement in HRQOL is also associated with higher ASA score and lower functional status. Thus patients at the highest risk for complications also often have the greatest potential for benefit.

Hazard of Delay in Therapeutic Bronchoscopy Versus Procedural Risks

In patients with obstruction <50% who are asymptomatic, options include observation versus proceeding with therapeutic bronchoscopy. The benefit of observation is that it avoids procedural risk, and if there are other treatment alternatives (e.g., radiation therapy or chemotherapy), it provides time for these treatments to take effect, and if the patient responds to those treatments and the airway obstruction improves, the risk of the procedure may ultimately be avoided altogether. The risk of observation is that the malignant airway obstruction will worsen, symptoms will develop, the procedural difficulty will increase, the risk of complications will increase, and the probability of technical success will go down. In essence, the hazard of delay in asymptomatic patients is that the window of opportunity when it is possible to intervene with a low-risk procedure will be missed.

Balancing the hazard of delay versus the risks of immediate intervention in these patients therefore requires a global and multidisciplinary perspective. In patients who are treatment naive with tumors that are likely to respond rapidly to treatment, it is often reasonable to proceed with chemotherapy and radiation first, provided that the patient is followed closely as an outpatient. There should be a low threshold to change strategy and intervene with therapeutic bronchoscopy if dyspnea develops or there is radiographic worsening. Conversely, in patients who are not treatment naive and are unlikely to have a rapid dramatic response to chemotherapy and radiation, early intervention is often the more prudent strategy, since it will minimize the aggregate risk of procedural complications and disease progression while maintaining HRQOL.

PREPROCEDURAL MANAGEMENT

The decisions to intervene and the preprocedural management of the patient, although discussed separately, really are performed simultaneously and in parallel. The decision to intervene and the preparation for the procedure are closely interlinked, and each process informs the other. Preprocedural management should take into account factors that impact technical success, as noted earlier. The goal is to optimize care and position everything to maximize the chances of technical success while mitigating risk as much as possible.

Imaging is fundamental to proper preparation. Imaging facilitates planning of the procedure and allows identification of the extent of disease. Obtaining old computed tomography (CT) images is a vital part of this process. A key determinant of both technical success and the impact of bronchoscopy on HRQOL is the extent of disease in the lung distal to the obstruction. If the distal lung is nonviable, then reopening the airway to that lung is not likely to have a meaningful impact on HRQOL. Often patients will present with significant atelectasis and collapse of either a lobe or an entire lung. The extent of disease in the lung distal to the obstruction may not be visible on CT imaging after this occurs, since it will be impossible to distinguish atelectasis from diseased lung. It will also not be visible bronchoscopically prior to intervention. However, old imaging can be very helpful in identifying how much viable lung remains distal to the obstruction. If recent prior CT scans demonstrate viable lung distal to the obstruction without significant disease, intervention is probably warranted. In addition, old scans may be able to show the origin of the obstruction (e.g., whether a polypoid lesion in the left mainstem bronchus grew out of the superior segment of the left lower lobe or from the left upper lobe), which will be useful information when resecting the lesion.

Patients should be optimized from a medical perspective, with special attention to cardiac risk factors and hemostasis considerations. Standard preoperative laboratories include prothrombin time (i.e., international normalized ratio [INR]), partial thromboplastin time (PTT), complete blood count (CBC), chemistries, and a type and screen. Anesthesia preoperative clearance is usually prudent, especially in difficult cases.

Careful preparation prior to the procedure is essential, and communication between the interventional pulmonologist and bronchoscopy technicians and nurses is vital. This should be done prior to the case so that all the necessary equipment is set up ahead of time and is within easy reach in case there is an emergency. Most cases of malignant airway obstruction should be approached with the rigid bronchoscope (with flexible bronchoscopy being done through the rigid as needed). Occasionally simpler cases (e.g., an endobronchial lesion that is only 10% obstructing a segment that requires APC for intermittent hemoptysis) may be performed with the flexible bronchoscope through an endotracheal tube. However, the ability to rapidly escalate the level of care when required is essential. In the event of an airway emergency, there may not be time to get and set up the necessary equipment. So even when doing "simple" cases with the flexible bronchoscope through an endotracheal tube, the rigid bronchoscope should be set up and ready to go within arm's reach. Careful communication with bronchoscopy technicians and nurses can facilitate this. All of the required equipment should be set up prior to the start of the procedure and tested as appropriate. At a minimum, this should typically include:

- Rigid bronchoscope and rigid bronchoscope equipment (e.g., suction, forceps)
- A large therapeutic bronchoscope and a smaller scope (for getting through narrow openings to visualize the airways distal to the lesion)
- Tools for rapid thermal ablation of endobronchial lesions (e.g., electrocautery probe, yttrium aluminum garnet [YAG] laser, yttrium aluminum perovskite [YAP] laser)
- Stents of appropriate sizes and fluoroscopy readily available if metal stents are planned
- Cryotherapy probe for removal of clots in case bleeding occurs
- Bronchial blocker readily available.

In addition, communication between the interventional pulmonology team and the anesthesia team is essential. General anesthesia is usually preferred. Although therapeutic bronchoscopy can be done using moderate sedation, it is associated with higher complication rates.[2,4] Prior to the procedure, there should be a review of the management plan for the patient with anesthesia and interventional pulmonology teams. This should include a clear airway plan (e.g., intubation with an endotracheal tube vs. laryngeal mask airway for airway inspection vs. intubation with the rigid broncho-scope from the beginning), the method of ventilation planned (e.g., jet ventilation via the rigid bronchoscope vs. volume cycled), the types of ablative techniques that are likely to be used (e.g., electrocautery probe vs. APC vs. laser), whether or not stenting is likely to be required, and contingency plans for difficult airways and emergencies.

INTRAPROCEDURAL MANAGEMENT

The initial portion of the procedure should in general follow the plan that was carefully developed and com-municated with the anesthesia and bronchoscopy teams as outlined earlier. Establishment of an airway will be achieved, usually with either the rigid bronchoscope or an endotracheal tube. Next the airway examina-tion should be completed, and the malignant airway obstruction should be evaluated and classified by the bronchoscopist as either being due to endobronchial disease, extrinsic compression, or a mixed pattern, as described earlier. After careful consideration of the full medical context (e.g., is the patient treatment naive or is this purely palliative), severity of dyspnea, probability

of technical success, and probability of having a mean-ingful improvement in HRQOL, the bronchoscopist will have to reach a final decision as to whether or not inter-vention is warranted.

Assuming that intervention is indeed warranted, intraprocedural decision-making and management will follow an iterative algorithm consisting of:
1. Assessment of obstruction type and severity
2. Application of an appropriate interventional modal-ity (e.g., electrocautery)
3. Analysis of response/success as the modality is applied
4. Determining whether ongoing intervention is still required
5. If intervention is still needed, return to step 1.

Assessment of obstruction type will drive interven-tion selection. For endobronchial lesions, ablative ther-apies will be the best option. Often a variety of different ablative therapies will be used in the same case, with the bronchoscopy team switching between modalities. For example, initial tumor ablation might begin with YAG laser therapy for a polypoid lesion obstructing the bronchus intermedius (Fig. 14.2). As the tumor is ablated, the bronchoscopist might switch to contact

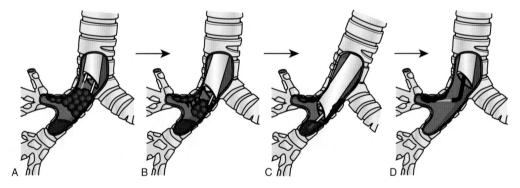

Fig. 14.2 Rigid bronchoscopy for treatment of endobronchial malignant central airway obstruction using multiple abla-tive techniques. (A) Rigid bronchoscope inserted, the lesion identified, and a laser is passed through the channel as well as a suction catheter. The laser is used to ablate the target, causing coagulation of the blood in the target. (B) After coagulating the tumor, mechanical debridement is done to remove coagulated tumor tissue. This can be done with suc-tion (as shown here) or with forceps or microdebriders or cryotherapy or coring out. (C) The process is iterative—after initial mechanical removal of tissue in panel (B), there is more tumor visible as well as secretions and blood. This por-tion of the tumor has not been adequately coagulated, since the initial laser in (A) could not penetrate far enough. So the blood is drained with suction (C) and then a decision is made on whether ablation is needed. (D) After removal of blood, additional ablation can be done. Often a different type of ablative modality is used. In this case, since the tumor is on the side at a difficult angle for the rigid scope, the flexible bronchoscope is passed through the rigid, and a flexible laser is passed through the bronchoscope working channel to coagulate the residual tumor. After coagulation of this tumor, it will be resected (panel B), excess blood and mucus will be removed (panel C), and the process starts again.

electrocautery with the rigid electrocautery suction probe for particularly difficult-to-reach areas in order to achieve tumor ablation and in order to suction blood that might be oozing from the tumor. The rigid electrocautery suction probe offers the benefit of both suctioning out blood while simultaneously coagulating the tumor. The bronchoscopist might then proceed with mechanical debridement until the cauterized tissue was removed. At that point additional oozing of blood might indicate the need for additional hemostasis (since the coagulated tumor has been removed, revealing untreated tumor below it) and another cycle of ablation might begin, this time starting with the electrocautery suction probe. Eventually, with good control of hemostasis and good coagulation and debridement, the distal side of the obstruction might be visible enough that mechanical coring out could be done with the rigid

scope, reestablishing a secure patent airway (Fig. 14.3). Note the iterative pattern: hemostasis and coagulation with an ablation tool followed by mechanical resection, reassessment, and repeat as needed. It is critical to achieve good coagulation with an ablation device prior to mechanical resection in order to avoid bleeding complications.

For purely extrinsic disease, stenting will be the best option. The choice of stent depends on the location of the obstruction, the anatomy, the clinical context, and consideration of long-term risks. Silicone stents currently are the only Y-shaped stent available in the United States. So for patients with extrinsic compression involving the main carina, a Y-shaped silicone stent will often be required. For mainstem obstructions or obstruction of the bronchus intermedius, either silicone or metal stents will be feasible.

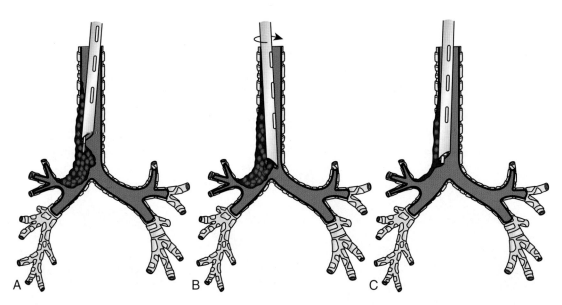

Fig. 14.3 The ablation-resection cycle with coring out to achieve mechanical resection. The key for successful coring out of a lesion is to (A) first achieve good hemostasis through coagulation. In this image laser bronchoscopy is used for coagulation, but other rapid ablative modalities could be used. Before deciding on coring out, it is important to be able to "see the other side" where you will want to get to. In this case the other side is the distal trachea. (B) After good coagulation of the tumor is achieved, the rigid scope is advanced using a rotating motion to "core out" the coagulated tumor. Not all the tumor has to be removed, but enough of the tumor has to be removed so that the rigid scope can be passed to the "other side." The rigid scope does not have to get into the right lower lobe in this example, but it does need to be able to reach into the distal trachea past the first portion of the tumor. Once the tissue has been cored out, *do not remove the rigid scope immediately.* (C) Instead the barrel of the rigid scope is left in position to tamponade the tumor base, which will ooze blood. Suction and tamponade along with the prior coagulation performed in step A will achieve hemostasis. Once hemostasis is good, the rigid scope is repositioned, the obstruction is reassessed, and a new cycle begins.

Self-expandable metal stents offer the benefit of being more conformable to tortuous airways and can be passed through narrow stenotic airways, since they are deployed using guidewires with catheter-based systems using the Seldinger technique and have a low profile (Fig. 14.4). Silicone stents in contrast must be deployed through the rigid scope, and they typically have a fairly large profile (i.e., they cannot easily be pushed through a tight stenosis). So for many tight stenotic lesions caused by malignant extrinsic compression in the mainstem bronchi and bronchus intermedius, expandable metal

stents may be easier to place. In general, for malignant airway obstruction being treated with expandable metal stents, covered stents (as opposed to uncovered) should be used, since tumors can quickly grow through uncovered stents.

When selecting stents it is also useful to consider long-term complication rates. When the obstruction is at the carina, Y-shaped silicone stents are often required. The benefit of silicone Y-stents in terms of long-term complications is that they do not usually migrate. However, they are more apt to develop granulation

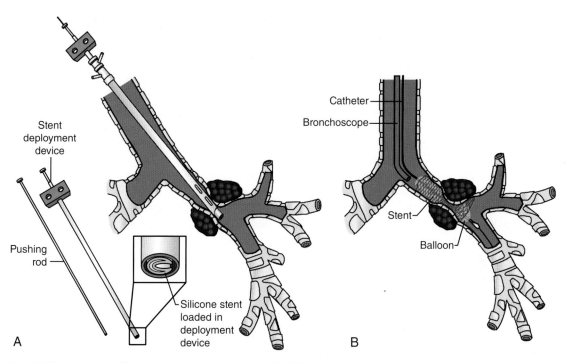

Fig. 14.4 Differences in silicone versus metal stents. (A) Silicone stent through rigid scope, (B) expandable metal stent. (A) Silicone stents are high profile—they require a relatively open lumen for deployment since they are pushed out through the rigid bronchoscope using a rigid stent deployment system that has a large diameter. Once the rigid bronchoscope is within the stenosis, the stent deployment system is passed through the rigid scope. The stent deployment system is essentially a hollow metal tube with a stent inside the tube. A pushing rod is used to push the silicone stent into the airway. Note that the rigid bronchoscope must be able to pass into the stenotic area in order for the stent to be deployed. If the stenosis is too tight, such that the rigid bronchoscope cannot pass through it, the high-profile silicone stent deployment system will also not be able to pass the stenosis and the stent will deploy proximal to (above) the stenosis rather than opening the stenosis. (B) Expandable metal stents have a low profile. They are typically deployed using a Seldinger technique. A guidewire is passed through the stenosis. The stent is on a flexible catheter that passes over the guidewire. The proximal end of the stent is positioned just above the stenosis and the distal end is just past the stenosis. Note the catheter diameter is very small—it can be passed through a very tight stenosis. When the stent is deployed, it opens up in a radial fashion along its entire length, pushing the airway outward from the center. Because it is low profile and it opens radially outward, metal stents are more practical for tight stenosis.

tissue and develop mucus plugging.[5,6] When stenting the mainstem bronchi or bronchus intermedius, stents with a simple tube shape will be used so both silicone and metal stents can be used. Silicone tube stents are more likely to migrate than metal stents and are also more likely to plug with mucus.[5,6] Importantly all stents increase the risk of subsequent respiratory infections,[6,7] and such respiratory infections are associated with significant morbidity and mortality.

For mixed lesions, it is usually best to begin with ablative interventions, and once the endobronchial component is treated the airway should be reassessed. If there is persistent significant extrinsic compression with residual narrowing of the airway to >50% even after elimination of the endobronchial component, stenting should be considered. The benefits of stenting in such cases must be weighed against the long-term risks of mucus plugging, granulation tissue, migration, and infection. If the patient is treatment naive and there is a good chance of the tumor responding to treatment, then it is often better to hold off on stenting if the patient has sufficient respiratory function.[8] Conversely, if the patient has limited pulmonary reserve and/or is unlikely to respond to chemotherapy/radiation, then it may be worth stenting in cases with residual persistent extrinsic compression.

Throughout the procedure the bronchoscopist is continuously reassessing the obstruction in order to select the appropriate tool as well as to decide when to stop. One of the key decisions intraoperatively is when to quit. This requires an assessment of the magnitude of the possible benefits to be gained by additional interventions as compared to the marginal risk of complications if the procedure is continued. This is why having a deep understanding of the indications for the procedure and the predictors of success is so vital. How much marginal benefit, in terms of dyspnea and HRQOL, is likely to be obtained by continuing the procedure, is a question that must be asked repeatedly throughout the procedure. Early in a procedure the risks of ablation are relatively low—the lesion is typically big, anatomic landmarks are clear, and risks are low. But as the procedure goes on, especially if the tumor is more extensive than anticipated, it may be that the risks of continuing the procedure increase, such that they outweigh the benefits. This is especially true if the lung distal to the obstruction is found to have tumor involvement. In such cases stopping the procedure and limiting the

risk of complications is often the best option. Similarly, once the airway is open to >50%, it may be reasonable in some circumstances to stop once a moderate degree of success has been achieved, rather than continuing on since the magnitude of the functional benefit of further reopening of the airway may be modest relative to the marginal risk incurred. The key concept here is that risk-benefit assessment should be done continuously throughout the procedure in an iterative pattern, since the probability of complications and the probability of accruing additional benefit from further interventions will change during the course of the procedure.

POSTPROCEDURAL MANAGEMENT

For patients with stents, the main long-term risks are mucus plugging, stent migration, infection, fracture, and granulation tissue. Twice-daily nebulized albuterol and hypertonic saline should be used to mitigate the risk of mucus plugging. Patients should be instructed to seek prompt medical attention for any evidence of respiratory infection, such as worsening cough with purulent sputum or increasing shortness of breath or fevers.

Malignant lesions will frequently recur, requiring repeat intervention. Careful follow-up with the interventional pulmonology team is therefore warranted. Follow-up should include a routine clinic visit, typically 2–4 weeks after the initial intervention. CT imaging of the chest at 1 month postprocedure is also warranted to evaluate for evidence of recurrence. Routine bronchoscopy in all patients is not warranted. Instead use of bronchoscopy for follow-up evaluation should be based on symptoms, clinical findings, and CT imaging. While routine bronchoscopy is not warranted, physicians should have a low threshold to perform a follow-up bronchoscopy if there is any worsening of dyspnea, cough, postobstructive pneumonia, or evidence of recurrence on CT.

REFERENCES

1. Ernst A, Simoff M, Ost D, Goldman Y, Herth FJF. Prospective risk-adjusted morbidity and mortality outcome analysis after therapeutic bronchoscopic procedures: results of a multi-institutional outcomes database. *Chest.* 2008;134(3):514–519.
2. Ost DE, Ernst A, Grosu HB, et al. Therapeutic bronchoscopy for malignant central airway obstruction: success

rates and impact on dyspnea and quality of life. *Chest.* 2015;147(5):1282–1298.

3. Ong P, Grosu HB, Debiane L, et al. Long-term quality-adjusted survival following therapeutic bronchoscopy for malignant central airway obstruction. *Thorax.* 2019;74(2):141–156.

4. Ost DE, Ernst A, Grosu HB, et al. Complications following therapeutic bronchoscopy for malignant central airway obstruction: results of the AQuIRE registry. *Chest.* 2015;148(2):450–471.

5. Ost DE, Shah AM, Lei X, et al. Respiratory infections increase the risk of granulation tissue formation following airway stenting in patients with malignant airway obstruction. *Chest.* 2012;141(6):1473–1481.

6. Grosu HB, Eapen GA, Morice RC, et al. Stents are associated with increased risk of respiratory infections in patients undergoing airway interventions for malignant airways disease. *Chest.* 2013;144(2):441–449.

7. Agrafiotis M, Siempos II, Falagas ME. Infections related to airway stenting: a systematic review. *Respiration.* 2009;78(1):69–74.

8. Dutau H, Di Palma F, Thibout Y, et al. Impact of silicone stent placement in symptomatic airway obstruction due to non-small cell lung cancer - a French multicenter randomized controlled study: the SPOC trial. *Respiration.* 2020;99(4):344–352.

15

Multimodality Approach to Benign Central Airway Obstruction

George Z. Cheng and Momen M. Wahidi

INTRODUCTION

Central airway obstruction (CAO) is the narrowing of central airways (trachea, mainstem bronchi, and bronchus intermedius) due to benign and malignant diseases. In this chapter we focus on CAO due to benign diseases; it is important to note that "benign" here refers to the cause of the CAO (not caused by malignancy), but the consequences of benign CAO can be devastating and not benign in nature. The etiology of benign causes of CAO can be grouped into several large categories: mechanical/iatrogenic, inflammatory, infectious, dynamic, and idiopathic.[1] The management of benign CAO depends on the etiology, type of lesion, and patient's characteristics.

CLASSIFICATION SYSTEMS

Benign CAO can be classified into simple and complex. Simple CAO lesions are less than 1 cm in length, shaped like a web, and have no associated malacia or damage to cartilaginous tissue. Complex CAO lesions are longer than 1 cm, can involve the cartilage, and have more complex shapes like hourglass or irregular thickening.

ETIOLOGY OF BENIGN CENTRAL AIRWAY OBSTRUCTION

Lung Transplant

Airway complication rates after lung transplantation range from 2% to 33%. Complication rate is related to surgical technique, donor ventilation time, donor bronchus length, donor-recipient height mismatch, and prolonged periods of ischemia. Airway complications from transplantation include bronchial infection, necrosis, anastomotic dehiscence, fistula formation, granulation tissue, malacia, stenosis, or complete obstruction of the airway (vanishing airway). The location of the lesion can be at the anastomotic site or distal to it.[2]

PITS/PTTS

Postintubation/posttracheostomy tracheal stenosis (PITS/PTTS) are manifestations of mechanical injury to central airway. PITS usually develops due to prolonged intubation (>7 days) with an overinflated cuff (pressure >20 cm H_2O). PTTS occurs due to cartilage damage during initial tracheostomy, infection, bleeding, or an overinflated cuff.[3]

Chemical Injury

Chemical injury to the airway can result from a variety of caustic gases (hydrochloric acid, ammonia, aldehydes), thermal injury from fire exposure in poorly ventilated areas, and pill aspiration (such as iron, potassium chloride, metformin).[4] These injuries result in tracheobronchitis and extensive airway mucosal sloughing that ultimately leads to granulation, stricture, and stenosis.

Systemic/Inflammatory Disease
Cartilaginous Processes

Relapsing polychondritis (RP) is an immune-mediated disease that targets cartilage (collagen type II, IX, XI) in the eyes, ears, nose, joints, and large airways. Both malacia and stenosis can occur. RP spares the posterior tracheal membrane because it has no cartilage. The resulting tracheobronchomalacia/excessive dynamic airway collapse can be focal or diffused.[5]

Tracheobronchopathia osteochondroplastica (TO) presents as calcified nodules due to accumulation of calcium phosphate in the airway cartilage. These lesions are characteristically located on the cartilages only. They are mainly asymptomatic and found incidentally but can be extensive in some patients and can lead to symptomatic airway stenosis.[6]

Granulomatous Processes

Granulomatosis with polyangiitis (GPA) is an antineutrophil cytoplasmic antibody (ANCA)-associated necrotizing granulomatous vasculitis that can lead to airway inflammation and stenosis. The airway involvement is usually more resistant to systemic treatment.[7]

Sarcoidosis is a systemic nonnecrotizing granulomatous disorder that almost always involves the pulmonary system, including the airways. Stenosis can occur due to unchecked inflammation. Enlarged lymph nodes may cause extrinsic compression and airway stenosis.[8]

Inflammatory bowel disease (ulcerative colitis and Crohn's disease) can lead to a necrotizing granulomatous infiltrative process in the airways that may result in inflammation and stenosis.[9]

Infiltrative Process

Amyloidosis results from extracellular amyloid fibril deposition that is usually due to a beta-pleated sheet conformation of proteins. Light chain amyloidosis is due to plasma cell dyscrasia. Amyloid A amyloidosis is due to chronic inflammation with excess amyloid A deposition. Airway involvement is notable for infiltration and stenosis.[10]

Infections

Recurrent respiratory papillomatosis (RRP), due to human papillomavirus (HPV) type 6 and 11 (with potential to transform to squamous cell cancer), presents as papilloma that can affect the entire upper and lower airways; the characteristic appearance is a "bunch of grapes."[11]

Tuberculosis (TB) can cause endobronchial infection that can appear in various forms bronchoscopically, including edematous-hyperemic, fibrostenotic, tumorous, granular, or ulcerative form. Endobronchial TB usually involves lobar airways and airways >2 cm in length. These airway lesions can be highly contagious, and bronchoscopy should be done with strict respiratory precautions when TB is suspected.[12]

Fungal infections (*Aspergillus*, *Fusarium*, mucormycosis, and *Cryptococcus*) can also present as airway stenosis. The presentation of fungal infection–related airway stenosis is extremely variable, and so care and caution should be noted when evaluating CAO to ensure ruling out concurrent fungal infection.[13]

Idiopathic

After exclusion of all other causes, the diagnosis may be idiopathic subglottic stenosis—a disease that usually affects middle-aged women who also suffer from gastroesophageal reflux disease. Idiopathic CAO usually involves short segments of the subglottic area and can be recurrent over many years.[1]

CLINICAL PRESENTATION

Patient presentation is dependent on etiology and severity of CAO. Commonly, patients will report dyspnea on exertion that can progress to shortness of breath at rest, wheezing, or stridor. Patients may also develop chronic cough or recurrent respiratory infections due to inability to clear secretions at the site of CAO. The degree of dyspnea typically correlates with the diameter of the affected airway, with dyspnea on exertion appearing when central airway luminal size is less than 25% to 50% of normal, with stridor occurring at a lumen less than 5 mm in diameter.[1]

DIAGNOSTIC TESTS

Pulmonary Function Tests With Flow-Volume Loops

Flow-volume loops can help differentiate CAO into three functional groups (fixed, variable extrathoracic, and variable intrathoracic) and may help with characterizing the CAO diagnosis. These are illustrated in Fig. 15.1.

Imaging

Computed tomography (CT) of the chest is a critical component to both diagnosis and treatment planning for benign CAO. High-resolution CT (0.6–1-mm slices with overlap) allows for accurate evaluation of the length and extent of the stenosis, assessment of the extraluminal component, and determination of distal airway patency. High-resolution CT also enables custom/

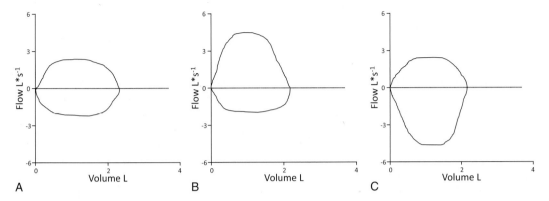

Fig. 15.1 Flow-volume curves in (A) fixed upper airway obstruction, (B) variable extrathoracic obstruction, and (C) variable intrathoracic obstruction. (Modified from West, John B., West's respiratory physiology: the essentials, Philadelphia, Wolters Kluwer, 2015.)

personalized stent design in appropriate situations.[14] If dynamic airway pathology is suspected, then CT images in both the inspiratory and expiratory phases should be performed.[15]

Bronchoscopy Evaluation

Bronchoscopic evaluation of CAO should be done with the goal being to fully characterize the lesion (visual evaluation and measurement) and determine if there is a reversible component such as infection (via washing, needle/brush/forceps biopsy).

A stand-alone diagnostic flexible bronchoscopy can be the first step, but it is discouraged if the airway stenosis is severe; if the lesion is severe, a simple diagnostic bronchoscopy can turn into an airway emergency, so the ability to escalate the level of care if required, even if doing a "simple" diagnostic bronchoscopy, is important. Often it is better for the interventional pulmonologist to perform one bronchoscopic evaluation that is both diagnostic and possibly therapeutic, starting with a flexible bronchoscope but with the rigid bronchoscope standing by, so that if warranted the procedure can be switched from diagnostic to therapeutic intervention as warranted.[16]

BENIGN CENTRAL AIRWAY OBSTRUCTION MANAGEMENT

Successful benign CAO management rests on three fundamental principles. First, a multidisciplinary approach to the disease is essential to ensure all treatment modalities are considered. Thoracic surgery, otolaryngology, and interventional pulmonology should all be involved. Second, systemic treatment of the underlying disease is often more effective than local bronchoscopic treatment alone, so an integrated therapeutic approach is often warranted. Finally, in patients with minimal to no symptoms, it is often best to resort to a watchful waiting approach as interventions may make the lesion worse by precipitating additional inflammation and trauma.

BRONCHOSCOPIC TREATMENTS

Mechanical Dilation

Dilation of the airway stricture can be accomplished using a balloon or rigid bronchoscope. Various types of balloons are available for dilation in the airway. The key is to use a balloon of the appropriate diameter and length. The diameter of the balloon is selected based on the airway size proximal to the stenotic segment as measured on CT scan. The length of the balloon is typically at least 0.5 cm longer than that of the stenotic segment, thus flanking the stenosis. Time of inflation is usually 30 s to 120 s. Repeated dilation and longer duration of dilation are suggested if the patient is able to tolerate the longer inflation times. Caution should be exercised in benign airway disease, as some airways can be very inflamed and fragile, and overdilation can result in rupture across a large area. It is usually prudent to start dilating with smaller balloons and then progressively increase balloon diameters during subsequent dilations as the airways permit, making sure to reassess tissue effects after each dilation. Never inflate the balloon against significant pressure that can be felt by the assistant inflating the balloon and communicated to the operator.[17]

Of note, a rigid bronchoscope can be used as a dilation tool. In order to circumvent the need for repeated intubation of the patient, the operator can use a larger rigid tracheoscope to intubate the patient, then remove the universal head from the scope and insert smaller but longer rigid ventilating scopes through the tracheoscope. Smaller rigid ventilating scopes are used to dilate the stricture initially. Subsequently, progressively larger rigid ventilating bronchoscopes are passed through the rigid tracheoscope and across the stenotic segment. This telescope technique allows for ventilation and sequential dilation without the need for repeated intubation through the vocal cords.[18]

Electrocautery

Radial cuts at 4, 8, and 12 o'clock location using an electrocautery knife or lasers (neodymium-doped yttrium aluminum garnet [Nd:YAG], potassium titanyl phosphate [KTP], carbon dioxide [CO_2]) can be performed prior to balloon dilation for tight, circumferential strictures. These cuts allow for more effective dilation (Fig. 15.2)[19] of simple weblike strictures.

Cryospray

Cryospray ablation (cryotherapy, liquid nitrogen–based) is a noncontact method that uses supercooling to cause cryonecrosis at the treatment site. This approach allows for both immediate softening of the scar tissue that allows for improved balloon dilation and also preserves extracellular matrix in tissues to form a scaffold for subsequent healing with minimal fibrotic response. However, care must be taken to ensure there is effective gas egress. The liquid nitrogen is released under conditions for rapid expansion (1 mL of liquid nitrogen expands to occupy 700 mL of volume in the form of nitrogen gas). The rapid increase in volume can result in barotrauma and potentially fatal pneumothorax and pneumomediastinum as well as air embolism if there is no effective gas egress/evacuation. Effective gas egress can be achieved by using a rigid scope with an open system, an endotracheal tube (ETT) with a deflated cuff, and by avoiding spray near severely obstructed lesions.[20]

Mitomycin C

As an antineoplastic agent, mitomycin C inhibits fibroblast proliferation. Mitomycin C has been used topically (0.4 mg/mL in 5 mL for total of 2 mg) to treat stenotic segments applied with a cotton pledget. It can also be

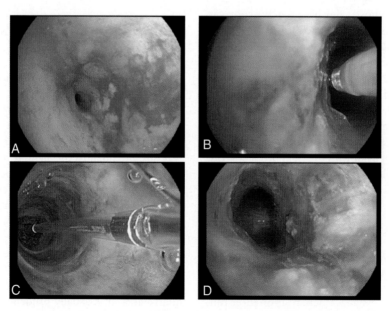

Fig. 15.2 Left main stem stenosis in a patient with granulomatosis with polyangiitis (A). After failure to respond to initial balloon dilation, radial cuts were performed (B), followed by successful balloon dilation (C, D).

given as a local injection in the airways with a transbronchial needle aspiration (TBNA) needle.[21]

Steroids

Steroids are thought to suppress inflammation in the posttraumatic, proliferative phase of inflammation and may prevent progression to the fibrotic stage. However, there is no consensus on the timing, dosage, and route of administration, and efficacy remains largely unproven for many diseases. Usually, 80 mg of Depo-Medrol is mixed with 6 mL of normal saline and injected into the stenotic segment using a TBNA needle. Injections are usually given at multiple sites in the stenotic areas.[22]

Stent

Airway stents (silicone, hybrid, or covered self-expanding metallic) can be used in the treatment of benign CAO. Uncovered self-expanding metallic stents should not be used for benign CAO, as they quickly become embedded in the airway epithelium, resulting in significant difficulty when removing the stent. Airway stents

in benign airways are typically left in place for short periods of time (3–12 months) while systemic treatments are administered or surgical options are contemplated. In rare occasions, airway stents can be the only options for some difficult lesions and can be left for years. In these situations, surveillance bronchoscopies are required every 6–12 months and stent replacement may be required (Fig. 15.3).[23]

Surgery

It is important to discuss benign CAO in a multidisciplinary conference. In the appropriate patients, surgery can be a definitive treatment option. Bronchoscopic treatment for benign CAO can lengthen the stenotic lesion if there are complications, thus risking converting a surgical lesion to a nonsurgical one. Bronchoscopic treatment should be considered as a bridge treatment or used in patients with no surgical options. Always consult with your surgery team and document your multidisciplinary treatment decision in patients with benign CAO.[23]

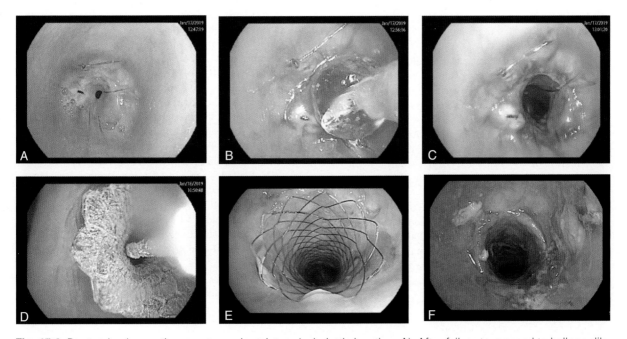

Fig. 15.3 Posttracheal resection anastomosis stricture (subglottic location, A). After failure to respond to balloon dilation (B, C), a Bonastent was placed at the subglottic location (D). Follow up bronchoscopy after 1 month showed good response (E). Stent was removed at 9 months with resolution of stenosis (F).

SUMMARY

In summary, benign central airways obstruction can result in significant morbidity; if left untreated, it can lead to increased mortality. There is a wide range of disease entities that lead to benign CAO, and treatments should be tailored in a multidisciplinary fashion to address each disease entity. Therapeutic bronchoscopy is one component of this multidisciplinary approach, but it is important to treat the underlying disease.

REFERENCES

1. Ernst A, Feller-Kopman D, Becker HD, Mehta AC. Central airway obstruction. *Am J Respir Crit Care Med.* 2004;169(12):1278–1297.
2. Machuzak M, Santacruz JF, Gildea T, Murthy SC. Airway complications after lung transplantation. *Thorac Surg Clin.* 2015;25(1):55–75.
3. Shin B, Kim K, Jeong BH, et al. Clinical significance of differentiating post-intubation and post-tracheostomy tracheal stenosis. *Respirology.* 2017;22(3):513–520.
4. Küpeli E, Khemasuwan D, Lee P, Mehta AC. "Pills" and the air passages. *Chest.* 2013;144(2):651–660.
5. Ernst A, Rafeq S, Boiselle P, et al. Relapsing polychondritis and airway involvement. *Chest.* 2009;135(4):1024–1030.
6. Ulasli SS, Kupeli E. Tracheobronchopathia osteochondroplastica: a review of the literature. *Clin Respir J.* 2015;9(4):386–391.
7. Martinez Del Pero M, Jayne D, Chaudhry A, Sivasothy P, Jani P. Long-term outcome of airway stenosis in granulomatosis with polyangiitis (Wegener granulomatosis): an observational study. *JAMA Otolaryngol Head Neck Surg.* 2014;140(11):1038–1044.
8. Polychronopoulos VS, Prakash UBS. Airway involvement in sarcoidosis. *Chest.* 2009;136(5):1371–1380.
9. Camus P, Piard F, Ashcroft T, Gal AA, Colby TV. The lung in inflammatory bowel disease. *Med (Baltim).* 1993;72(3):151–183.
10. O'Regan A, Fenlon HM, Beamis Jr JF, Steele MP, Skinner M, Berk JL. Tracheobronchial amyloidosis. *Boston Univ experience 1984 1999 Med (Baltim).* 2000;79(2):69–79.
11. Fortes HR, von Ranke FM, Escuissato DL, et al. Recurrent respiratory papillomatosis: a state-of-the-art review. *Respir Med.* 2017;126:116–121.

12. Chung HS, Lee JH. Bronchoscopic assessment of the evolution of endobronchial tuberculosis. *Chest.* 2000;117(2):385–392.
13. Marchioni A, Casalini E, Andreani A, et al. Incidence, etiology, and clinicopathologic features of endobronchial benign lesions: a 10-year consecutive retrospective study. *J Bronchol Interv Pulmonol.* 2018;25(2):118–124.
14. Cheng GZ, San Jose Estepar R, Folch E, Onieva J, Gangadharan S, Majid A. Three-dimensional printing and 3D slicer: powerful tools in understanding and treating structural lung disease. *Chest.* 2016;149(5):1136–1142.
15. Ferretti GR, Jankowski A, Perrin MA, et al. Multidetector CT evaluation in patients suspected of tracheobronchomalacia: comparison of end-expiratory with dynamic expiratory volumetric acquisitions. *Eur J Radiol.* 2008;68(2):340–346.
16. Mahmood K, Wahidi MM, Thomas S, et al. Therapeutic bronchoscopy improves spirometry, quality of life, and survival in central airway obstruction. *Respiration.* 2015;89(5):404–413.
17. Carlin BW, Harrell 2nd JH, Moser KM. The treatment of endobronchial stenosis using balloon catheter dilatation. *Chest.* 1988;93(6):1148–1151.
18. Ernst A, Herth FJF. *Principles and practice of interventional pulmonology.* New York: Springer; 2013. xiv, 757.
19. Wahidi MM, Herth FJF, Chen A, Cheng G, Yarmus L. State of the art: interventional pulmonology. *Chest.* 2020;157(3):724–736.
20. Bhora FY, Ayub A, Forleiter CM, et al. Treatment of benign tracheal stenosis using endoluminal spray cryotherapy. *JAMA Otolaryngol Head Neck Surg.* 2016;142(11):1082–1087.
21. Madan K, Agarwal R, Aggarwal AN, Gupta D. Utility of rigid bronchoscopic dilatation and mitomycin C application in the management of postintubation tracheal stenosis: case series and systematic review of literature. *J Bronchol Interv Pulmonol.* 2012;19(4):304–310.
22. Bertelsen C, Shoffel-Havakuk H, O'Dell K, Johns 3rd MM, Reder LS. Serial in-office intralesional steroid injections in airway stenosis. *JAMA Otolaryngol Head Neck Surg.* 2018;144(3):203–210.
23. Oberg CL, Holden VK, Channick CL. Benign central airway obstruction. *Semin Respir Crit Care Med.* 2018;39(6):731–746.

Pleural Disease

16

Chest Tubes and Indwelling Pleural Catheters

Kevin Ross Davidson and Samira Shojaee

CHEST TUBES

Definition

Tube thoracostomy has been described since antiquity, with the earliest accounts of using a tube for drainage of empyema from the pleural cavity from Hippocrates.[1] Original chest tubes were implemented from fashioned reeds or metal tubes. Modern chest tubes are typically latex-free silicone or polyvinyl chloride (PVC) tubes ranging from size 6 to 40 French (Fr), with multiple proximal fenestrations to improve drainage (see Fig. 16.1). Multiple differing sizes and shapes such as right-angle or pigtail tubes are available. Additionally, several different insertion methods have been described, including a surgical cut-down approach, trocar insertion, and a percutaneous method. The purpose of all of these tubes is to evacuate air, pleural fluid, blood, or pus from the pleural space to allow apposition of the visceral and parietal pleura and enable normal respiratory mechanics. These tubes also afford the ability to instill fibrinolytics, agents for pleurodesis, antibiotics, or other medications into the pleural space as well.

History

Since the age of Hippocrates, ongoing controversy existed on whether thoracic injuries should be managed in an open or closed method. The first flexible chest tube with use of a water seal was described to treat empyema in 1873 by Playfair.[2] Subsequently, major conflicts and war propelled rapid advancement of surgical techniques to manage blast and penetrating chest injuries. World War I coincided with the influenza epidemic of 1918 leading to the Empyema Commission and increasing recognition of the importance of timely drainage of empyema.[3] At the time, open thoracic drainage with rib resection was associated with high mortality.[4] In the 1920s, closed pleural drainage gained recognition, and by the outbreak of World War II chest tubes were left in place after thoracotomy. Even after World War II, serial thoracentesis was still common as the primary management for hemothoraces. It was not until the Vietnam war when closed pleural drainage gained traction as the primary means to evacuate the pleural space in traumatic injuries such as hemothorax and pneumothorax.[5] Advances in medical and surgical techniques discovered on the battlefield were adopted to hospitals and civilian life and applied in routine clinical practice.

Anatomy and Physiology

With tidal respiration, the diaphragm and external intercostal muscles contract decreasing intrathoracic pressure within the thorax. Intrapleural pressure is typically -5 cm H_2O at functional residual capacity, slightly subatmospheric due to the recoil of the chest wall and lung elasticity.[6] With tidal respiration, the intrapleural pressure drops to about -8 cm H_2O as intrathoracic volume increases. These oscillations in pressure are responsible for restful tidal respiration. A defect within the lung or chest wall can cause loss of pressure and inadequate ventilation. Accumulation of fluid or air within the pleural space can compress lung parenchyma and impair respiratory mechanics.[6]

Chest tubes connected to a closed drainage system allow for continuous drainage without influx of air into the chest. Several closed thoracic drainage systems including smaller portable models are available, which follow the same general principles. Most drainage systems utilize a three-chamber closed system

165

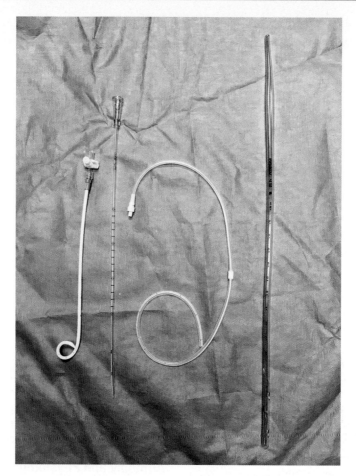

Fig. 16.1 Array of chest tube sizes and indwelling pleural catheter. From left to right: 14 Fr pigtail, 14 Fr chest tube, 15.5 Fr indwelling pleural catheter, 28 Fr chest tube.

(see Fig. 16.2). The first collection chamber closest to the patient is a reservoir where pleural fluid collects and can be measured. The second water-seal chamber is connected in-line and functions as a one-way valve. Air escapes out of the first collecting reservoir beyond the water seal but cannot return to the chest. Escaping air that travels through the water seal can be seen as bubbles. The third suction chamber allows regulated negative pressure to be applied, typically −20 cm H_2O but ranging up to −40 cm H_2O. If no suction is applied, then the system is said to be on water seal. Because the second chamber functions as a one-way valve, the maximum pressure in the pleural space cannot exceed the height of the column of water in the water-seal chamber, typically 2 cm.

Intermittent or continuous air leaks can be identified by the presence of air bubbles within the water-seal chamber. Note that in some older systems, the third suction control chamber that regulates the amount of negative pressure had water in it, which, when connected to wall suction, would bubble. This is not to be mistaken for the water-seal chamber, which is different. It is air bubbles coming through the water-seal chamber that indicates whether an air leak is present. Air leaks can be caused by leaks at any point in the drainage system, whether they are due to true lung disease or to loose connections, dislodgement of the chest tube, or equipment malfunction.

Air leaks caused by incomplete or loose connections between the chest tube and the closed drainage

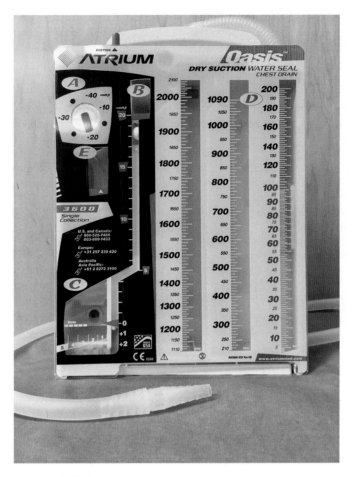

Fig. 16.2 Closed thoracic drainage system.

system or a tube that has migrated out of the chest and is entraining ambient air will generally cause continuous air leaks in the water-seal chamber if the system is on suction. If the system is not on suction (i.e., it is on water seal), such leaks may not be apparent. When a patient is on water seal, tidal variations in pleural pressure can be observed by movement of pleural fluid within the tubing if the system is closed and working properly. Lack of "tidaling" while on water seal without visible bubbles can indicate either an occluded chest tube or evacuation of all pleural fluid such that the lung has expanded completely to cover all fenestrations. Air leaks due to lung disease (such as bronchopleural fistulas) may be intermittent and flow rates may vary both over time and with phases of the respiratory cycle.

Cerfolio devised a classification system to grade the degree of air leaks (see Box 16.1). Newer collection systems incorporate digital monitoring that can detect and quantify air leaks more precisely in addition to monitoring fluid output. The magnitude of the airflow through an air leak predicts time to air leak closure, with higher flow rates being associated with longer time until closure. Continuous monitoring, by informing physicians about flow rates, indirectly informs them about the probability of air leak closure, and may facilitate better management decisions and lead to earlier chest tube removal, which in turn may decrease hospital length of stay.[8,9] For pneumothorax or prolonged air leak not accompanied by blood or pleural effusion, a rubber one-way Heimlich valve can also be considered as a less cumbersome alternative to water seal.[10]

BOX 16.1   Cerfolio Classification of Air Leaks[7]

- Grade 1, FE. Air leak present during forced exhalation or coughing only
- Grade 2, E. Air leak present during expiratory phase
- Grade 3, I. Air leak present during inspiratory phase
- Grade 4, C. Continuous air leak during both inspiration and exhalation

Chest tube insertion can be a life-saving procedure with several established indications (see Box 16.2). In these circumstances, the risk and complications are low, although serious injury and death may occur from accidental complications during placement (see Box 16.3). No absolute contraindications exist for this possibly life-saving procedure, although relative contraindications include prior pleurodesis, large pulmonary blebs, severe coagulopathy, or severe thrombocytopenia.

BOX 16.2   Indications for Chest Tube Insertion

- Empyema
- Hemothorax
- Penetrating chest trauma
- Pleurodesis via chest tube (talc slurry)
- Pneumothorax
- Postoperative in cardiothoracic surgery
- Symptomatic or complicated parapneumonic effusions

BOX 16.3   Complications of Chest Tube Insertion

- Fistula formation
- Hemorrhage
- Infection
- Lung laceration and intraparenchymal tube placement
- Malpositioning into abdominal cavity
- Pneumomediastinum
- Pneumothorax
- Occlusion, kinking, or fracture of tubing
- Vascular or mediastinal injury

Procedural Technique

An anatomic triangle of safety is defined for safe insertion of chest tubes using the perimeter outlined by the lateral edge of the pectoralis major, lateral edge of the latissimus dorsi, and the fifth intercostal space (see Fig. 16.3). In emergencies, chest tubes should be inserted within this region to decrease risks of placement complications. Aside from emergent circumstances, ultrasound with Doppler is very useful to confirm underlying pleural fluid or pneumothorax at a selected insertion site, exclude any intervening vascular structures, and also measure the thickness of the chest wall.[11] Review of prior imaging is highly valuable to determine if there is an elevated hemidiaphragm or

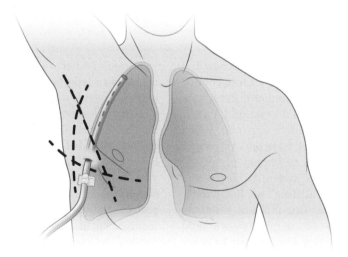

Fig. 16.3 Anatomic triangle of safety for chest tube insertion is demarcated laterally by latissimus dorsi, medially by pectoralis major, and inferiorly by the fifth intercostal space. (Special thank you to Lauren Hugdahl for creation of this image.)

diaphragmatic hernia as well as loculations of fluid. Generally, lateral insertion sites are preferred over posterior locations to afford patient comfort while in bed or in a chair, although loculated pleural fluid collections may dictate limited options for tube insertion location. Procedure sites should never be selected overlying regions of cellulitis or concerning rashes. Tube insertion sites should be selected immediately above each rib to avoid damage to the intercostal nerve and vasculature, which are typically shielded immediately inferior to each rib. Extremely posterior paraspinal approaches should also be approached with caution given evidence that the intercostal artery often runs within the intercostal space unshielded by the ribs within the first 6 cm lateral to the spine.[12]

After informed consent is obtained, an appropriate site is selected and marked, and a time-out is performed to verify the patient's identity, laterality of the procedure, and relevant clinical data. The skin is cleansed and prepped with topical antiseptics such as chlorhexidine or povidone-iodine. Proceduralists don sterile attire including a sterile gown, gloves, bouffant cap, mask, and protective eyewear. The site is then draped with a sterile field. Local anesthesia is injected within the skin and deeper levels of the chest wall down to the parietal pleura. Adequate analgesia can be accomplished with local anesthesia alone, although an intercostal nerve block or intravenous sedation and analgesia may be considered in some cases.

For surgical chest tube insertion, scalpel incision is made parallel to the rib through the skin. Subcutaneous fat, fascia, and intercostal muscles of the chest wall are then bluntly divided. The parietal pleura is also entered bluntly immediately over the rib with the closed end of a pair of curved Kelly forceps. This tract is then dilated and a gloved finger is used to enter the rent within the parietal pleura and the finer is then used to sweep circumferentially to ensure there are no pleural adhesions. Next, using curved Kelly forceps, the chest tube is guided through the tract into the pleural space. An alternative method of surgical chest tube placement is to use a preloaded chest tube over a sharp trocar rather than the Kelly forceps.

Once the chest tube has successfully entered the pleural space, it may be directed either apically or toward the base of the thorax depending on indication. Apical chest tubes are warranted for pneumothorax, while a more basal position may be required for pleural effusions and empyema. The chest tube is anchored into position with sutures, covered with gauze, and secured to the chest wall with tape. Attention should be paid to ensure all connections are tight and secured. Chest tubes should be connected to a closed drainage system on either water seal or continuous suction (typically −20 cm H_2O) initially.

Alternatively, chest tubes can also be placed percutaneously over a wire utilizing a Seldinger technique similar to that used for central venous catheter placement. With this technique, ultrasound use, site location, prepping, draping, and steps for anesthesia remain the same. A needle is then advanced immediately over the rib into the pleural space with confirmation of correct location either by aspiration of pleural fluid or air in the case of pneumothorax. Next, a flexible wire is introduced into the pleural space via the needle and then the needle is withdrawn leaving just the flexible guidewire. One or more dilators are then passed over the wire until the passage is large enough for the chest tube to pass. For a small chest tube that might be used for a pneumothorax, typically only one dilator will be needed, whereas for larger chest tubes, progressively larger dilators would be used. Once the tract is dilated sufficiently, the chest tube is loaded with a stiffening trocar inside of it and the chest tube/trocar unit is passed over the wire into the pleural space. At this point the trocar and wire are removed and the chest tube is secured as described earlier. Proponents of this method favor the ease of insertion, minimally invasive technique, and smaller incision at entrance site.

Selection of chest tube size remains a controversial topic, although use of small-bore (≤14 Fr) chest tubes is increasing. Procedural indication should guide the choice of chest tube size. Larger chest tubes are preferred by some physicians in cases of hemothorax, empyema, or large air leaks in patients on positive-pressure ventilation because they may in theory be less likely to clog, kink, or become dislodged.[13] For these reasons they are often selected in trauma settings. However, small-bore chest tubes are tolerated better by patients, with less pain and splinting.[14] In addition, studies suggest that small percutaneous chest tubes are as efficacious in management of intrapleural infections, including empyema, as larger tubes are.[15] Smaller chest tubes can be flushed routinely with sterile saline to preserve patency.

Once in place, chest x-ray is obtained to verify location. The insertion depth at the skin should be noted in case there is a concern for tube migration or dislodgement. In particular, the distance of the most proximal fenestration to the chest wall should be noted, as any outward migration of the tube can dislodge this fenestration into the tissues of the chest wall. In the case of drainage of infection or instillation of medications into the chest, extrathoracic fenestrations may seed these tissues with infection or allow unintended medication administration. The cumulative fluid drainage through the tube and presence of an air leak should also be charted. A practical step is to mark the date and time next to the fluid level within the drainage system with each nursing shift. In the case of pneumothorax, ongoing air leak is evaluated by the presence of air bubbles during the respiratory cycle in the water-seal chamber (Fig. 16.4).

Medication Administration Via Chest Tube for Pleural Space Infections

Once in place, chest tubes can be used to deliver medications into the pleural space. An in-line three-way stopcock can simplify instillation of medications. Fibrinolytics in combination with dornase alfa are used in pleural space infections to disrupt complex fluid collections with septations and thin infected fluid to afford drainage. The combination of 10-mg tissue plasminogen activator (tPA) and 5-mg dornase alfa twice daily with 1-h dwell time for 3 days has demonstrated benefit in resolution of pleural space opacification on chest x-ray and decreased need for surgical intervention when combined with antibiotic therapy.[16] However, patients with

pleural sepsis who fail antibiotics and chest tube drainage with fibrinolytics should be considered for surgical management.

Medication Administration Via Chest Tube for Pleurodesis

A similar method using a three-way stopcock can be used for delivering sclerosing agents for pleurodesis. Talc is the most common sclerosant used for chemical pleurodesis; however, many other agents such as bleomycin, povidone-iodine, and tetracycline antibiotics have been used and have shown varying degrees of efficacy.[17] The goal of chemical pleurodesis is obliteration of the pleural space by achieving symphysis of the parietal and visceral pleura. Chemical pleurodesis is a definitive therapy for the management of reexpandable recurrent malignant pleural effusion (MPE) and some nonmalignant etiologies. Guidelines for management of MPE suggest that talc slurry delivered via chest tube and talc poudrage via thoracoscopy are similar in terms of their ability to promote pleurodesis.[18] Prior to administering sclerosant medication for pleurodesis, lidocaine can be administered via chest tube to decrease pain associated with pleurodesis. Typically, 10–20 mL of 1% lidocaine without epinephrine is used (not to exceed maximum total recommended lidocaine dosage of 4.5 mg/kg). Additional analgesics may be needed to ensure patient comfort. Other therapies such as intrapleural saline

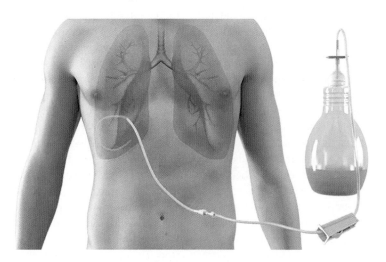

Fig. 16.4 Diagram of tunneled pleural catheter. (Image use approved by Beckton Dickinson, Franklin Lakes, New Jersey.)

irrigation, antibiotic instillation, and intrapleural chemotherapeutic administration have also been described, but there are limited data regarding their efficacy.[19,20]

Troubleshooting and Removal of Chest Tubes

On examination, the connections between the chest tube, tubing, closed drainage system, and suction should be examined for discontinuity or leakage, obstruction, or kinking. If a chest tube becomes clogged, it can be cleared by flushing with sterile saline with attention to maintaining sterile techniques to avoid introducing any contaminants into the chest. For small chest tubes, a three-way stopcock can be placed in-line to facilitate access. Routine stripping or milking of chest tubes is not recommended.[21]

Patients with chest tubes in place should be encouraged to maintain their activity level with physical therapy, time out of bed, and daily walking to prevent deconditioning and reduce risks of venous thrombosis. In addition to anchoring sutures and securing tubing to the chest wall with tape, patients and nursing personnel should be cautioned to be mindful of tubing to prevent accidental dislodgement.

A small amount of physiologic pleural fluid, ~12 mL, exists based on an equilibrium of inflow and egress based on Starling forces.[6,22] Removal of a chest tubes is determined by several clinical and radiographic factors. For example, after lobectomy, a chest tube can be removed in the absence of an air leak when drainage tapers to 300–450 mL/day.[23,24] Evacuation of an effusion, rate of ongoing drainage, presence of any air leak, and reexpansion of lung on chest imaging all need to be taken into account. Although a controversial topic, most doctors use a target volume of 50–100 mL daily drainage as the appropriate time for chest tube removal. Protocols for removal of chest tubes vary and should be tailored to each patient's circumstances. Very small chest tubes can be removed with placement of a small dressing. In patients with a very thin chest wall or larger chest tube, an occlusive dressing such as petroleum gauze is recommended to prevent air entry into the chest. Removal of large chest tubes occasionally necessitates sutures to close the defect/tract in the chest wall at the skin. As a practical tip to simplify removal of larger tubes, a horizontal mattress anchoring stitch can be sutured into the skin at the time of insertion, which enables a simple purse-string-like closure at time of removal, without need for an additional suturing step.[25]

The patient is directed to hum or Valsalva while tubes are being removed to reduce risk of entraining ambient air through the defect in the chest wall.

Future Horizons for Chest Tubes

Tube thoracostomy remains a proven procedure and at times can be a life-saving technique with verified efficacy. Use of ultrasound reduces risk of malpositioned tubes and smaller tubes can be tolerated better by patients. Digital monitoring systems may have a role in minimizing the duration chest tubes stay in place in postsurgical patients, which may in turn help shorten hospital length of stay.[26]

INDWELLING PLEURAL CATHETERS

Definition

Indwelling pleural catheters (IPCs), also referred to as tunneled pleural catheters (TPCs), are a useful tool in the management of recurrent pleural effusions. They are flexible silicone 15.5 Fr or 16 Fr chest tubes with fenestrations along the tubing length and tip, inserted into the pleural space via a tunneled insertion site (see Fig. 16.4). A 1-cm long polyester cuff attached to the outside surface of the catheter is positioned within the tunneled portion, which granulates into tissues of the chest wall thereby decreasing risk of dislodgement. IPCs can be left in place indefinitely while draining recurrent pleural effusions with a low infection risk.[27]

General Considerations

Formerly, patients with MPEs were treated with serial thoracentesis or pleurodesis in cases with reexpandable lung. In 1994, Robinson et al. described a series of patients with recurrent MPE who were palliated with a pleural Tenckhoff catheter, usually used in the abdomen for peritoneal dialysis.[28] Thereafter, IPCs gained in popularity as a potentially useful tool to allow ambulatory patients the ability to drain recurrent pleural effusions independently for several indications (see Box 16.4). Possible complications of IPC placement are similar to chest tube placement (see Box 16.5). Multiple studies assessing the efficacy, safety, impact on patient-centric outcomes such as dyspnea score, days out of hospital, and quality of life have confirmed their positive impact in the care of recurrent symptomatic pleural effusions.[29–31] For MPEs, IPCs have been shown to decrease

> **BOX 16.4 Indications for IPC placement**
>
> - Recurrent symptomatic malignant pleural effusion
> - Recurrent symptomatic nonmalignant effusions refractory to medical management

> **BOX 16.5 Complications of IPC placement**
>
> - Catheter tract metastasis
> - Hemorrhage
> - Infection (including pleural space infection, tunnel-site infection, exit-site infection, cellulitis)
> - Leakage around tubing
> - Lung laceration
> - Malpositioning
> - Mediastinal injury
> - Obstruction, kinking, or fracture of tubing
> - Pneumomediastinum
> - Pneumothorax

hospital length of stay, improve quality of life, and have a low rate of malfunction while also being cost-effective as compared to alternative strategies such as serial thoracentesis.[32]

Procedural Technique

IPCs can be placed either as an outpatient bedside percutaneous procedure or at the time of medical or surgical thoracoscopy.

Steps in identifying an appropriate site for percutaneous insertion are similar to chest tube placement described earlier. More anterolateral positioning is preferred to afford patients the ability to monitor both the exit site and tunneled portions for signs of infection or leakage. Ultrasound is recommended to confirm a satisfactory position, evaluate for any intervening vessels, and estimate the thickness of the chest wall. Once a pleural insertion site is selected, the planned tunneled portion and tube exit site should be planned in a region more anteromedial, which will be easy to access and dress while being mindful to avoid being too close to the nipple, breast tissue, axilla, or around ostomies, tunneled ports, ventriculoperitoneal shunt, or other implanted devices. The tunneled length can vary but should be planned to span a palm's width ~8–12 cm.

Informed consent is obtained and a time-out is performed. The patient is prepped and draped in sterile fashion with a full-length drape exposing the pleural insertion site, planned tunnel, and exit site for the IPC. The skin is anesthetized with local anesthesia. A needle is advanced immediately over the rib at the planned insertion site into the pleural space until pleural fluid can be aspirated. Then a wire is advanced through the needle into the thorax and the needle is removed leaving the wire behind. Additional local anesthesia with lidocaine is given at the insertion site and at the planned exit site/cuff site as well as along the planned tunnel that will connect the two sites. Two small parallel incisions are made with a scalpel nick, one at the insertion site (which has the guidewire in place) and another one at the planned exit site/cuff site. The blunt-ended dilator is loaded onto the IPC to guide tunneling through subcutaneous tissues that connect the exit site/cuff site to the insertion site. The tunneling will start at the exit site/cuff site and move toward the insertion site where the wire currently is placed. The blunt dilator is advanced along the previously planned tunnel until it emerges from the insertion site incision. At that point, the blunt dilator is pulled through the tunnel, bringing the loaded IPC with it. Once the IPC comes out of the insertion site, it can be disconnected from the blunt dilator and pulled further through the tunnel. The IPC is pulled just far enough that the cuff of the IPC is adjusted to within 1 cm from the exit site at the skin (not the insertion site). Next, serial dilators are loaded onto the wire and advanced into the pleural space and then removed. A final peel-away trocar with an internal dilator is advanced all the way into the pleural space, and the inner dilator and wire are removed. Special attention during dilation over the wire is critical to ensure only the chest wall tissues are being dilated. Advancing stiff dilators deeper into the chest can result in lung or vascular injury or mediastinal perforation. The proximal end of the IPC is then advanced through the peel-away trocar into the chest with attention to avoid any kinking or coiling of the tubing. Thereafter, the peel-away catheter is withdrawn with attention to keeping the IPC in place and preventing dislodgement during the peeling process. After the peel-away catheter is fully removed, the remainder of the IPC should be gently pushed into the pleural space and any kinks in the tubing should be fixed by application of appropriate gentle pressure. If the IPC bends too sharply at the insertion site the tube may kink, blocking fluid drainage. Appropriate tube placement is verified by hooking the IPC to suction to confirm the flow of pleural fluid. If there is kinking of the catheter obstructing fluid flow, additional gentle pressure to the catheter at the insertion site to straighten out the turn in the catheter will usually suffice. Putting gentle back tension on the skin surrounding the catheter at the cuff site may help facilitate working out the kink. The two chest wall incisions are then closed with suture and the catheter is anchored with suture to the skin. A sterile foam pad is applied to the skin and the IPC is coiled in place under a second sterile bandage. An occlusive dressing is then applied over these dressings to secure the IPC to the chest wall. In 2 weeks, the sutures are removed and the IPC is held in place by granulation tissue surrounding the polyester cuff.

Care and Drainage of Indwelling Pleural Catheters

Patients and their caretakers are educated on how to perform drainage with aseptic technique, dressing changes, and to monitor for signs and symptoms of infection. Patients are directed to drain until fluid stops flowing or they develop discomfort in their chest, or pain or pressure radiating to their neck, jaw, or shoulder. Handwashing and diligent aseptic techniques are emphasized to decrease infectious complications. With each drainage, the prior dressing is removed and discarded and a new sterile dressing is applied. Development of fever, swelling, erythema over the entry site, tunnel, or exit site, or change in character and color of the fluid drainage should prompt further evaluation. Patients with IPC are advised against immersion in baths, swimming, or hot tubs, or other situations in which the catheter would be underwater.

The goal of IPC placement in MPE is palliation of symptoms such as dyspnea and chest discomfort. Patients are directed to drain daily, every other day, or when symptomatic. The rate of pleural fluid accumulation can vary, and some patients require more frequent drainage than others. A randomized controlled trial of daily drainage versus every other day demonstrated shorter time to autopleurodesis and catheter removal with daily drainage as compared to draining every other day—median time 54 days with daily drainage versus 90 days with every other day.[33]

Removal of Indwelling Pleural Catheters

IPCs are considered for removal once drainage has decreased to ≤150 mL on three consecutive drainages. Depending on the patient's drainage schedule, the frequency of drainage can then be reduced. If drainage remains ≤150 mL for three occurrences on an every-other-day schedule, the IPC can be considered for removal. Chest x-ray or chest ultrasound should be performed prior to removal to rule out a persistent nondraining effusion due to either IPC occlusion or kinking (see section on Troubleshooting Indwelling Pleural Catheters). IPCs that have been in place for shorter durations may be removed with steady traction. Otherwise the patient can be given local anesthesia with 1% lidocaine so adherent tissue to the polyester cuff can be dissected away with the tip of Kelly forceps. Fracture of IPCs on removal is rarely described in case series where fragments of the catheter may break off during removal. If the catheter is in sight and tissue dissection can result in retrieval of the catheter, the IPC can be removed; however, if there are no concerns for infection, abandonment of the fractured portion of the IPC can be considered, especially in light of the limited prognosis and palliative goal of care for most recipients of IPCs.[34]

Benefits of Indwelling Pleural Catheters Versus Mechanical/Chemical Pleurodesis

Recurrent symptomatic pleural effusions can be treated with pleurodesis or placement of an IPC with similar success rates.[35] However, if the underlying lung is unexpandable, IPCs can still alleviate symptoms of dyspnea by reducing weight and pressure on the diaphragm, whereas pleurodesis has a higher rate of failure due to lack of pleural apposition in these instances.[36]

IPC has been compared to talc pleurodesis in a head-to-head randomized controlled trial demonstrating fewer hospitalization days from treatment to death with no significant difference in improvement in breathlessness or quality of life between two groups.[30]

Talc Slurry Pleurodesis Via Indwelling Pleural Catheter

IPCs are proven to be effective for delivery of talc slurry pleurodesis.[37] The pleural space is drained completely via IPC, then patients are premedicated with intrapleural lidocaine without epinephrine, typically 3 mg/kg up to 250 mg (maximum total recommended dosage from all sources ≤4.5 mg/kg of lidocaine), followed by talc slurry containing 4 g of sterile-graded talc combined with 50 mL of 0.9% sterile saline followed by a saline flush of the tubing.[37] The rate of successful pleurodesis was increased from 23% (IPC alone) to 43% (IPC plus talc) by day 35 with this intervention without significant increase in blocked IPCs. By day 70, the rate of successful pleurodesis was increased from 27% to 51% with talc. Furthermore, IPC talc pleurodesis was also associated with statistically significant improvements in questionnaire-reported quality-of-life scores as well.

Management of Indwelling Pleural Catheter Complications

Multicenter trials have demonstrated a relatively low IPC infection rate of 5%.[27] Similar rates of infection have also been described among immunocompromised patients with IPC undergoing chemotherapy.[38] Infections can manifest as cellulitis surrounding the exit site, infection and abscess overlying the tunneled portion, or pleural space infection (see Table 16.1). The most common causative organism is *Staphylococcus aureus*, although nosocomial and drug-resistant organisms are also described.[27] There are no randomized trial or prospective studies that inform the management of IPC-related pleural space infections and controversy remains regarding catheter removal, continuous drainage through existing IPC, or placement of new chest tubes. However, oftentimes infection may not necessitate removal of the catheter. The IPC can be connected in-line to a closed pleural drainage system to allow continuous drainage under water seal or suction. If there is suspicion for infection, cell count with differential and culture can be obtained from the IPC, although pleural fluid acquisition via thoracentesis is an option when IPC bacterial colonization is considered. Among patients who are treated for an IPC-associated pleural space infection, there is a higher rate of subsequent pleurodesis.[27]

Metastatic seeding of the catheter tract is a rare event, occurring in less than 5% of cases. The one exception to this is malignant mesothelioma, which is associated with a higher incidence of catheter tract metastasis—up to 26% of cases as observed in a single-center study.[41] A randomized controlled trial evaluating prophylactic radiation for prevention of procedure tract metastasis following pleural interventions in mesothelioma patients failed to demonstrate any benefit.[42] However, only 25 out of 183 patients in the trial had IPCs—the majority of patients had other pleural interventions that were short-term like thoracoscopy or video-assisted thoracoscopic surgery (VATS). Incidence of tract

TABLE 16.1   Infectious Complications and Management of IPCs

	Clinical Signs and Symptoms	Management
IPC exit-site cellulitis	Erythema, swelling, or pain surrounding IPC exit site	Often oral antibiotics alone can overcome local infection. Removal of IPC infrequently indicated.[39,40]
IPC tunnel-site infections	Erythema, swelling, or pain overlying tunneled portion of IPC	Antibiotics may be sufficient, but IPC removal may be needed if there is abscess formation.
IPC pleural space infections	Fever, chest pain, malaise, or change in character of fluid drainage that becomes cloudier or frank pus	Continuous IPC drainage with intravenous antibiotics. Intrapleural fibrinolytics can be considered; however, if treatment fails IPC can be removed followed by chest tube placement.[27] Surgical interventions may be considered for refractory infections.

IPC, Indwelling pleural catheter.

metastasis may be related to both the specific form of cancer and the duration in which an indwelling tube remains in place. Providers should be aware of and vigilant to monitor this complication, especially in cases of malignant mesothelioma.

Troubleshooting Indwelling Pleural Catheters

If drainage slows or stops and imaging reveals a persistent pleural effusion, the IPC can be flushed with sterile saline to ensure adequate function. There are no clear guidelines or clinical trials to address the management of nondraining IPCs. Based on limited existing literature, however, if saline flushing does not lead to improved drainage, 2–4 mg of tPA can be instilled via the IPC followed by 20-mL sterile saline flush and allowed to dwell for 1 h.[43] For patients with persistent dyspnea with symptomatic loculations that prevent adequate draining, intrapleural tPA can also be considered, although with a small increased risk of bleeding.[34]

Utility of Indwelling Pleural Catheters in Nonmalignant Pleural Effusions

Congestive heart failure is the most common cause of pleural effusions. Effusions can become refractory to therapy necessitating serial thoracentesis. Symptomatic patients can undergo IPC placement with improvement in symptoms and may also achieve eventual pleurodesis with subsequent removal.[44,45]

Hepatic hydrothorax is another morbid condition that can cause rapidly reaccumulating symptomatic pleural effusion. If patients develop refractory symptomatic effusions despite sodium restriction, diuretic therapy, or consideration for transjugular intrahepatic portosystemic shunt (TIPS), IPC can be considered in a multidisciplinary approach in selected patients as either a bridge to liver transplantation or to palliate symptoms; although caution should be exercised as these patients are shown to have a higher risk of IPC-related infection.[46] A multicenter study of hepatic hydrothorax treated with IPC observed a 10% infection risk and 2.5% mortality.[47]

Pleural effusions are also common in patients with end-stage renal disease. In a small case series of eight patients, IPCs have a similar rate of efficacy and can achieve pleurodesis in this population when used for refractory effusions.[48]

Future Horizons of Indwelling Pleural Catheters

Since their inception, IPCs have gained rapid acceptance in their efficacy for palliation of MPE. Their utility as a route of pleurodesis is also encouraging as a minimally invasive means to palliate recurrent pleural effusions. IPCs are well tolerated by patients, cost-effective in cases of MPE and limited life expectancy, and removable in some cases.[49] A newer generation of IPCs coated with sclerosants such as silver nitrate is being evaluated.

REFERENCES

1. Hippocrates *Genuine Works of Hippocrates*. London: Sydenham Society; 1847.
2. Playfair GE. Case of empyema treated by aspiration and subsequently by drainage: recovery. *Br Med J*. 1875;1:45.
3. Walcott-Sapp S., Sukumar M. A history of thoracic drainage: from ancient Greeks to wound sucking drummers to digital monitoring. Retrieved from <https://www.ctsnet.org/article/history-thoracic-drainage-ancient-greeks-wound-sucking-drummers-digital-monitoring>; 2018.
4. Churchill E. Wound surgery encounters a dilemma. *J Thorac Surg*. 1958;35:279–290.
5. McNamara J, Messersmith J, Dunn R, Molot MD, Stremple JF. Thoracic injuries in combat casualties in Vietnam. *Ann Thorac Surg*. 1970;10:389–401.
6. Mason R, Broaddus V, Martin T, eds. *Murray & Nadel's Textbook of Respiratory Medicine*. 5th ed. Philadelphia: Elsevier Saunders; 2010.
7. Cerfolio RJ. Advances in thoracostomy tube management. *Surg Clin North Am*. 2002;82(4):833–848.
8. Shintani Y, Funaki S, Ose N, et al. Air leak pattern shown by digital chest drainage system predict prolonged air leakage after pulmonary resection for patients with lung cancer. *J Thorac Dis*. 2018;10(6):3714–3721.
9. Zhou J, Lyu M, Chen N, et al. Digital chest drainage is better than traditional chest drainage following pulmonary surgery: a meta-analysis. *Eur J Cardiothorac Surg*. 2018;54(4):635–643.
10. Gogakos A, Barbetakis N, Lazaridis G, et al. Heimlich valve and pneumothorax. *Ann Transl Med*. 2015;3(4):54.
11. Liu YH, Lin YC, Liang SJ, et al. Ultrasound-guided pigtail catheters for drainage of various pleural diseases. *Am J Emerg Med*. 2010;28:915–921.
12. Helm EJ, Rahman NM, Talakoub O, Fox DL, Gleeson FV. Course and variation of the intercostal artery by CT scan. *Chest*. 2013;143(3):634–639. https://doi.org/10.1378/chest.12-1285.
13. McCracken DJ, Psallidas I, Rahman NM. Chest drain size: does it matter? *Eurasian J Pulmonol*. 2018;20:1–6.
14. Mahmood K, Wahidi MM. Straightening out chest tubes: what size, what type, and when. *Clin Chest Med*. 2013;34:63–71.
15. Rahman NM, Maskell NA, Davies CW, et al. The relationship between chest tube size and clinical outcome in pleural infection. *Chest*. 2010;137(3):536–543. https://doi.org/10.1378/chest.09-1044. Epub 2009 Oct 9.
16. Rahman NM, Maskell NA, West A, et al. Intrapleural use of tissue plasminogen activator and DNase in pleural infection. *N Engl J Med*. 2011;365(6):518–526.

17. Clive AO, Jones HE, Bhatnagar R, Preston NJ, Maskell N. Interventions for the management of malignant pleural effusions: a network meta-analysis. *Cochrane Database Syst Rev.* 2016;5(5):CD010529. https://doi.org/10.1002/14651858.CD010529.pub2.

18. Feller-Kopman DJ, Reddy CB, DeCamp MM, et al. Management of malignant pleural effusions: an official ATS/STS/STR clinical practice guideline. *Am J Respir Crit Care Med.* 2018;198(7):839–849.

19. Hooper CE, Edey AJ, Wallis A, et al. Pleural irrigation trial (PIT): a randomized controlled trial of pleural irrigation with normal saline versus standard care in patients with pleural infection. *Eur Respir J.* 2015;46:456–463.

20. Hu R, Jiang H, Li H, Wei D, Wang G, Ma S. Intrapleural perfusion thermo-chemotherapy for pleural effusion caused by lung carcinoma under VATS. *J Thorac Dis.* 2017;9(5):1317–1321.

21. Day TG, Perring RR, Gofton K. Is manipulation of mediastinal chest drains useful or harmful after cardiac surgery? *Interact Cardiovasc Thorac Surg.* 2008;7(5):888–890.

22. Zocchi L. Physiology and pathophysiology of pleural fluid turnover. *Eur Respir J.* 2002;20:1545–1558.

23. Zhang Y, Li H, Hu B, et al. A prospective randomized single-blind control study of volume threshold for chest tube removal following lobectomy. *World J Surg.* 2014;38(1):60–67.

24. Motono N, Iwai S, Funasaki A, Sekimura A, Usuda K, Uramoto H. What is the allowed volume threshold for chest tube removal after lobectomy: a randomized controlled trial. *Ann Med Surg (Lond).* 2019;43:29–32.

25. Maritz D, McLauchlan C. A novel way to secure a chest drain. *Ann R Coll Surg Engl.* 2014;96(1):82.

26. Pompili C, Detterbeck F, Papagiannopoulos K, et al. Multicenter international randomized comparison of objective and subjective outcomes between electronic and traditional chest drainage systems. *Ann Thorac Surg.* 2014;98(2):490–496.

27. Fysh ETH, Tremblay A, Feller-Kopman D, et al. Clinical outcomes of indwelling pleural catheter-related pleural infections: an international multicenter study. *Chest.* 2013;144(5):1597–1602.

28. Robinson RD, Fullerton DA, Albert JD, Sorensen J, Johnston MR. Use of pleural Tenckhoff catheter to palliate malignant pleural effusion. *Ann Thorac Surg.* 1994;57:286–828.

29. Tremblay A, Michaud G. Single-center experience with 250 tunneled pleural catheter insertions for malignant pleural effusion. *Chest.* 2006;129(2):362–368.

30. Thomas R, Fysh ETH, Smith NA, et al. Effect of an indwelling pleural catheter vs talc pleurodesis on hospitalization days in patients with malignant pleural effusion: the AMPLE randomized clinical trial. *JAMA.* 2017;318(19):1903–1912.

31. Rahman NM, Pepperell J, Rehal S, et al. Effect of opioids vs NSAIDS and larger vs smaller chest tube size on pain control and pleurodesis efficacy among patients with malignant pleural effusion: the TIME1 randomized clinical trial. *JAMA.* 2015;314(24):2641–2653.

32. Boshuizen R, Thomas R, Lee YCG. Advantages of indwelling pleural catheters for management of malignant pleural effusions. *Curr Respir Care Rep.* 2013;2:93–99.

33. Wahidi MM, Reddy C, Yarmus L, et al. Randomized trial of pleural fluid drainage frequency in patients with malignant pleural effusions: the ASAP trial. *Am J Crit Care Med.* 2017;195:1050–1057.

34. Thomas R, Piccolo F, Miller D, et al. Intrapleural fibrinolysis for the treatment of indwelling pleural catheter-related symptomatic loculations: a multicenter observational study. *Chest.* 2015;148(3):746–751.

35. Kheir F, Shawwa K, Alokla K, Omballi M, Alraiyes AH. Tunneled pleural catheter for the treatment of malignant pleural effusion: a systematic review and meta-analysis. *Am J Ther.* 2016;23(6):e1300–e1306.

36. Roberts ME, Neville E, Berrisford RG, Antunes G, Ali NJ, BTS Pleural Disease Guideline Group Management of a malignant pleural effusion: British Thoracic Society pleural disease guideline 2010. *Thorax.* 2010;65(Suppl 2):ii32–ii40.

37. Bhatnagar R, Keenan EK, Morley AJ, et al. Outpatient talc administration by indwelling pleural catheter for malignant pleural effusion. *N Engl J Med.* 2018;378:1313–1322.

38. Gilbert CR, Lee HJ, Skalski JH, et al. The use of indwelling tunneled pleural catheters for recurrent pleural effusions in patients with hematologic malignancies: a multicenter study. *Chest.* 2015;148(3):752–758.

39. Faiz SA, Pathania P, Song J, et al. Indwelling pleural catheters for patients with hematologic malignancies. A 14-year, single-center experience. *Ann Am Thorac Soc.* 2017;14(6):976–985.

40. Skalski JH, Pannu J, Sasieta HC, Edell ES, Maldonado F. Tunneled indwelling pleural catheters for refractory pleural effusions after solid organ transplant. A case-control study. *Ann Am Thorac Soc.* 2016;13(8):1294–1298.

41. Mitchell MA, Li P, Pease C, et al. Catheter tract metastasis in mesothelioma patients with indwelling pleural catheters. *Respiration.* 2019;97:428–435.

42. Clive AO, Taylor H, Dobson L, et al. Prophylactic radiotherapy for the prevention of procedure-trace metastases after surgical and large-bore pleural procedures in malignant pleural mesothelioma (SMART): a multicenter, open-label, phase 3, randomized controlled trial. *Lancet Oncol.* 2016;17(8):1094–1104. https://doi.org/10.1016/S1470-2045(16)30095-X.

43. Vial MR, Ost DE, Eapen GA, et al. Intrapleural fibrinolytic therapy in patients with nondraining pleural catheters. *J Bronchol Interv Pulmonol.* 2016;23(2):98–105.

44. Srour N, Potechin R, Amjadi K. Use of indwelling pleural catheters for cardiogenic pleural effusions. *Chest.* 2013;144(5):1603–1608.

45. Patil M, Dhillon SS, Attwood K, Saoud M, Alraiyes AH, Harris K. Management of benign pleural effusions using indwelling pleural catheters: a systematic review and meta-analysis. *Chest.* 2017;151:626–635.

46. Kniese C, Diab K, Ghabril M, Bosslet G. Indwelling pleural catheters in hepatic hydrothorax: a single-center series of outcomes and complications. *Chest.* 2019;155(2):307–314.

47. Shojaee S, Rahman N, Haas K, et al. Indwelling tunneled pleural catheters for refractory hepatic hydrothorax in patients with cirrhosis: a multicenter study. *Chest.* 2019;155(3):546–553.

48. Potechin R, Amjadi K, Srour N. Indwelling pleural catheters for pleural effusions associated with end-stage renal disease: a case series. *Ther Adv Respir Dis.* 2015;9:22–27.

49. Olfert JA, Penz ED, Manns BJ, et al. Cost-effectiveness of indwelling pleural catheter compared with talc in malignant pleural effusion. *Respirology.* 2016;22(4):764–770.

17

Medical Thoracoscopy

Pyng Lee

INTRODUCTION

Thoracoscopy, video-assisted thoracic surgery (VATS), medical thoracoscopy (MT), and pleuroscopy are minimally invasive procedures that provide access to the pleural space. They differ only in the approach to anesthesia. In this review, the focus is on diagnostic MT.

VATS is performed by a surgeon in the operating room, typically with single lung ventilation, three entry ports, and rigid instruments. Stapled lung biopsy, resection of pulmonary nodules, lobectomy, pneumonectomy, esophagectomy, and pericardial windows are performed with VATS, in addition to guided parietal pleural biopsy, drainage of pleural effusion or empyema, and pleurodesis[1,2] (Table 17.1). MT on the other hand is conducted by a pulmonologist in an endoscopy suite under local anesthesia and moderate sedation. MT allows biopsy of the parietal pleura under direct visualization with good accuracy. In addition, it facilitates therapeutic interventions such as fluid drainage, guided chest tube placement, and pleurodesis.[3] Practitioners in Europe perform MT sympathectomy for essential hyperhidrosis and lung biopsy for diffuse lung disease.[4]

In 1910 Hans Christian Jacobaeus, a Swedish internist, described examination of the thoracic cavity with a rigid cystoscope attached to an electric lamp as "thorakoscopie." He later advanced the technique to include lysis of pleural adhesions by galvanocautery, also known as the Jacobaeus operation, to facilitate collapse of the tuberculous lung because at that time there was no effective antituberculous therapy.[5,6] At a presentation to the American College of Surgeons, Jacobaeus opined that "in making a differential diagnosis between tumors and pleurisy of other origin, thoracoscopy is of no small value." He was a strong advocate for thoracoscopic-guided biopsies in the evaluation of pleural effusions of unknown etiology and applied thoracoscopy as a diagnostic and therapeutic tool.[7]

EQUIPMENT

Rigid Instruments

Historically, rigid instruments such as stainless steel trocars and telescopes were central to the technique.[3–9] Rigid thoracoscopy requires a cold xenon light source, an endoscopic camera attached to the eyepiece of the telescope, a video monitor, and recorder (Fig. 17.1). The 0-degree telescope is useful for direct viewing while the oblique (30- or 50-degree) and periscope (90-degree) telescopes provide a panoramic view of the pleural cavity.[8,9] Selection of trocars of varying sizes (5–13 mm in diameter) and made of disposable plastic or reusable stainless steel, as well as rigid telescopes of different angles of vision, depends on the operator's preference and patient consideration. A large trocar that accommodates a larger telescope with better optics improves the quality of examination; however, compression of the intercostal nerve during manipulation of the trocar can cause greater discomfort, especially if MT is conducted under local anesthesia and moderate sedation. A 7-mm trocar, 0-degree viewing 4-mm or 7-mm telescope, and 5-mm optical forceps will often allow for effective pleural biopsy without the need for a second port and frequently is often the initial approach used for rigid thoracoscopy.[4,8,9]

Tassi and Marchetti reported excellent views of the pleural space using a 3.3-mm telescope for a group of patients with small loculated pleural effusions that were

TABLE 17.1   VATS Versus Medical Thoracoscopy (Pleuroscopy)

Procedure	VATS	Medical Thoracoscopy
Where	Operating room (OR)	Endoscopy suite or OR
Who	Surgeons	Trained nonsurgeons
Anesthesia	General anesthesiaDouble-lumen intubationSingle lung ventilation	Local anesthesiaConscious sedationSpontaneous respiration
Indications	Parietal pleural biopsy, pleurodesis, decortication, stapled lung biopsy, lung nodule resection, lobectomy, pneumonectomy, pericardial window, esophagectomy, lung	Parietal pleural biopsy, pleurodesis, chest tube placement under direct visualization

VATS, Video-assisted thoracoscopic surgery.

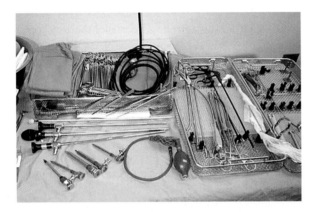

Fig. 17.1 Rigid trocars, telescopes, and accessories.

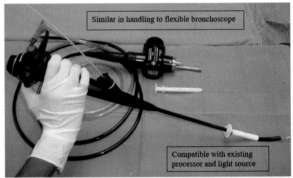

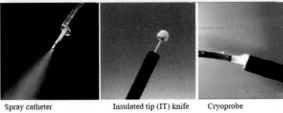

Fig. 17.2 Flex-rigid pleuroscope (LTF 160/240, Olympus, Tokyo, Japan). Spray catheter, insulated tip knife, and cryoprobe.

inaccessible to standard-sized instruments. Two 3.8-mm trocars were used: one for a 3.3-mm telescope and the other for a 3-mm biopsy forceps. Diagnostic yield of 93.4% was comparable with that achieved using conventional 5-mm biopsy forceps.[10]

Flex-Rigid Pleuroscope

The flex-rigid pleuroscope represents an advance in the field of MT as it is fashioned like a bronchoscope, making it easier to learn for physicians who have previously mastered bronchoscopy. The autoclavable flex-rigid pleuroscope (LTF 160 or 240, Olympus, Tokyo, Japan) has a handle and a shaft that measures 7 mm in outer diameter and 27 cm in length. The proximal 22 cm is rigid, whereas the distal 5 cm is flexible with two-way angulation (160 degrees up and 130 degrees down). It has a 2.8-mm working channel that can accommodate biopsy forceps, needles, cryo- and electrosurgical accessories (Fig. 17.2), as well as interfaces with existing processors

(CV-160, CLV-U40) and light sources (CV-240, EVIS-100 or 140, EVIS EXERA-145 or 160) made by the same manufacturer available in most endoscopy units at no additional cost.[3,11,12] The procedure is typically performed in the bronchoscopy suite using local anesthesia and moderate sedation.[3,12] A single 1-cm skin incision to accommodate the disposable flexible trocar is required to perform flex-rigid pleuroscopy. The flex-rigid pleuroscope is also equipped with narrow band imaging (NBI), a technology that highlights mucosal abnormalities and vascular patterns associated with malignancy. NBI can aid in the detection and biopsy of early pleural lesions.[3]

CONTRAINDICATIONS

The only contraindication is the lack of pleural space due to adhesions. However, Marchetti and colleagues have demonstrated that MT can be safely performed by trained practitioners in patients without pleural effusions over sites where lung sliding is observed on thoracic ultrasound (US).[13] Since MT is performed under moderate sedation in spontaneously breathing patients with partial or near-total lung collapse, the patient must not have hypoxia unrelated to pleural effusion, unstable cardiovascular status, bleeding diathesis, refractory cough, or allergy to medications that are administered during MT.

PATIENT PREPARATION

History and physical examination are vital components of any preoperative evaluation. The entry site is selected after careful review of chest radiographs (CXR), decubitus films, US imaging, and computed tomography (CT). Prior to MT 200 to 300 mL of fluid is aspirated from the pleural cavity using a needle, angiocatheter, thoracentesis catheter, or Boutin pleural puncture needle. A pneumothorax is induced by opening the needle to air until stable equilibrium is achieved. Air causes the lung to collapse away from the chest wall to facilitate trocar insertion. The operator may choose to do MT directly with US imaging, which has been shown to reduce access failure as well as the need for iatrogenic pneumothorax.[13,14]

ANESTHESIA

Benzodiazepines (midazolam) combined with opioids (demerol, fentanyl, morphine) provide good analgesia and sedation. Meticulous administration of local anesthesia to the epidermis, aponeurosis, intercostal muscles, and parietal pleura at the entry site ensures patient comfort during manipulation of the thoracoscope.[15]

There is increasing utilization of propofol in recent years to enhance patient comfort during talc poudrage. Propofol use, however, requires monitoring by anesthesiologists in many countries. In patients who received propofol titrated according to comfort, 64% developed hypotension, of which 9% required corrective measures.[16] When propofol was compared against midazolam, more hypoxemia (27% vs. 4%) and hypotension (82% vs. 40%) were observed in the propofol group,

which led to the authors' conclusion that propofol should not be the first choice of sedation for MT.[17]

Good pain control for talc poudrage was achieved by combining opioids, benzodiazepines, and anesthetizing the pleura with up to 250 mg of 1% lidocaine by spray catheter.[18] Preoperative anesthesia should be individualized according to the patient's general condition and expectations; however, physicians must be aware of potential adverse events associated with anesthetic drugs and be ready to manage them.

TECHNIQUE

The patient is positioned in the lateral decubitus position with the affected side up. Continuous monitoring of the electrocardiogram, blood pressure, and pulse oximetry is performed throughout the procedure. Although the site of entry depends on the location of effusion or pneumothorax, hazardous sites such as the anterior chest where the internal mammary artery courses, axilla with lateral thoracic artery, infraclavicular area with subclavian artery, and diaphragm should be avoided. A single port between the fourth and seventh intercostal spaces of the chest wall and along the midaxillary line is preferred for diagnostic MT. A second port may be necessary to facilitate adhesiolysis, drainage of complex fluid collections, lung biopsy, or sampling of pathologic lesions located around the first entry site. Double port access may be necessary if rigid instruments are used, particularly around the posterior and mediastinal aspects of the hemithorax that are inaccessible due to partial collapse of lung, or when the lung parenchyma is adherent to the chest wall.[4,8]

A single port will often suffice for the flex-rigid pleuroscope as its flexible tip allows easy maneuverability within a limited pleural space and around adhesions.[11,12,18] A chest tube is inserted at the end of diagnostic MT and residual air is aspirated. The tube is removed as soon as the lung has reexpanded, and the patient may be discharged after a brief observation period in the recovery area.[19] If talc poudrage or lung biopsy is performed, the patient is hospitalized for a period of monitoring, chest tube drainage, and to optimize pain control.[4,12]

Thoracoscopic-Guided Biopsy of Parietal Pleura Table 17.2

It is desirable to perform biopsy of the parietal pleura over a rib to avoid the neurovascular bundle (Fig. 17.3).

TABLE 17.2 Indications for Rigid Thoracoscopy or Flex-Rigid Pleuroscopy

Clinical Scenario	Type of Procedure
Diagnostic thoracoscopy for indeterminate, uncomplicated pleural effusion where suspicion of mesothelioma is not high	Flex-rigid pleuroscopy[a] or use of rigid telescopes under local anesthesia
Trapped lung with radiographically thickened pleura	Rigid optical biopsy forceps[a] or flex-rigid pleuroscopy with flexible forceps performing multiple bites over the same area to obtain specimens of sufficient depth or use of flexible forceps, IT knife[a], or cryobiopsy[a]
Mesothelioma is suspected	Rigid optical biopsy forceps[a] or flex-rigid pleuroscopy with IT knife[a] or cryobiopsy[a]
Pleuropulmonary adhesions	Fibrous: rigid optical biopsy forceps[a] or flex-rigid pleuroscopy with electrocautery accessoriesThin, fibrinous: flex-rigid pleuroscopy with flexible forceps
Empyema, split pleural sign, loculated pleural effusion	Rigid instruments (VATS)[a] or conversion to thoracotomy for decortication
Pneumothorax with bulla or blebs	Rigid instruments (VATS)[a] for staple bullectomy

[a]Denotes procedure preferred.
IT, insulated tip; *VATS*, video-assisted thoracoscopic surgery.

The forceps probe for the rib, grasp the overlying parietal pleura, and tear the pleura off, moving roughly parallel to and along the wall rather than "grab and pulling" perpendicular to the wall. Specimens obtained with the rigid forceps are larger than those obtained with the Abrams or Cope needle. Biopsies using the flex-rigid pleuroscope are smaller since they are limited by the size of the flexible forceps, which in turn depends on the diameter of the working channel. The flexible forceps also lack the mechanical strength necessary to obtain

deep pleural specimens, which might pose a challenge if mesothelioma is suspected. This problem can overcome by taking multiple biopsies (8–12) of the abnormal area as well as several "bites" of the same area to obtain more representative tissue.

Comparative studies show no difference in diagnostic yield between biopsies by flexible and rigid forceps even in mesothelioma if pleural biopsies could be successfully performed.[20,21] Full-thickness parietal pleural biopsies can be obtained with the insulated tip (IT) diathermic knife during flex-rigid pleuroscopy. In one study, the reported diagnostic yields were 85% and 60% with IT knife and flexible forceps, respectively. The IT knife was notably useful when smooth, thickened parietal pleura was encountered, of which nearly half were malignant mesothelioma.[22] Cryobiopsy is another method that achieves bigger specimens and better preserved cellular architecture and tissue integrity.[23]

Management of Hemorrhage

The principal danger is hemorrhage from inadvertent biopsy of an intercostal vessel. External finger compression of the intercostal space over the bleeding site is the first intervention while another access port is made. The physician then uses two entry sites to examine and cauterize tissues at the same time. Direct pressure with gauze mounted on forceps can be applied from the inside to also tamponade the bleeding site. Connecting the chest tube to underwater seal can also reexpands the lung, serving to tamponade the bleeding site. If the bleeding does not cease with the aforementioned measures, thoracic surgery consultation is warranted. Surgical options include ligating the bleeding vessels with endoclips, enlarging the incision to facilitate repair, or even thoracotomy.

Thoracoscopic Talc Poudrage

Since malignant pleural effusion (MPE) tends to recur unless the primary tumor is chemosensitive, chemical pleurodesis plays an integral role in management of recurrent MPE. Recurrence prevention by chemical pleurodesis is also a primary goal for secondary spontaneous pneumothorax. Chemical pleurodesis is performed via instillation of sclerosant through intercostal tube or small-bore catheter or via talc poudrage during thoracoscopy. Thoracoscopic talc poudrage is performed after fluid aspiration and pleural biopsy, and can be administered by various delivery devices such as talc

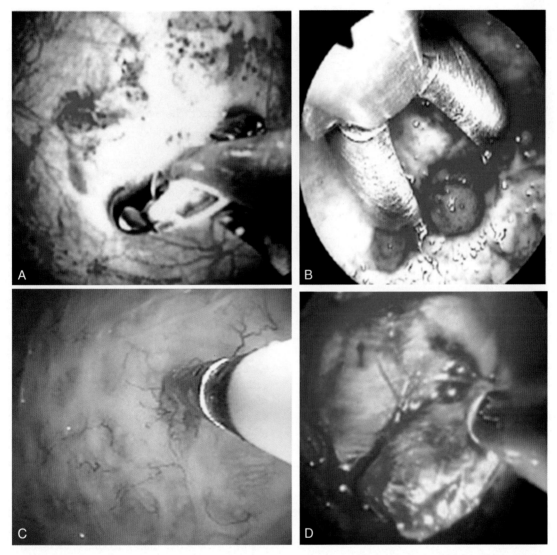

Fig. 17.3 Biopsy of parietal pleura with (A) flexible forceps, (B) rigid optical forceps, (C) cryoprobe, and (D) insulated tip knife.

spray atomizer or bulb syringe, where talc is administered via the trocar without visualization but sprayed in different directions within the pleural space (Fig. 17.4).

COMPLICATIONS

Mortality from rigid thoracoscopy ranges between 0.09% and 0.34%.[24]

Major complications such as prolonged air leak, hemorrhage, empyema, pneumonia, and port site tumor growth occur in 1.8%, whereas minor complications that include subcutaneous emphysema, wound infection, fever, hypotension, and cardiac arrhythmias are observed in 7.3% of MT.[25,26]

A serious but rare complication in association with pneumothorax induction is air embolism (<0.1%).[23] During MT, liters of pleural fluid can be removed with minimal risk of reexpansion pulmonary edema due to immediate equilibration of pressures provided by entry of air through the trocar into the pleural space. Fever

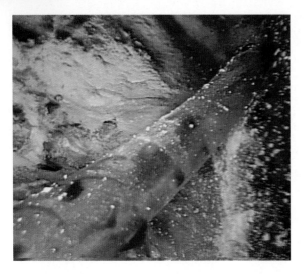

Fig. 17.4 Thoracoscopic talc poudrage.

may occur after talc poudrage that resolves within 48 h, whereas bronchopleural fistula requiring prolonged chest drain and suction may occur after thoracoscopic lung biopsy for interstitial lung disease. Wound infection, pneumonia, and empyema can develop from long-term tube drainage.[25,26] In cases of mesothelioma, tumor growth may occur at the incision sites that can be managed with radiotherapy.[27]

Complications associated with the flex-rigid pleuroscope are rare. Although no mortality was reported in a recent meta-analysis of 755 patients undergoing flex-rigid pleuroscopy,[11,28] training in the proper techniques cannot be overemphasized. Table 17.2 describes the type of patient suitable for rigid or flex-rigid pleuroscopy.

CLINICAL APPLICATIONS

Pleural Effusion of Unknown Etiology

Thoracentesis is the first step in the evaluation of a pleural effusion. Since more than half of exudative effusions are due to malignancy in developed countries, pleural fluid cytology can be a simple definitive test. Diagnostic sensitivity of thoracentesis depends on the nature of the primary malignancy and extent of disease.[29] A single pleural aspiration is diagnostic of malignancy in 60% of cases and 30% of mesothelioma.[30,31] A second sample increases the yield by 15% and the third sample is noncontributory even when large volumes (>50 mL) are submitted.[32]

"Blind" or closed pleural biopsy is positive in 40% of MPE due to patchy pleural involvement. Malignancy tends to affect the costophrenic recess and diaphragm, which are inaccessible to closed pleural biopsy, so adding closed pleural biopsy to pleural fluid cytology increases the yield by only 7%–27% for malignancy and 20% for mesothelioma.[33,34] Contrast-enhanced thoracic CT is superior to standard CT for characterizing MPEs, and nodularity, irregularity, and pleural thickness measuring >1 cm are highly suggestive of malignancy.[30,35,36] Pleural imaging with bedside US is now the standard of care for the selection of appropriate sites for thoracentesis, tube thoracostomy, and MT. As US has been shown to improve safety and decrease access failure, national guidelines recommend use of US to guide all pleural procedures.[12,13,30] US features such as pleural nodularity, pleural thickening >10 mm, and diaphragmatic thickening >7 mm are suggestive of malignancy, with 73% sensitivity and 100% specificity.[37] An "echogenic swirling pattern," described as numerous free-floating echogenic particles swirling in the pleural cavity during respiration or heartbeat, is another sign suggestive of MPE.[38] CT and US features may suggest pleural metastasis but pathologic diagnosis is necessary, and where MT is not readily available, CT- or US-guided pleural biopsy is superior to core needle biopsy (CNB). In a randomized trial, CT-guided biopsy of pleural thickening measuring >5 mm achieved 87% yield for malignancy versus 47% with CNB using the Abrams needle.[39] US-guided biopsy of pleural lesions >20 mm in size with a 14-gauge cutting needle gave 85.5% yield for malignancy, 100% for malignant mesothelioma, and a 4% pneumothorax rate.[40] The type of needle appeared important; Tru-Cut needles were better than a modified Menghini needle for malignancy (95.4% vs. 85.8%),[41] and Abrams needles were also superior for tuberculous effusions.[42]

Abnormal pleural appearances are not always seen on contrast-enhanced CT. In a study where CT-reported diagnoses were compared against histologic results by MT, sensitivity for CT report of malignancy was 68%, which implied that a significant number of patients had malignancy despite negative CT findings. So CT findings alone are not sufficient to rule out malignancy, and studies defining the diagnostic pathway are therefore required.[43,44]

About 20% of pleural effusions remain undiagnosed despite repeated thoracentesis and image-guided needle biopsy. This is where MT plays an important role[25,45] to enhance our diagnostic capabilities when other minimally invasive tests fail. If a neoplasm is strongly suspected, the diagnostic sensitivity of thoracoscopic exploration and biopsy approaches 90%–100%.[10,11,19,20,25,28] Endoscopic characteristics such as nodules, polypoid masses, and "candle wax drops," are highly suggestive of malignancy (Fig. 17.4) but early stage mesothelioma can resemble pleural inflammation (Fig. 17.5).[45,46]

Chrysanthidis and Janssen conducted a study to determine if autofluorescence mode (Richard Wolf GmbH, Knittlingen, Germany) could differentiate early

malignant lesions from nonspecific inflammation in order to help target sites for biopsy during thoracoscopy and to help delineate tumor margins for more precise staging. Using a 300 W xenon lamp in the violet blue range (390–460 nm) a color change from white/pink to red was demonstrated in all cases of malignant pleuritis (100% sensitivity). They were easily identified and their margins better delineated with autofluorescence thoracoscopy. However, color change from white/pink to orange/red was also observed in two cases of chronic pleuritis, so the specificity of autofluorescence

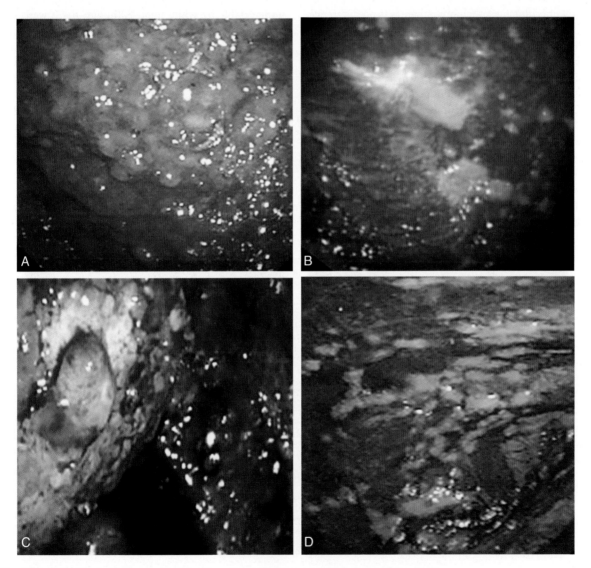

Fig. 17.5 Endoscopic findings of polypoid masses (A,B) and candle wax nodules (C,D).

thoracoscopy was 75% for malignancy. The authors concluded that there was little value in autofluorescence thoracoscopy for patients with extensive pleural involvement due to malignancy that was easy to diagnose with white light thoracoscopy, but that autofluorescence mode might be useful for early pleural malignancies.[47]

NBI is a feature of the flex-rigid pleuroscope (Olympus LTF-160). NBI uses unfiltered narrow bands in the blue (415 nm) and green (540 nm) light wavelengths that coincide with the peak absorption of oxyhemoglobin and thereby enhance the vascular architecture of tissues. In 26 patients with malignant involvement of the pleura (nine mesothelioma), there was no difference in the diagnostic accuracy between NBI and white light videopleuroscopy (Fig. 17.6).[48] Similar observations were made in 45 patients (unpublished data, National University Hospital, Singapore) of which 32 had pleural metastases, 12 with tuberculous pleuritis, and 1 nonspecific pleuritis. Although pleural vasculature was imaged well with NBI, it was difficult to discriminate tumor neovascularization from inflammation based on vascular patterns. In patients with metastatic pleural malignancy, NBI demarcated tumor margins clearly but failed to improve the quality of the biopsies obtained.

Baas and colleagues investigated if prior administration of 5-aminolevulinic acid (ALA) before VATS could lead to improved detection and staging of thoracic malignancy. 5-ALA was administered by mouth 3–4 h before VATS and the pleural cavity was examined first with white light followed by fluorescence thoracoscopy (D light Autofluorescence System, Karl Storz, Tuttlingen, Germany). Tissue sampling of all abnormal areas was performed, and histologic diagnoses were compared against thoracoscopic findings. Although fluorescence imaging-guided thoracoscopy was not superior to white light thoracoscopy, it led to upstaging in 4 out of 15 patients with mesothelioma due to better visualization of visceral pleural lesions that were otherwise undetectable by white light. Although there were several postoperative complications reported, the authors concluded that fluorescence thoracoscopy using 5-ALA was feasible with minimal side effects, and it could have potential applications in the diagnosis and staging of mesothelioma.[49]

Probe-based confocal laser endomicroscopy (pCLE) provides real-time images of the airways, alveoli, lung tumors, pleura, and lymph nodes with a resolution of 3.5 μm, a depth of 70 μm, and field of view of 600 μm. It is compatible with the bronchoscope and medical thoracoscope and can be inserted into a needle for transthoracic needle-based interventions. A fiberoptic probe is advanced through the working channel of the

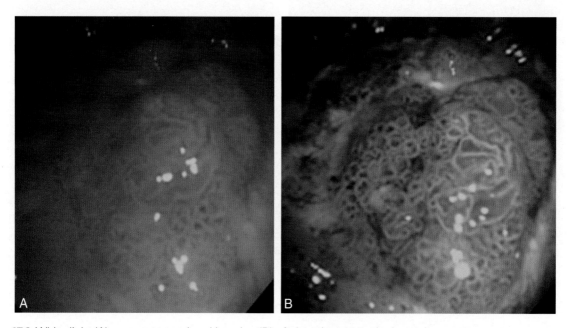

Fig. 17.6 White light (A) versus narrow band imaging (B) of pleural metastasis due to breast cancer.

bronchoscope, thoracoscope, or needle (nCLE), and directed to the area of interest where it illuminates the tissue with laser light (488 nm). Reflected light in focus will pass through the pinhole, resulting in high-resolution images. Moving the laser beam vertically or horizontally enables reconstruction of 3D images by special software.

Both pCLE and nCLE have been used to assess pleural lesions. Bonhomme and colleagues[50] showed pCLE images of normal pleura, non–small cell lung cancer pleural metastasis, and mesothelioma. pCLE was able to differentiate normal from malignant involvement of pleura. A subsequent study was undertaken demonstrating that pCLE and nCLE could differentiate malignant mesothelioma from pleural fibrosis to guide biopsy.[51] Another ex vivo study has found high sensitivity and specificity for pleural malignancy with pCLE in pleural effusion.[52]

Lung Cancer

Cancer-related pleural effusions occur due to direct invasion, tumor embolization to visceral pleura with secondary seeding of the parietal pleura, hematogenous, or lymphangitic spread. Elastin staining and careful examination for invasion beyond the elastic layer of the visceral pleura should be carried out for lung cancer resections as visceral pleural invasion is important for staging in the absence of nodal involvement. It is rare to find resectable lung cancer in the setting of an exudative pleural effusion despite negative cytologic examination. MT can assess surgical operability by determining if the pleural effusion is paramalignant or due to metastases.[25] If pleural metastases are found they denote disseminated disease with reduced life expectancy and talc poudrage or tunneled pleural catheter can be performed at the same setting.[53]

Malignant Mesothelioma

The average survival of a patient diagnosed with malignant mesothelioma is 6 to 18 months, and death occurs from respiratory failure.[53] Malignant mesothelioma is suspected in a patient with asbestos exposure and characteristic CXR of a pleural effusion without contralateral mediastinal shift. Diagnosis by pleural fluid cytology, even with closed pleural biopsy, is difficult, which prompts some physicians to advocate open biopsy by mini or lateral thoracotomy in order to obtain specimens of sufficient size and quantity for immunohistochemical stains.[54] Pleural fluid mesothelin (>2 nmol/L) and megakaryocyte potentiating factor (MPF, >12.4 ng/mL), which originate from a common precursor protein, have shown 65% sensitivity and 95% specificity for pleural mesothelioma in a large study of 507 patients.[55]

MT is favored over thoracotomy as the pleural specimens obtained with 5- or 7-mm rigid forceps are comparable with open biopsies.[56] MT allows staging to be performed in a minimally invasive manner with good sensitivity. 5-ALA-fluorescence VATS should be viewed as experimental but may be able to improve staging accuracy.[49] Adequacy of tissue sampling obtained with the flexible forceps is a concern in cases of mesothelioma, so biopsy with the rigid 5-mm optical forceps, IT knife, or cryobiopsy is recommended to establish the diagnosis.[21,22,55-57] Since mesothelioma is notorious for seeding, biopsy, MT, and chest tube sites should be chosen carefully to avoid tumor involvement and seeding. Boutin and colleagues recommended prophylactic irradiation of 7 Gy for three consecutive days within 2 weeks of MT[58]; however, a recent randomized trial comparing immediate drain site radiotherapy (21 Gy in three fractions) to best supportive care in 61 patients failed to show any difference in the occurrence of tract metastases.[59] Thus prophylactic radiotherapy to MT and drain sites remains controversial.[60] As only 5% of patients are suitable for curative surgery,[61] a palliative approach toward aggressive relief of dyspnea by removing pleural fluid, talc poudrage, pain control, and prophylactic irradiation of incision sites has conferred good symptom control.[62] In recurrent symptomatic pleural effusions, tunneled pleural catheters may represent a viable option.[60]

Tuberculous Pleural Effusion

The diagnostic yield of closed pleural biopsy in tuberculous pleural effusions is variable. In a prospective study of 100 tuberculous effusions in Germany, an immediate histologic diagnosis was established in 94% by MT compared with 38% by closed pleural biopsy (Fig. 17.7). A positive yield from tissue cultures was also higher with MT-guided biopsies than with closed pleural biopsy tissue and pleural fluid combined.[63] Similar results were reported by another study performed in a tuberculosis (TB) endemic country, where MT-guided pleural biopsies achieved superior yield over closed pleural biopsy with Abrams needle (98% vs. 80%). On balance, it appears that MT is superior to closed pleural biopsy for TB diagnosis, and can be the first choice if drug-resistant

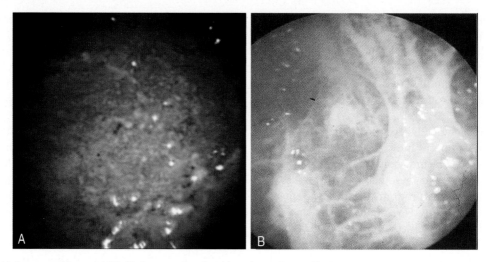

Fig. 17.7 (A) Sago nodules and (B) fibrinous adhesions in tuberculous effusion.

TB is a concern as large quantities of pleural tissue can be obtained via MT for culture. In addition, adhesiolysis can also be performed to promote drainage of fluid loculations.[64]

SUMMARY

Diagnostic MT is effective in the evaluation of pleural and pulmonary diseases when routine fluid analysis and cytology fail. In many institutions where facilities for MT are available, it is used after a first thoracentesis fails to establish a diagnosis and demonstrates an exudative effusion of unknown etiology. MT can also be used to break down loculations in complicated parapneumonic effusions. For patients with recurrent MPEs, MT combined with talc poudrage can be used to effectively drain the effusion and establish pleurodesis. This is also useful in cases of pneumothorax when pleurodesis is warranted.

Training in MT is required; the American College of Chest Physicians recommend 20 supervised procedures before operators are considered competent and 10 each year to maintain competency.[65] The flex-rigid pleuroscope is a significant invention in the era of minimally invasive pleural procedures and is likely to replace traditional biopsy methods.[66] The future of MT will define "when and how" to apply flex-rigid and rigid instruments for the evaluation of pleuropulmonary diseases.

REFERENCES

1. McKenna Jr. RJ. Thoracoscopic evaluation and treatment of pulmonary disease. *Surg Clin North Am.* 2002;80:1543–1553.
2. Yim AP, Lee TW, Izzat MB, Wan S. Place of video-thoracoscopy in thoracic surgical practice. *World J Surg.* 2001;25:157–161.
3. Lee P, Mathur PN, Colt HG. Advances in thoracoscopy: 100 years since Jacobaeus. *Respiration.* 2010;79:177–186.
4. Tassi GF, Davies RJ, Noppen M. Advanced techniques in medical thoracoscopy. *Eur Respir J.* 2006;28:1051–1059.
5. Moisiuc FV, Colt HG. Thoracoscopy: origins revisited. *Respiration.* 2007;74:344–355.
6. Jacobaeus HC. Uber die Möglichkeit, die Zystoskopie bei Untersuchungen seröser Höhlungen anzuwenden. *MunchMed Wschr.* 1910;40:2090–2092.
7. Jacobaeus HC. The practical importance of thoracoscopy in surgery of the chest. *Surg Gynecol Obstet.* 1922;34:289–296.
8. Loddenkemper R. Thoracoscopy-state of the art. *Eur Respir J.* 1998;11:213–221.
9. Rodriguez-Panadero F, Janssen JP, Astoul P. Thoracoscopy: general overview and place in the diagnosis and management of pleural effusion. *Eur Respir J.* 2006;28:409–421.
10. Tassi G, Marchetti G. Minithoracoscopy: a less invasive approach to thoracoscopy- minimally invasive techniques. *Chest.* 2003;124:1975–1977.
11. Munavvar M, Khan MA, Edwards J, Waqaruddin Z, Mills J. The autoclavable semi-rigid thoracoscope: the way forward in pleural disease? *Eur Respir J.* 2007;29:571–574.

12. Lee P, Hsu A, Lo C, Colt HG. Prospective evaluation of flex-rigid pleuroscopy for indeterminate pleural effusion: accuracy, safety and outcome. *Respirology.* 2007;12:881–886.

13. Marchetti G, Valsecchi A, Indellicati D, Arondi S, Trigiani M, Pinelli V. Ultrasound-guided medical thoracoscopy in the absence of pleural effusion. *Chest.* 2015;147:1008–1012.

14. Medford AR, Agarwal S, Bennett JA, Free CM, Entwisle JJ. Thoracic ultrasound prior to medical thoracoscopy improves pleural access and predicts fibrous septation. *Respirology.* 2010;15:804–808.

15. Migliore M, Giuliano R, Aziz T, Saad RA, Sgalambro F. Four-step local anesthesia and sedation for thoracoscopic diagnosis and management of pleural diseases. *Chest.* 2002;121:2032–2035.

16. Tschopp JM, Purek L, Frey JG, et al. Titrated sedation with propofol for medical thoracoscopy: a feasibility and safety study. *Respiration.* 2011;82:451–457.

17. Grendelmeier P, Tamm M, Jahn K, Pflimlin E, Stolz D. Propofol versus midazolam in medical thoracoscopy: a randomized, noninferiority trial. *Respiration.* 2014;88:126–136.

18. Lee P, Colt HG. A spray catheter technique for pleural anesthesia: a novel method for pain control before talc poudrage. *Anesth Analg.* 2007;104:198–200.

19. DePew ZS, Wigle D, Mullon JJ, Nichols FC, Deschamps C, Maldonado F. Feasibility and safety of outpatient medical thoracoscopy at a large tertiary medical center: a collaborative medical-surgical initiative. *Chest.* 2014;146:398–405.

20. Rozman A, Camlek L, Marc-Malovrh M, Triller N, Kern I. Rigid versus semi-rigid thoracoscopy for the diagnosis of pleural disease: a randomized pilot study. *Respirology.* 2013;18:704–710.

21. Dhooria S, Singh N, Aggarwal AN, Gupta D, Agarwal R. A randomized trial comparing the diagnostic yield of rigid and semirigid thoracoscopy in undiagnosed pleural effusions. *Respir Care.* 2014;59:756–764.

22. Sasada S, Kawahara K, Kusunoki Y, et al. A new electrocautery pleural biopsy technique using an insulated-tip diathermic knife during semirigid pleuroscopy. *Surg Endosc.* 2009;23:1901–1907.

23. Shafiq M, Sethi J, Ali MS, Ghori UK, Saghaie T, Folch E. Pleural cryobiopsy: a systematic review and meta-analysis. *Chest.* 2020;157(1):223–230.

24. Viskum K, Enk B. Complications of thoracoscopy. *Poumon-Coeur.* 1981;37:25–28.

25. Rahman NM, Ali NJ, Brown G, et al. Local anaesthetic thoracoscopy: British Thoracic Society Pleural Disease Guideline 2010. *Thorax.* 2010;65(Suppl 2):ii54–ii60.

26. Colt HG. Thoracoscopy: a prospective study of safety and outcome. *Chest.* 1995;108:324–329.

27. Kindler HL, Ismaila N, Armato 3rd SG, et al. Treatment of malignant pleural mesothelioma: American Society of Clinical Oncology Clinical Practice Guideline. *J Clin Oncol.* 2018;36(13):1343–1373.

28. Agarwal R, Aggarwal AN, Gupta D. Diagnostic accuracy and safety of semirigid thoracoscopy in exudative pleural effusions: a meta-analysis. *Chest.* 2013;144:1857–1867.

29. Hsu C. Cytologic detection of malignancy in pleural effusion: a review of 5, 255 samples from 3, 811 patients. *Diag Cytopathol.* 1987;3:8–12.

30. Hooper C, Lee YC, Maskell N, BTS Pleural Guideline Group Investigation of a unilateral pleural effusion in adults: British Thoracic Society Pleural Disease Guideline 2010. *Thorax.* 2010;65(Suppl 2):ii4–ii17.

31. Renshaw AA, Dean BR, Antman KH, Sugarbaker DJ, Cibas ES. The role of cytologic evaluation of pleural fluid in the diagnosis of malignant mesothelioma. *Chest.* 1997;111:106–109.

32. Abouzgheib W, Bartter T, Dagher H, Pratter M, Klump W. A prospective study of the volume of pleural fluid required for accurate diagnosis of malignant pleural effusion. *Chest.* 2009;135:999–1001.

33. Canto A, Ferrer G, Ramagosa V, Moya J, Bernat R. Lung cancer and pleural effusion: clinical significance and study of pleural metastatic locations. *Chest.* 1985;87:649–651.

34. Whitaker D, Shilkin KB. Diagnosis of pleural malignant mesothelioma in life: a practical approach. *J Pathol.* 1984;143:147–175.

35. Leung AN, Müller NL, Miller RR. CT in differential diagnosis of diffuse pleural disease. *AJR Am J Roentgenol.* 1990;154:487–492.

36. Traill ZC, Davies RJ, Gleeson FV. Thoracic computed tomography in patients with suspected malignant pleural effusions. *Clin Radiol.* 2001;56:193–196.

37. Qureshi NR, Rahman NM, Gleeson FV. Thoracic ultrasound in the diagnosis of malignant pleural effusion. *Thorax.* 2009;64:139–143.

38. Chian CF, Su WL, Soh LH, Yan HC, Perng WC, Wu CP. Echogenic swirling pattern as a predictor of malignant pleural effusions in patients with malignancies. *Chest.* 2004;126:129–134.

39. Maskell NA, Gleeson FV, Davies RJ. Standard pleural biopsy versus CT-guided cutting-needle biopsy for diagnosis of malignant disease in pleural effusions: a randomised controlled trial. *Lancet.* 2003;361:1326–1330.

40. Diacon AH, Schuurmans MM, Theron J, Schubert PT, Wright CA, Bolliger CT. Safety and yield of ultrasound-assisted transthoracic biopsy performed by pulmonologists. *Respiration.* 2004;71:519–522.

41. Tombesi P, Nielsen I, Tassinari D, Trevisani L, Abbasciano V, Sartori S. Transthoracic ultrasonography-guided core needle biopsy of pleural-based lung lesions:

prospective randomized comparison between a Tru-Cut-type needle and a modified Menghini-type needle. *Ultraschall Med.* 2009;30:390–395.

42. Koegelenberg CF, Bolliger CT, Theron J, et al. Direct comparison of the diagnostic yield of ultrasound-assisted Abrams and Tru-Cut needle biopsies for pleural tuberculosis. *Thorax.* 2010;65:857–862.

43. Hallifax RJ, Haris M, Corcoran JP, et al. Role of CT in assessing pleural malignancy prior to thoracoscopy. *Thorax.* 2015;70:192–193.

44. Dixon G, de Fonseka D, Maskell N. Pleural controversies: image guided biopsy vs. thoracoscopy for undiagnosed pleural effusions? *J Thorac Dis.* 2015;7:1041–1051.

45. Boutin C, Cargnino P, Viallat JR. Thoracoscopy in the early diagnosis of malignant pleural effusions. *Endoscopy.* 1980;12:155–160.

46. Weissberg D, Kaufman M, Zurkowski Z. Pleuroscopy in patients with pleural effusion and pleural masses. *Ann Thorac Surg.* 1980;29:205–208.

47. Chrysanthidis MG, Janssen JP. Autofluorescence videothoracoscopy in exudative pleural effusions: preliminary results. *Eur Respir J.* 2005;26:989–992.

48. Schönfeld N, Schwarz C, Kollmeier J, Blum T, Bauer TT, Ott S. Narrow band imaging (NBI) during medical thoracoscopy: first impressions. *J Occup Med Toxicol.* 2009;4:24–28.

49. Baas P, Triesscheijn M, Burgers S, van Pel R, Stewart F, Aalders M. Fluorescence detection of pleural malignancies using 5 aminolaevulinic acid. *Chest.* 2006;129. 718–724.

50. Bonhomme O, Duysinx B, Heinen V, Detrembleur N, Corhay JL, Louis R. First report of probe based confocal laser endomicroscopy during medical thoracoscopy. *Respir Med.* 2019;147:72–75.

51. Wijmans L, Baas P, Sieburgh TE, et al. Confocal laser endomicroscopy as a guidance tool for pleural biopsies in malignant pleural mesothelioma. *Chest.* 2019;156(4):754–763.

52. Zirlik S, Hildner K, Rieker RJ, Vieth M, Neurath MF, Fuchs FS. Confocal laser endomicroscopy for diagnosing malignant pleural effusions. *Med Sci Monit.* 2018;24:5437–5447.

53. Roberts ME, Neville E, Berrisford RG, BTS Pleural Disease Guideline Group Management of a malignant pleural effusion: British Thoracic Society Pleural Disease Guideline 2010. *Thorax.* 2010;65(Suppl 2):ii32–ii40.

54. Ceresoli GL, Locati LD, Ferreri AJ, et al. Therapeutic outcome according to histologic subtype in 121 patients with malignant pleural mesothelioma. *Lung Cancer.* 2001;34:279–287.

55. Hollevoet K, Nackaerts K, Thimpont J, et al. Diagnostic performance of soluble mesothelin and megakaryocyte potentiating factor in mesothelioma. *Am J Respir Crit Care Med.* 2010;181:620–625.

56. Herbert A, Gallagher PJ. Pleural biopsy in the diagnosis of malignant mesothelioma. *Thorax.* 1982;37:816.

57. Chan HP, Liew MF, Seet JE, Lee P. Use of cryobiopsy during pleuroscopy for diagnosis of sarcomatoid malignant mesothelioma. *Thorax.* 2016;72:193–195.

58. Boutin C, Rey F, Viallat JR. Prevention of malignant seeding after invasive diagnostic procedures in patients with pleural mesothelioma: a randomized trial of local therapy. *Chest.* 1995;108:754–758.

59. O'Rouke N, Garcia JC, Paul J, Lawless C, McMenemin R, Hill J. A randomized controlled trial of intervention site radiotherapy in malignant pleural mesothelioma. *Radiother Oncol.* 2007;84:18–22.

60. Scherpereel A, Astoul P, Baas P, et al. Guidelines of the European Respiratory Society and the European Society of Thoracic Surgeons for the management of malignant pleural mesothelioma. *Eur Respir J.* 2010;35:479–495.

61. Sugarbaker DJ, Garcia JP, Richards WG, et al. Extrapleural pneumonectomy in the multimodality therapy of malignant pleural mesothelioma. Results in 120 consecutive patients. *Ann Surg.* 1996;224:288–294.

62. Parker C, Neville E. Management of malignant mesothelioma. *Thorax.* 2003;58:809–813.

63. Loddenkemper R, Mai J, Scheffeler N, Brandt HJ. Prospective individual comparison of blind needle biopsy and of thoracoscopy in the diagnosis and differential diagnosis of tuberculous pleurisy. *Scand J Respir Dis.* 1978;102:196–198.

64. Diacon AH, Van de Wal BW, Wyser C, et al. Diagnostic tools in tuberculosis pleurisy: a direct comparative study. *Eur Respir J.* 2003;22:589–591.

65. Ernst A, Silvestri GA, Johnstone D, American College of Chest Physicians Interventional pulmonary procedures: guidelines from the American College of Chest Physicians. *Chest.* 2003;123:1693–1717.

66. Lee P, Colt HG. Steps to flex-rigid pleuroscopy. In: Lee P, Colt HG, eds. *Flex-Rigid Pleuroscopy: Step by Step.* Singapore: CMP Medica Asia; 2005:77–111.

Additional IP Topics

18

Percutaneous Tracheostomy

Tenzing Phanthok, Crystal Ann Duran and Shaheen Islam

INTRODUCTION

Tracheostomy is derived from the Latin words "trachea arteria" and "ostium," which means "creating an opening in the trachea." The earliest documentation of tracheostomy is a description of the healing of a throat incision in the Rig Veda.[1] Hippocrates described intubation of the trachea to support ventilation.[1] Tracheostomy to resolve upper airway obstruction was first mentioned in hieroglyphics by Imhotep.[2] The first documented case of a successful tracheostomy was performed in a patient with tonsillar obstruction by Antonio Brassavola in 1546.[1] In 1620, Nicolas Habicot successfully resuscitated a boy who was initially pronounced dead after sustaining a stab wound to the neck, following an emergent tracheostomy and release of a tracheal blood clot.[2] In 1833, Trousseau saved more than 200 patients with diphtheria by performing a tracheostomy.[3]

Tracheostomy techniques available today are surgical tracheostomy (ST) and percutaneous dilational tracheostomy (PDT).

ST is usually performed in the operating room under general anesthesia and entails surgical dissection of the neck tissue to create a stoma. Conversely, in PDT, a needle is placed percutaneously and then, using a modified Seldinger technique, a stoma is created by dilation.

PDT has a smaller incision size, shorter procedural duration, less postoperative bleeding, and faster healing time compared to ST.[4] Several meta-analyses and randomized controlled trials (RCTs) comparing ST and PDT have also confirmed that PDT is associated with significantly shorter operative time, lower cost, lower incidence of perioperative bleeding, shorter sedation time, accelerated wound healing, and lower risk of stoma infections. However, there is no difference in mortality between ST and PDT.[5–9]

In this chapter, we will primarily focus on PDT in the intensive care unit (ICU) setting.

SURGICAL TRACHEOSTOMY TECHNIQUE

ST is ideally performed in the operating room under general anesthesia, although ST may be performed at the bedside. Landmarks should be identified preoperatively, including the thyroid cartilage, cricoid cartilage, and sternal notch. Local anesthetic with 1% lidocaine with epinephrine is infiltrated at the incision site if not performing under general anesthesia. A 2–3-cm long transverse skin incision is made about a centimeter below the cricoid cartilage. The midline raphe is located, and retractors are used on either side of the strap muscles to expose the trachea. The endotracheal tube (ETT) is slightly withdrawn to allow stoma creation. An incision is made in the interspaces between the first and the second tracheal rings and is extended laterally. Stay sutures are placed through the skin, around the tracheal ring, and then back through the skin.[10] Often a Bjork flap is made. The tracheostomy tube (TT) is then placed through the tracheostomy stoma, the cuff inflated, and the ventilator circuit connected. The TT is secured with sutures in the neck and ventilation is then transferred from the ETT to TT.

TYPES OF PERCUTANEOUS DILATIONAL TRACHEOSTOMY

The first tracheostomy technique described in 1955 required a special needle to enter the trachea and involved a one-stage insertion of the TT using a cutting trocar.[11]

Percutaneous tracheostomy has been modified over the years. The Ciaglia technique, introduced in 1985, is one of the most widely used techniques in North America.[12, 13] In 1990, the Griggs guidewire dilating forceps (GWDF) was developed, where a special forceps is threaded over the guidewire into the trachea, and a tracheal aperture is created by opening the forceps.[14] In 1997, Fantoni and Ripamonti[15] described the translaryngeal method where the dilator and the TT are pulled in a retrograde fashion through the stoma. Another single-dilator technique called the PercuTwist, developed by Frova and Quintel in 2002, utilizes a single dilator, which is advanced over the guidewire into the soft tissue using a clockwise rotation to create a stoma.[16]

Since these latter techniques do not exert pressure over the tracheal wall during dilation, they were thought to minimize the risk of posterior tracheal wall injury.

INDICATIONS

Indications for PDT are similar to ST (Box 18.1). ST is primarily performed in patients with upper airway obstruction from laryngeal or cervical malignancies or in emergencies. It is also done in patients undergoing neck surgery, total laryngectomy, and in patients with ineffective swallowing or cough mechanisms resulting in an inability to protect their airway.

In the medical ICU, tracheostomy is commonly performed in patients requiring prolonged ventilation[17] or for airway protection. Transitioning from oral intubation to tracheostomy helps to minimize sedation requirements, decrease the incidence of lung infections, reduce dead space ventilation, improve respiratory work, and aid in tracheobronchial toileting while protecting the airways.[18]

CONTRAINDICATIONS

Although when first introduced there were suggested contraindications related to body habitus, today it is recognized that PDT is a viable alternative to ST and there are no absolute contraindications for PDT as compared to ST.

Relative contraindications (Box 18.1) to PDT include trauma resulting in an unstable cervical spine, uncontrollable coagulopathy, or prior neck surgery. In addition, PDT can be performed with caution in patients with difficult anatomy (enlarged thyroid gland, local malignancy, short neck, tracheal deviation, previous

---

> ### BOX 18.1 Indications and Contraindications
>
> **Indications**
> - Prolonged ventilator dependence with failure to wean
> - Inability to protect airway (stroke, encephalopathy, etc.)
> - Obstruction of proximal trachea or upper airways
>
> **Relative Contraindications**
> - Gross distortion of neck anatomy due to tumor, high innominate artery, thyromegaly
> - Soft-tissue infection on anterior neck
> - Anatomic landmarks
> - Medically uncorrected bleeding disorders
> - High positive end-expiratory pressure (PEEP) of more than 20 cm of water
> - Emergent airway
> - Major head and neck surgery or trauma
> - Overwhelming systemic infection

---

tracheostomy), high ventilator support (FIO_2 >70% or positive end-expiratory pressure [PEEP] >10 cm H_2O), and radiation therapy to the cervical region within the previous 4 weeks.[19] Other contraindications include infection at the insertion site or palpable but obscured neck anatomy. Recent data suggest that PDT is largely dependent on operator experience[20] and can be safely performed in patients with relative contraindications.

PDT has been performed in patients with an average PaO_2/FIO_2 of 130 and an average PEEP of 17 cm H_2O without any significant deterioration in oxygen saturation.[21] PDT has also been done in patients with acute respiratory distress syndrome (ARDS) on high-frequency oscillatory ventilation without any significant hemodynamic or respiratory compromise.[22]

ST is often preferred over PDT in patients with a body mass index (BMI) >30 kg/m² in neck trauma, and in head and neck malignancy.[23] However, PDT can be safely performed in the obese population.[24-26] A retrospective study found no significant difference between PDT and ST in malpositioning of TT, loss of airway, or bleeding in patients with BMI >35 kg/m².[25] Another prospective study comparing PDT in ICU patients with BMI ≥30 kg/m² versus lower BMI revealed significantly higher major complication rates (12% vs. 2%, $P < 0.04$) in obese patients.[27] The creation of a false passage due to the increased distance from skin to trachea was a major complication in morbidly obese patients.[28] The risk of complications can be minimized with proper evaluation, appropriate patient selection, operator experience, and concurrent bronchoscopic visualization to avoid unrecognized false passages.

TIMING OF TRACHEOSTOMY

In general the consensus for appropriate time to perform tracheostomy is around 10–20 days after intubation. Early tracheostomy (within 7 days after intubation) in critically ill patients is associated with a reduction in weaning time, complications, and morbidity and mortality.[29–31]

Early tracheostomy, performed within 4–7 days of admission, is associated with a significant increase in ventilator-free days (VFD).[32] A systematic review of RCTs comparing outcomes of early versus late tracheostomy confirmed more VFD, shorter ICU stays, a shorter duration of sedation, and reduced long-term mortality in patients with early tracheostomy.[33] However, although early tracheostomy reduced hospital length of stay and cost, it did not affect in-hospital mortality.[34]

TRACHEOSTOMY TUBES AND TYPES

The main components of the TT are an outer cannula, the flange, and an inner cannula (Fig. 18.1).

The curved outer cannula (Fig. 18.1a,b) is attached to the flange and has a cuff attached to the distal end to provide a seal within the trachea for ventilation.

The flange is attached to the proximal end or is a part of the TT, which is used to secure the TT on the neck with a tracheostomy tie or suture. The flange is commonly labeled with the tube size, type, and length.

The inner cannula (Fig. 18.1c) snugly fits inside the outer cannula and often has a 15-mm adapter for connecting to the ventilator circuit. The inner cannula can be reusable or disposable. Reusable inner cannulas need to be cleaned at least twice a day. Some TTs do not have the provision of an inner cannula and the inner aspect is specially coated with water-repellent material to prevent mucus plugging.

The obturator (Fig. 18.1d) is a firm guide with a rounded tip designed to be placed inside the outer cannula of the TT for easy placement through a matured stoma during tracheostomy tube replacement.

Patients on a ventilator or those with risk of aspiration usually require a cuffed TT. The cuff is connected to a pilot balloon (Fig. 18.1b) that provides information on the cuff inflation. When patients are weaned off mechanical ventilation, they can be transitioned to a cuffless TT in preparation for decannulation. Cuff pressures should be checked periodically to avoid ischemic injury of the tracheal mucosa.

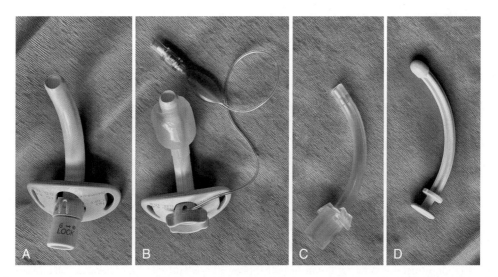

Fig. 18.1 Common tracheostomy tubes (Shiley tracheostomy, Medtronic, Minneapolis, MN, USA). From left to right: *a*, Cuffless tracheostomy tube with inner cannula. Inner cannula has 15-mm adapter. *b*, Cuffed tracheostomy tube. *c*, Inner cannula with 15-mm adapter. *d*, Obturator.

The TTs come in different sizes and shapes depending on the length, curvature, thickness, and a detailed discussion is beyond the scope of this chapter.

A modified TT is available for placement with the PDT technique (Fig. 18.2b), which has a tapering distal end to make it easier to insert through the newly created stoma by dilation.

A longer TT is used in obese patients to accommodate the longer skin to tracheal distance so the distal tip of the TT (Fig. 18.2a) remains parallel to the long axis of the trachea. Various commercially available TTs are available that are extra long.

PERCUTANEOUS TRACHEOSTOMY KIT

The two well-known commercially available kits in the United States that use a single-stage dilator include the Ciaglia Blue Rhino (Cook Medical Inc, Bloomington, IN, USA) and Portex Ultraperc (Smiths Medical, Dublin, OH, USA).

BRONCHOSCOPY

Bronchoscopic guidance is an important adjunct in proper placement of TTs during PDT to avoid posterior wall trauma or puncture, and is especially important in patients with obesity, difficult anatomy, or those with cervical fixation or an unstable cervical spine. A more detailed procedural description is provided later, including how bronchoscopy can be utilized to confirm placement of the guidewire, and to avoid false lumen formation and tracheal injury.

There is conflicting evidence, with some studies failing to demonstrate a benefit for concurrent bronchoscopy, whereas others have found that bronchoscopic visualization during PDT reduces complications. For example, a retrospective analysis of PDT with and without bronchoscopy in the trauma population revealed no significant difference in safety and efficacy with experienced operators.[35] However, over time other studies have shown the benefits of routinely utilizing bronchoscopy when performing PDT. For example, a prospective study reported significantly lower rates of major complications including bleeding, subcutaneous emphysema, or pneumothorax (20% vs. 40%); higher rate of first-time successful needle puncture; and significantly shorter procedural duration with bronchoscopic guidance.[36] On balance, given that false lumens and unrecognized tracheal lacerations are the most significant major complications of PDT, concurrent bronchoscopy during PDT should be considered an essential element of PDT in terms of safety. At present, bronchoscopic guidance is used routinely by almost all interventional pulmonologists.

ULTRASOUND GUIDANCE DURING PERCUTANEOUS DILATIONAL TRACHEOSTOMY

Ultrasound guidance during PDT can assist with localizing anatomic landmarks and to identify the appropriate point of entry by examining the pretracheal area for aberrant vasculature, tracheal rings, neck mass, and the thyroid gland. Real-time ultrasound can be used to

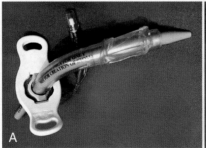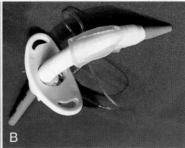

Fig. 18.2 *a*, Extra-long tracheostomy tube with a cuff (Shiley XLT, Medtronic, Minneapolis, MN, USA) loaded on a straight dilator. Note the raised distal end of the tube creating a sharp rise on the dilator. *b*, Regular tracheostomy tube with tapered end for easy placement during percutaneous tracheostomy, loaded onto a straight dilator. Note the flush distal end of the tracheostomy tube with the dilator (Shiley PERC, Medtronic, Minneapolis, MN, USA).

follow the needle path during tracheal puncture and to determine the final position of the TT.[37, 38] However, injury to the posterior tracheal wall cannot be assessed with ultrasound due to the inability to visualize the posterior wall.[39] In our practice, we do not routinely use ultrasound guidance.

A randomized prospective study comparing efficacy, safety, and incidence of complications between bronchoscopic guidance and ultrasound guidance revealed no significant differences between the two groups in terms of technical difficulty of the procedure or the number of needle interventions. Interestingly, the risk of hemorrhage was higher and the mean duration of procedure was longer in the bronchoscopy group.[40] A network meta-analysis found that bronchoscopy or ultrasound-guided percutaneous tracheostomy has similar rate of procedure-related complications.[9] Ultrasound guidance may not be an alternative to bronchoscopic guidance, but rather an adjunct to bronchoscopy to potentially improve the safety profile in select cases.

EVALUATION OF PATIENT FOR TRACHEOSTOMY

A thorough clinical and anatomic evaluation should be performed before planning a PDT. Review of the clinical history including medication use, previous tracheostomy or neck surgery, bleeding disorders, evaluation of the neck anatomy for palpable cricoid cartilage or tracheal rings, palpable isthmus of the thyroid gland, cricoid to sternal distance, and ability to extend the neck are essential.

Hemodynamically unstable, coagulopathic, and obese patients need careful risk stratification to avoid any complications. Depending on the clinical context, PDT on obese patients can be done safely by a skilled operator.[12, 41] In select patients with mild hemodynamic instability, PDT may be feasible, depending on the alternatives. Coagulopathy should in general be corrected prior to PDT, but if it is mild and cannot be corrected, then with a skilled operator and appropriate surgical backup it may be done if there are no alternatives.

History of sedation tolerance is helpful to plan the procedural sedation. Platelet count and coagulopathy should be reviewed 24 h prior to procedure.

There is a high risk of aerosolization of SARS-CoV-2 (severe acute respiratory syndrome coronavirus 2) during tracheostomy. Delaying the procedure for 10

days or until the patient is stable and able to tolerate apnea during creation of the stoma and insertion of TT may minimize risk of aerosolization.[42] We perform PDT in COVID-19 (Coronavirus disease 2019) patients in a negative airflow room wearing full personal protective equipment with a powered air-purifying respirator (PAPR).

After a decision for tracheostomy is made, informed consent should be obtained from the patient (if able), durable power of attorney (DPOA), or family for tracheostomy, bronchoscopy, and ultrasound examination (if planned). Risks, benefits, potential complications, and alternative options should be clearly explained to the patient or family.

ANTICOAGULATION OR ANTIPLATELET THERAPY MANAGEMENT IN PERCUTANEOUS DILATIONAL TRACHEOSTOMY

There are no specific guidelines on anticoagulation and antiplatelet management in patients undergoing PDT. The incidence of major bleeding requiring blood transfusions directly related to PDT is extremely low.[43] However, general guidelines for perioperative management of antithrombotic therapy can be applied to PDT.[44]

The incidence of major and minor bleeding following PDT, in patients on extracorporeal membrane oxygenation (ECMO) receiving systemic heparinization, was 1.7% and 31.4%, respectively,[45] with a median platelet count of 126, 000/μL and international normalized ratio (INR) 1.1, when heparin infusion was held 1 h before the procedure. Even with coagulation disorders (activated partial thromboplastin time [aPTT] >50 s, prothrombin time [PT] <50%, INR >1.4, or platelet <50, 000/μL) there was mild bleeding without any need for surgical intervention or transfusion.[46] Thus PDT is relatively safe in patients with coagulopathy and severe thrombocytopenia after correction.[47–49]

We recommend holding the heparin drip at least 3 h prior to the procedure and resuming heparin 3 h postprocedure. Subcutaneous heparin and enoxaparin should be held at least 12 h prior if they are receiving BID dosing. If they are receiving once-a-day therapeutic dosing of enoxaparin, it should be held for 24 h. Dual antiplatelet therapy preferably should be held for 3–5 days. However, in the setting of recent cardiac stenting, PDT can be performed safely on clopidogrel[50] with appropriate informed consent. Direct oral anticoagulation agents (DOAC) and vitamin K antagonists (VKA) should be bridged with unfractionated heparin if possible. DOAC should be held for two to three drug half-lives in cases with low risk of bleeding and four to five drug half-lives in high risk of bleeding. Renal dysfunction is also a key factor and desmopressin (DDAVP) can be used in uremic patients since platelets can be dysfunctional. There is no specific guidance on the use of antiangiogenic agents such as bevacizumab or other oral VEGF (vascular endothelial growth factor) TKI (tyrosine kinase inhibitor) such as sunitinib or cabozantinib during PDT. A French guideline recommends a delay of 2 days between implantation of an intravenous device and the initiation of bevacizumab, a delay of at least 5 weeks between the last dose of bevacizumab and invasive surgery, and a delay of 4 weeks between surgery and the initiation of bevacizumab treatment.[51]

PREPARATION FOR PERCUTANEOUS DILATIONAL TRACHEOSTOMY

Once the decision for bedside PDT is made, the plan should be communicated to the primary team, the nursing staff in the ICU, and the bronchoscopy team. A procedural checklist (Box 18.2) ensures that all necessary supplies, medications, and equipment are available at the bedside. Tube feeding should be held, or patients should be NPO for at least 4–6h prior to the procedure. Anticoagulation should be managed as described earlier.

Extra tubing for IV lines should be arranged to access the IV line during the procedure for medication administration without compromising the sterile field. The size of the ETT is verified to determine the appropriate size of the bronchoscope to be used during the procedure.

SETUP AND TECHNIQUE

Personnel

A primary operator and an assistant usually stand on either side of the patient (Fig. 18.3). Ideally the tracheostomy operator (if right-handed) stands on the right side of the patient or vice versa if left-handed, and the

> **BOX 18.2 Equipment and Supplies for Percutaneous Dilational Tracheostomy**
>
> **Bronchoscopy**
> - Flexible bronchoscope with monitor and other equipment
>
> **Medications**
> - Fentanyl, midazolam, propofol, dexmedetomidine
> - Rocuronium or succinylcholine for neuromuscular block
> - Additional saline available in case of hypotension
> - Norepinephrine
>
> **Tracheostomy Kit**
> - Percutaneous tracheostomy kit
> - Tracheostomy tube
> - Extra-long tracheostomy tube (if deep neck or BMI >35 kg/m²)
>
> **Miscellaneous**
> - Sterile gowns
> - Sterile gloves
> - Face shield and caps
> - Chlorhexidine
> - Large drape
> - Lubricant jelly
> - Electrocautery or thermocautery
> - Split sponge dressing
> - Tracheostomy ties
> - Lidocaine with epinephrine
> - Gauze
> - Razor
> - Tape

assistant on the opposite side. The bronchoscope operator usually stands at the head of the bed and the respiratory therapist (RT) managing the ETT next to the bronchoscopist closer to the ventilator.

The ventilator and bronchoscopy tower need to be placed closer to the bronchoscopist for easy access. The bronchoscope tower is positioned near the head of the bed and the bronchoscopy technician stands next to the tower. A circulating nurse is present to monitor the vitals and to administer medicine. A second nurse may be available depending on the institutional policy for documentation. All personnel in the room should wear appropriate personal protective equipment. The tracheostomy operator and the assistant, in addition, should wear sterile gloves and gown.

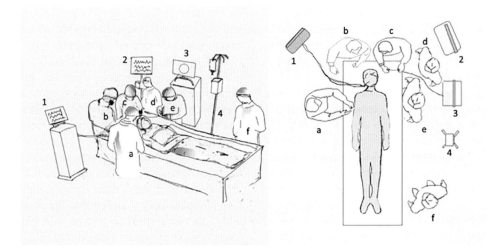

Fig. 18.3 Personnel and equipment setup for bedside percutaneous dilational tracheostomy. *a*, Primary operator; *b*, respiratory therapist managing the airway; *c*, bronchoscope operator; *d*, bronchoscopy technician; *e*, assistant; *f*, circulating nurse to monitor vitals, administer medications, and document procedure; *1*, ventilator; *2*, vital sign monitor; *3*, bronchoscopy tower; *4*, IV pole. *PDT*, Percutaneous dilational tracheostomy.

Patient Monitoring, Airway, and Ventilator Management

During the PDT, patients are sedated and paralyzed and placed on controlled mechanical ventilation on 100% F_{IO_2}. Continuous monitoring of blood pressure (BP), heart rate, and oxygen saturation is done during the procedure. BP should be checked every 2 min unless continuous arterial BP monitoring is available.

Patients may become hypotensive after sedation and neuromuscular blockade. Phenylephrine or norepinephrine can be used if hypotension is unresponsive to saline bolus.

Participation of an experienced RT is mandatory to avoid loss of the airway, especially during retraction of the ETT and securing the ETT when it is gently wedged into the glottis opening. Adequate ventilation is confirmed by monitoring the exhaled tidal volume and pulse oximetry. An alveolar recruitment maneuver may be needed if adequate oxygen saturation cannot by maintained during PDT on patients requiring PEEP >12 mmHg or high F_{IO_2}.

Technique

After informed consent is verified, a time-out is performed, and the patient is laid supine. The bed is maximally inflated. The neck is usually hyperextended to bring the cricoid cartilage superiorly above the sternal notch by placing a roll of towels under the shoulders (provided no contraindication like rheumatoid arthritis or neck fusion is present). Beard or hair from the anterior neck area will need to be shaved. The F_{IO_2} is increased to 100% for the duration of the procedure. A checklist (Box 18.2) assures that all necessary equipment and supplies are readily available prior to the procedure.

Landmarks such as the cricoid cartilage, sternal notch, and the tracheal rings are identified and marked. The distance between the cricoid and sternal notch is estimated. It is helpful to mark the anatomy and the incision site prior to the procedure, especially if trainees are involved. If the trachea can be palpated but is deep, we recommend using an extra-long TT.

The anterior neck area is then sterilized using chlorhexidine swabs. A sterile drape is placed over the neck and the rest of the body.

After adequate sedation is achieved, 2% lidocaine is instilled through the ETT to further anesthetize the airways. A bronchoscope is introduced through the ETT for a quick airway examination. The airway is suctioned and cleared of any mucus or secretions prior to the PDT to avoid hypoxia.

Lidocaine (1%) with 1:10,000 epinephrine is administered in the skin and subcutaneous tissue ideally against the first to third tracheal rings in between the cricoid cartilage and the sternal notch for topical anesthesia and hemostasis.

After adequate sedation is achieved, a short-acting paralytic is given. The bronchoscopist then inserts the bronchoscope and places it near the distal tip of the ETT. Both the bronchoscope and the ETT are retracted by the RT as one unit very slowly to avoid accidental loss of the airway. The bronchoscopist observes the bronchoscope monitor to identify the location of the ETT.

Once the ETT is retracted to the level of the cricoid cartilage, the cricothyroid membrane is identified with the bronchoscope. It is important to accurately identify the cricoid cartilage (Fig. 18.4A-B) so the first and second tracheal rings can be correctly distinguished from the rest of the cartilaginous interspaces. The cuff is then reinflated at the level of glottis and the RT stabilizes the ETT. The RT should be reassured that there may be tidal volume leak at this point, as complete seal may not be achieved. Often rostral traction is applied

on the laryngeal cartilage to bring the cricoid cartilage and the proximal tracheal rings superior to the sternal notch, when the cricoid cartilage is too deep or if the cricoid cartilage to sternal distance is less than 1 cm. The bronchoscope can also be pointed anteriorly at the interspace between cartilaginous rings and then used to transilluminate the proper entry site. This can help the tracheostomy operator identify and verify the proper insertion site.

Once the insertion site is selected, a 1.5-cm long vertical skin incision is made along the midline. It is very critical not to make a deep incision initially to avoid damage to the deeper structures. The pretracheal tissue and deep fascia are then cleared with blunt dissection using a small mosquito Kelly clamp (Fig. 18.4C). After the deep fascia and tissue are cleared, the tracheal rings including the cricoid cartilage are identified by palpation from outside. The cricoid cartilage is usually the most prominent cartilage.

The tracheostomy operator then stabilizes the tracheal cartilage with the nondominant hand (Fig. 18.4B). The tip of the closed Kelly clamp can be used to press on the

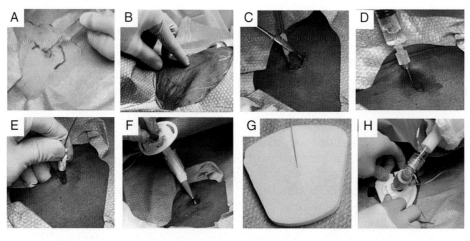

Fig. 18.4 Technique of percutaneous dilational tracheostomy. (A) Surface anatomy showing the laryngeal cartilage, cricoid cartilage, and the sternal notch marked. Injecting lidocaine with epinephrine. (B) Stabilization of the tracheal cartilage with the nondominant hand using the thumb and the third finger to hold the laryngeal cartilage and the second finger to identify the tracheal rings before inserting the introducer needle. (C) Blunt dissection of the pretracheal tissue to expose the tracheal rings. (D) Verification of the introducer needle tip in the trachea by observing aspiration of air bubbles inside the syringe. (E) Advancing the punch dilator over the guidewire. (F) Advancing the tracheostomy tube and dilator assembly over the guiding sheath and guidewire. (G) Split-foam tracheostomy sponge to protect skin from friction with the tracheostomy flange. (H) Connecting the tracheostomy tube to the ventilator circuit after placement of the tracheostomy tube. Bronchoscope adapter is still connected for bronchoscopic examination of the airways.

anterior wall to locate the exact location of possible needle insertion, which can be verified by watching the bronchoscope monitor while pressing on the trachea. Once the ideal location is identified, the introducer needle is loaded on a syringe with 1 cm³ saline and is inserted between the first and the second or the second and the third cartilaginous interspaces in the midline (Figs. 18.4D and 18.5B). Entry into the trachea is visualized with the bronchoscope.

Ideally, the introducer needle will enter the trachea along the midline at 12 o'clock or at least between 11 o'clock and 1 o'clock position (Fig. 18.6). Bronchoscopic guidance is crucial to confirm that the needle tip is not going through the posterior wall of the trachea. Aspiration of free air bubbles (Fig. 18.4D) confirms that the needle tip is within the airway and not in soft tissue. If entry into the trachea occurs outside of the 11 to 1 o'clock position, the needle should be withdrawn and another insertion attempted, in order to have a more midline entry site for the tracheostomy. Trainees should have a limited number of attempts to avoid potential complications.

Once optimal midline position is verified, a Seldinger technique is used. A J-tipped guidewire is inserted through the introducer needle and directed toward the distal trachea under bronchoscopic visualization (Fig. 18.5C). The introducer needle is then removed over the guidewire. A punch dilator is then advanced over the guidewire to dilate the stoma (Fig. 18.5D).

A guidesheath is then placed over the guidewire and the curved tapered dilator (Figs. 18.4D and 18.5E) is inserted over the guidewire to dilate the stoma. Soaking the tapering dilator in saline activates the hydrophilic surface coating, making it slippery and easier to insert through the stoma. The guiding sheath on the guidewire minimizes the likelihood of accidental kinking of the guidewire. The dilator is then removed, leaving the guidewire and the guidesheath in place.

The TT is then loaded on to an appropriate size dilator and positioned in such a way that the tapering end of the dilator is flushed with the end of the TT (Fig. 18.2b). The TT and the dilator assembly are then inserted over the guiding sheath and the guidewire, and advanced into the trachea, through the newly created stoma (Fig. 18.4F).

It is important to use a curved motion of the wrist to insert the TT to avoid direct pressure on the posterior tracheal wall. The dilator assembly (dilator, guiding

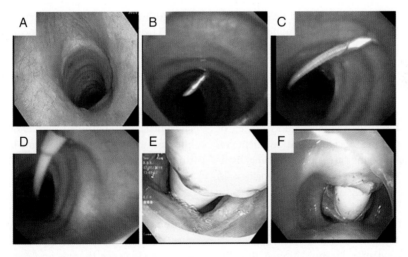

Fig. 18.5 Bronchoscopic view during percutaneous dilational tracheostomy. (A) Bronchoscopic view of the subglottic trachea showing cricothyroid membrane, cricoid cartilage (first prominence), and tracheal rings. (B) Introducer needle placed in between the first and the second tracheal rings. Note that although the bronchoscopic view is slightly rotated, the needle insertion appears to be at 11 o'clock position. Bronchoscopic guidance is valuable to avoid needle insertion through the posterior tracheal wall. (C) Guidewire inserted through the needle confirming that is going toward the distal trachea and not inserted through the posterior wall. (D) Placement of the tapering dilator over the guiding catheter. (E) Tracheostomy stoma being dilated with the tapering dilator. (F) Bronchoscopic view confirming good placement of the tracheostomy tube with the cuff before inflation.

sheath, and the guidewire) is then removed leaving the TT in the trachea (Fig. 18.5F).

The bronchoscope is then removed from the ETT and is introduced through the TT to confirm airway placement by visualizing the main carina. The distal end of the TT should be at least 2–4 cm or more proximal to the main carina.

Once placement is confirmed, the bronchoscope is removed, and the inner cannula with a 15-mm adapter is placed and connected to the ventilator circuit. The tracheostomy cuff is inflated, and tidal volume return is observed on the ventilator and used as a secondary confirmation of correct placement of the TT.

The TT is then secured with sutures or Velcro tracheostomy neck ties. We recommend flexing the head when securing the tracheostomy tie and prefer to place a split-foam dressing (Fig. 18.4G and H). The split-foam dressing cannot be placed if the TT is sutured to the neck.

Unless procedural difficulty was experienced during the procedure, there is no need to obtain a postprocedure chest radiograph.[52]

POST-TRACHEOSTOMY CARE

Institutional protocols assure uniform care by RT, nursing staff, house staff, and other providers. Postoperative complications such as accidental decannulation, bleeding, oxygen desaturation, and cuff leak should be brought to the attention of the appropriate service instantly.

Even if the TT is secured with sutures and tracheostomy tie, the TT can get dislodged. The most common signs of TT dislodgement are that there is unexplained hypoxia, the RT is unable to insert the inline suction catheter, or there is loss of tidal volume. Accidental dislodgment can happen during regular nursing care such as turning, bathing, or when the TT is removed by an agitated patient. In our practice, we do not usually suture the TT and use the tracheostomy tie to secure the tube. Split-foam dressings (Fig. 18.4G-H) avoid any skin injury from the flange and should be kept clean and dry to avoid infection.

In the event of accidental decannulation within the first 7 days, oral endotracheal intubation is recommended unless a provider experienced in tracheostomy management is available immediately. Attempting to reinsert the TT through a stoma in this context has a high risk of paratracheal placement in inexperienced hands.

Regular monitoring of cuff pressure avoids tracheal mucosal injury. Purulent secretion at the tracheostomy site should be cleaned daily with antiseptic wound care.

Sutures, if placed, should be removed in 5–7 days postprocedure, at the discretion of the provider.

LONG-TERM MANAGEMENT

Patients and their caregivers need to be educated on how to clean and care for the TT prior to the discharge unless the patient is transferred to a long-term acute care hospital or a ventilator weaning facility.

An alternative to cleaning the inner cannula regularly is the use of disposable inner cannulas. Thick, crusty secretions can form with loss of filtration, heat, and moisture blocking the TT. Use of heat and moisture exchange (HME) filters prevents mucus plugging.

Proper maintenance of TT mandates regular follow-up with a physician, respiratory therapist or speech therapist to assure optimal tracheostomy care. TT may be changed every 1–2 months (manufacturer recommendation is to change every 30 days), although no robust data are available to corroborate the recommendation.

COMMON PROCEDURAL COMPLICATIONS

PDT is a safe, reliable procedure with a low complication rate. Although PDT is becoming a routine procedure in the ICU setting, rare but serious complications can occur. It is strongly recommended that PDT be performed during the daytime, so surgical expertise and other resources are immediately available in the event of an emergency.

Technical complications include misplacement of the insertion needle; kinking of the guidewire; paratracheal placement of the TT with creation of a false lumen; and posterior tracheal wall injury involving the mediastinum, esophagus and rarely pleural spaces, and TT cuff rupture (Box 18.3).

The most common complication is bleeding. Usually it is venous, rarely arterial, and happens during neck dissection. Minor bleeding is controlled by applying pressure. On rare occasions, electro- or thermocautery can be used. However, there is an increased risk of fire with any cautery usage as the patient is on 100% FIO_2. Caution must be used to lower the FIO_2 prior to cautery usage. It is a good idea to inform all the team members about the fire hazard and to remind them to lower the FIO_2 to less than 40% prior to cautery use, if cautery use is absolutely necessary. Absorbable hemostat (Surgicel, Ethicon US, LLC, Cincinnati, OH, USA) can be applied locally for bleeding control. However, if major bleeding cannot

BOX 18.3 Complications of Percutaneous Dilational Tracheostomy

Early Complications <24 h

- Failure to insert tracheostomy tube
- Loss of airway during procedure
- Misplacement of the insertion needle, guidewire, or dilators
- Paratracheal placement
- Injury to tracheal wall or esophagus
- Tracheoesophageal fistula
- Tracheal tube cuff rupture
- Fracture of the tracheal ring
- Cuff leak
- Barotrauma
- Pneumothorax
- Pneumomediastinum
- Subcutaneous emphysema
- Premature decannulation
- Bleeding
- Thyroid injury
- Hypotension
- Cardiac or respiratory decompensation

Late Complications >24 h

- Delayed hemorrhage
- Granulation tissue formation
- Infections
- Skin breakdown
- Tracheal stenosis
- Tracheomalacia
- Tracheoinnominate artery
- Tracheoesophageal fistula

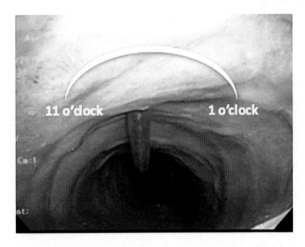

Fig. 18.6 Appropriate location for introducer needle entry between 11 o'clock and 1 o'clock.

be controlled, surgical intervention may be needed to explore the incision site to locate the bleeding vessel and ligate it. Anticipating the potential complications and understanding the anatomy and its variations are important to avoid bleeding from the brachiocephalic artery or a high-riding innominate artery.[53, 54]

The second most common difficulty encountered is the appropriate placement of the introducer needle. Ideally it should be midline in between the first and second or the second and third tracheal rings. Stabilizing the trachea with the nondominant hand (Fig. 18.4B) and confirming the location of the thyroid and the cricoid cartilage and the tracheal rings from outside by palpation facilitates accurate needle placement. Bronchoscopic transillumination can also help identify the proper site. Gentle tapping on the anterior wall with the needle prior to insertion is helpful to confirm the location with bronchoscopic

vision. Identifying the membranous trachea and maintaining orientation (anterior-posterior) during bronchoscopic examination assures proper needle placement (Fig. 18.6). Midline insertion of the needle avoids the risk of paratracheal placement of the TT during insertion.

Placement of the TT at or on the cricoid cartilage may lead to higher risk of subglottic stenosis, whereas placement below the third tracheal ring increases the risk of bleeding from the brachiocephalic trunk.

The skills and experience of the bronchoscopist are crucial to avoid complications. During retraction of the ETT, the airway may be lost by accidentally pulling the ETT out. Since the bronchoscope is already within the ETT, the best practice to correct this is to simply advance the bronchoscope through the vocal cords into the distal trachea and then reintubate by advancing the ETT over the bronchoscope into the mid-trachea. If this fails, direct laryngoscopy can be used to reintubate if the airway cannot be established immediately.

During retraction of the ETT, identification of the cricoid cartilage can often be challenging, as all the cartilaginous interspaces appear similar on bronchoscopic examination. The cricoid cartilage can be identified by its distinct appearance just below the cricothyroid membrane (Fig. 18.5A). We routinely identify the cricoid cartilage and the first tracheal ring just inferior to it using bronchoscopic guidance before inserting the percutaneous needle.

Bronchoscopic guidance is paramount to prevent posterior wall injury during needle placement or dilation. It is crucial to maintain constant visualization of the needle tip with the bronchoscope as the guidewire is inserted or when the dilator is inserted over the guidewire.

Subcutaneous emphysema occurs when air dissects through the trachea or subcutaneous tissue plane into the neck fascia and the mediastinum. A chest tube may be needed for pneumothorax, especially if the patient is mechanically ventilated. Thoracic surgery assistance may be needed in case of pneumomediastinum or tracheoesophageal fistula caused by posterior wall injury.

If there is any difficulty inserting the TT, it should be withdrawn, and the stoma dilated again. If a guidewire is found to be kinked, rapid reexploration of the wound and airway examination should be done with the bronchoscope, both through the ETT and through the stoma to rule out any airway injury.

In obese patients or in those with a deep neck but palpable trachea, a regular TT may be too short and may predispose to cuff leak. A longer TT (Fig. 18.2a) can be placed during the PDT to avoid tidal volume leak.

Other reported complications include fracture of the tracheal ring during the stoma dilation. Usually no intervention is needed for tracheal cartilage fracture.

Late complications occur after the first 24 h and include delayed hemorrhage, infection, skin breakdown, tracheal stenosis, tracheoinnominate artery fistula, or tracheoesophageal fistula.

Delayed hemorrhage can occur due to erosion of the anterior tracheal wall by the distal end of the TT. Any bleeding through the TT needs to be evaluated urgently to rule out tracheoinnominate artery fistula until proven otherwise. Computed tomography (CT) angiography may be needed to confirm the diagnosis. Otolaryngology and surgical consultation are mandatory.

Stable and slow bleeding can be managed with exploration of the stoma and careful examination of the trachea. Local cauterization controls mild stomal bleeding in most cases. In difficult cases, the patient may be intubated orally with an ETT, and the inflated cuff can tamponade the bleeding vessel temporarily to allow the patient to be transferred to a controlled setting like the operating room or procedure suite for exploration. Skin bleeders are controlled by cautery or packing with absorbable hemostat.

Local skin infections around the tracheostomy site, stoma infection, or tracheitis occur frequently. Wound infection extending into the mediastinum may result in mediastinitis. Prevention of tracheitis can be accomplished by frequent irrigation and suctioning of the tube. Overall, skin-related complications or infections occur less frequently in PDT compared to ST.[55] Management includes antiseptic stomal toileting, maintaining moisture, removal and cleaning of the inner cannula two to three times daily, and topical or systemic antibiotics.

Early tracheoesophageal fistula can be seen with posterior wall injury during the procedure and late tracheoesophageal fistula can occur due to erosion from prolonged use of an inflated cuffed tube. For immediate management, a longer TT passing beyond the distal end of the fistula can be used. However, tracheoesophageal fistula requires surgical correction with the closure of the defects.

Typical presentation of tracheal stenosis includes dyspnea on exertion, increasing cough, and stridor if the tracheal lumen narrowed by less than 50%. Obstruction by granulation tissue may be managed with cryotherapy, laser, or cautery. Switching to an uncuffed TT or deflating the cuff when no longer requiring the ventilator may be a practical option.

TRAINING AND PROCEDURAL COMPETENCY

Perioperative and late complications are lower after the first 20 procedures, suggesting a learning curve. Although the technique can be mastered after 5–10 supervised procedures, performance of at least 50 procedures assures exposure to rare complications.

SUMMARY

PDT is a minimally invasive, cost-effective, routine procedure done at the bedside on critically ill patients. Complication rates are operator dependent and minimal in expert hands. Bronchoscopic guidance minimizes procedural risk.[56] Appropriate patient selection and planning is the key to avoiding complications. The procedure can be done at the bedside in the ICU efficiently.

ACKNOWLEDGMENT

The authors acknowledge the contribution of Renaissance Islam from the School of Construction at Southern Alberta Institute of Technology for assistance with graphic arts.

REFERENCES

1. Colice G. Chapter 1. Historical Perspective on the Development of Mechanical Ventilation. In: Tobin MJ, ed. *Principles and Practice of Mechanical Ventilation*. 3rd ed. New York: McGraw Hill; 2013:1–37. https://accessmedicine.mhmedical.com/content.aspx?bookid=520&sectionid=41692236.

2. Rushman GB, Davies NJH, Atkinson RS. *Intubation of the trachea. A Short History of Anaesthesia*. Oxford: Butterworth-Heinemann; 1996:92–103.

3. Robertshaw F. Low resistance double-lumen endotracheal tubes. *Br J Anaesth*. 1962;34:576–579.

4. Zhao F, Zou Q, He X, Wang H. [The application of a small incision combined with improved percutaneous tracheostomy in difficult tracheostomy]. *Zhonghua Wei Zhong Bing Ji Jiu Yi Xue*. 2015;27(11):895–898.

5. Dulguerov P, Gysin C, Perneger TV, Chevrolet JC. Percutaneous or surgical tracheostomy: a meta-analysis. *Crit Care Med*. 1999;27:1617–1625.

6. Freeman BD, Isabella K, Lin N, Buchman TG. A meta-analysis of prospective trials comparing percutaneous and surgical tracheostomy in critically ill patients. *Chest*. 2000;118:1412–1418.

7. Delaney A, Bagshaw S, Nalos M. Percutaneous dilatational tracheostomy versus surgical tracheostomy in critically ill patients: a systematic review and meta-analysis. *Crit Care*. 2006;10(2):R55.

8. Johnson-Obaseki S, Veljkovic A, Javidnia H. Complication rates of open surgical versus percutaneous tracheostomy in critically ill patients. *Laryngoscope*. 2016;126:2459–2567.

9. Iftikhar IH, Teng S, Schimmel M, et al. A network comparative meta-analysis of percutaneous dilatational tracheostomies using anatomic landmarks, bronchoscopic, and ultrasound guidance versus open surgical tracheostomy. *Lung*. 2019;197(3):267–275. https://doi.org/10.1007/s00408-019-00230-7.

10. Walts PA, Murthy SC, DeCamp MM. Techniques of surgical tracheostomy. *Clin Chest Med*. 2003;24(3):413–422. https://doi.org/10.1016/s0272-5231(03)00049-2.

11. Sheldon C, Pudenz R, Tichy F. Percutaneous tracheostomy. *JAMA*. 1957;165:2068–2070. https://doi.org/10.1001/jama.1957.02980340034009.

12. Kost K. Endoscopic percutaneous dilatational tracheotomy: a prospective evaluation of 500 consecutive cases. *Laryngoscope*. 2005;115:1–30. https://doi.org/10.1097/01.MLG.0000163744.89688.E8.

13. Ciaglia P, Firsching R, Syniec C. Elective percutaneous dilatational tracheostomy. *Chest*. 1985;87:715–719.

14. Griggs WM, Worthley L, Gilligan J. A simple percutaneous tracheostomy technique. *Surg Gynecol Obstet*. 1990;170:543–545.

15. Fantoni A, Ripamonti D. A non-derivative, non-surgical tracheostomy: the translaryngeal method. *Intensive Care Med*. 1997;23:386–392.

16. Frova G, Quintel M. A new simple method for percutaneous tracheostomy: controlled rotating dilatation-a preliminary report. *Intensive Care Med*. 2002;28:299–303.

17. Plummer A, Gracey D. Consensus conference on artificial airways in patients receiving mechanical ventilation. *Chest*. 1989;96:178–180.

18. Griffiths J, Barber VS, Morgan L, Young JD. Systematic review and metaanalysis of studies of the timing of the tracheostomy in adult patients undergoing ventilation. *BMJ*. 2005;330(7502):1243. https://doi.org/10.1136/bmj.38467.485671.E0.

19. Huang C, Chen PT, Cheng SH, et al. Relative contraindications for percutaneous tracheostomy: from the surgeons' perspective. *Surg Today*. 2014;44:107–114. https://doi.org/10.1007/s00595-013-0491-y.

20. Pothmann W, Tonner PH, Schulte am Esch J. Percutaneous dilatational tracheostomy: risks and benefits. *Intensive Care Med*. 1997;23(6):610–612.

21. Beiderlinden M, Groeben H, Peters J. Safety of percutaneous dilational tracheostomy in patients ventilated with high positive end-expiratory pressure (PEEP). *Intensive Care Med*. 2003;29:944–948.

22. Shah S, Morgan P. Percutaneous dilation tracheostomy during high-frequency oscillatory ventilation. *Crit Care Med*. 2002;30:1762–1764.

23. Avalos N, Cataldo R, Contreras L. Unassisted percutaneous tracheostomy: a new flow chart decision making based on simple physical conditions. *Am J Otolaryngol*. 2019;40(1):57–60.

24. Mansharamani N, Koziel H, Garland R. Safety of bedside percutaneous dilatational tracheostomy in obese patients in the ICU *Chest*. 11720001426–1429.

25. Heyrosa M, Melniczek D, Rovito P. Percutaneous tracheostomy: a safe procedure in the morbidly obese. *J Am Coll Surg*. 2006;202:618–622.

26. Chambers D, Cloyes R, Abdulgadir A, Islam S, et al. Percutaneous tracheostomy in severe obesity: experience at a tertiary care center. *Chest*. 2013;144(66A).

27. Aldawood AS, Arabi YM, Haddad S. Safety of percutaneous tracheostomy in obese critically ill patients: a prospective cohort study. *Anaesth Intensive Care*. 2008;36(1):69–73.

28. Ahuja H, Mathai AS, Chander R, et al. Case of difficult tracheostomy tube insertion: a novel yet simple solution to the dilemma. *Anesth Essays Res*. 2013;7:402–404. https://doi.org/10.4103/0259-1162.123272.

29. Bouderka M, Fakhir B, Bouaggad A, et al. Early tracheostomy versus prolonged endotracheal intubation in severe head injury. *J Trauma*. 2004;57(2):251–254. https://doi.org/10.1097/01.ta.0000087646.68382.9a.

30. Arabi Y, Haddad S, Shirawi N, Al Shimemeri A, et al. Early tracheostomy in intensive care trauma patients improves resource utilization: a cohort study and literature review. *Crit Care.* 2004;8(5):R347–R352. https://doi:10.1186/cc2924.

31. Rumbak M, Newton M, Truncale T, et al. A prospective randomized study comparing early percutaneous dilatational tracheostomy to prolonged translaryngeal intubation in critically ill medical patients. *Crit Care Med.* 2004;32:1689–1694.

32. Elkbuli A, Narvel RI, Spano P, et al. Early versus late tracheostomy: is there an outcome difference? *Am Surg.* 2019;85(4):370–375. PMID 31043197.

33. Hosokawa K, Nishimura M, Moritoki E, Vincent JL, et al. Timing of tracheotomy in ICU patients: a systematic review of randomized controlled trials. *Crit Care.* 2015;19:424. https://doi:10.1186/s13054-015-1138-8

34. Chen W, Liu F, Chen J, Ma L, Li G, You C. Timing and outcomes of tracheostomy in patients with hemorrhagic stroke. *World Neurosurg.* 2019;131:e606–e613.

35. Jackson LS, Davis JW, Kaups KL, et al. Percutaneous tracheostomy: to bronch or not to bronch–that is the question. *J Trauma.* 2011;71(6):1553–1556. https://doi:10.1097/TA.0b013e31823ba29e.

36. Shen G, Hongzen Y, Cao Y, et al. Percutaneous dilatational tracheostomy versus fibre optic bronchoscopy-guided percutaneous dilatational tracheostomy in critically ill patients: a randomised controlled trial. *Ir J Med Sci.* 2019;188(2):675–681. https://doi:10.1007/s11845-018-1881-3.

37. Szeto C, Kost K, Hanley JA, et al. A simple method to predict pretracheal tissue thickness to prevent accidental decannulation in the obese. *Otolaryngol Head Neck Surg.* 2010;143:223–229. https://doi:10.1016/j.otohns.2010.03.007.

38. Ambesh S. *Principles and Practice of Percutaneous Tracheostomy.* New Delhi: Jaypee Brothers Medical Publisher; 2010.

39. Kundra P, Mishra S, Ramesh A. Ultrasound of the airway. *Indian J Anaesth.* 2011;55:456–462.

40. Sarıtaş A, Kurnaz MM. Comparison of bronchoscopy-guided and real-time ultrasound-guided percutaneous dilatational tracheostomy: safety, complications, and effectiveness in critically ill patients. *J Intensive Care Med.* 2017 885066617705641.

41. El A, Solh A, Jaafar W. Comparative study of the complications of surgical tracheostomy in morbidly obese critically ill patients. *Crit Care.* 2007;R3:11.

42. McGrath BA, Brenner MJ, Warrillow SJ, et al. Tracheostomy in the COVID-19 era: global and multidisciplinary guidance. *Lancet. Resp Med.* 2020;8(7):717–725. https://doi:10.1016/S2213-2600(20)30230-7.

43. Cabrini L, Greco M, Pasin L, et al. Preventing deaths related to percutaneous tracheostomy: safety is never too much! *Crit Care.* 2014;18(1):406.

44. Douketis JD, Spyropoulos A, Spencer F, et al. Perioperative management of antithrombotic therapy: antithrombotic therapy and prevention of thrombosis, 9th ed: American College of Chest Physicians Evidence-Based Clinical Practice Guidelines. *Chest.* 2012;141(2):e326S–e350S.

45. Braune S, Kienast S, Hadem J, et al. Safety of percutaneous dilatational tracheostomy in patients on extracorporeal lung support. *Intensive Care Med.* 2013;39:1792–1799.

46. Deppe A, Kuhn E, Scherner M, et al. Coagulation disorders do not increase the risk for bleeding during percutaneous dilatational tracheotomy. *Thorac Cardiovasc Surg.* 2013;61:234–239.

47. Kluge S, Meyer A, Kühnelt P. Percutaneous tracheostomy is safe in patients with severe thrombocytopenia. *Chest.* 2004;126:547–551.

48. Patel D, Devulapally K, Islam S. Safety of percutaneous tracheostomy in patients with coagulopathy and high ventilatory demand. *Chest.* 2009;136:50S-f1–50S-f2.

49. Dawood AA, Haddad S, Arabi Y, et al. The safety of percutaneous tracheostomy in patients with coagulopathy or thrombocytopenia. *Middle East J Anaesthesiol.* 2007;19:37–49.

50. Abouzgheib W, Meena N, Jagtap P, et al. Percutaneous dilational tracheostomy in patients receiving antiplatelet therapy: is it safe? *J Bronchol Interv Pulmonol.* 2013;20(4):322–325.

51. Gounant V, Milleron B, Assouad J, et al. Bevacizumab and invasive procedures: practical recommendations. *Rev Mal Respir.* 2009;26(2):221–226.

52. Tobler Jr WD, Mella JR, Ng J, Selvam A, Burke PA, Agarwal S. Chest x-ray after tracheostomy is not necessary unless clinically indicated. *World J Surg.* 2012;36(2):266–269.

53. Sharma S, Kumar G, Hill CS, et al. Brachiocephalic artery haemorrhage during percutaneous tracheostomy. *Ann R Coll Surg Engl.* 2015;97(2):e15–e17.

54. Ozlugedik S, Unal A. Surgical importance of highly located innominate artery in neck surgery. *Am J Otolaryngol.* 2005;26:330–332.

55. Brass P, Hellmich M, Ladra A, et al. Percutaneous techniques versus surgical techniques for tracheostomy. *Cochrane Database Syst Rev.* 2016;7:Cd008045.

56. Rashid AO, Islam S. Percutaneous tracheostomy: a comprehensive review. *J Thorac Dis.* 2017;9(Suppl 10): S1128–S1138.

19

How to Start an Interventional Pulmonology Program

Edward Kessler, Neeraj R. Desai, Kim D. French and Kevin L. Kovitz

INTRODUCTION

With ongoing advances in medical diagnostics and therapeutics, interventional pulmonology (IP) is playing an ever more impactful role in health care. This is becoming more evident with the increasing focus on costs and quality care, leading to the concept of value-based programs. Value-based programs are patient-centered and use a coordinated team-based approach with an overall goal to improve quality of care.[1] IP is well suited in this concept, as established and nascent IP programs continue to develop, providing more and more communities with access to expertise and efficient and quality care. In the effort to build and develop a new IP program, multiple factors should be considered and addressed.

NEEDS ASSESSMENT

When contemplating the initiation of a new service or product, a comprehensive needs assessment should be performed.[2,3] This would include evaluating specific factors in the intended community or region: the burden of disease of interest, competing and collaborating specialties (such as pulmonary, thoracic surgery, oncology, radiology, pathology, and others), associations (such as local or regional groups, professional societies), accessible equipment and supplies, and the focus and resources of the institution.[4] For example, if considering initiating an advanced diagnostic procedure such as endobronchial ultrasound (EBUS), one would need to consider the burden of lung cancer in the area of interest. This would help to guide expectations for the utility of the intended service. An area with a high burden of lung cancer would then be expected to generate a large number of EBUS referrals. Additionally, the current referral patterns for lung cancer would also need to be evaluated to ensure patients are directed to the appropriate service. Further, one would also need to assess if any other physicians (whether within the same group or even a competing practice) are already performing EBUS. Initiating a new service would ideally avoid undue competition or cannibalizing the practice to facilitate growth of the service. Lastly, one would need to consider available location(s) to perform and store equipment and supplies. Given the finite amount of space in most health care facilities, determining where the procedure will be performed (more details later) in addition to the areas for equipment and supply storage is essential. One would need to be sure the equipment is stored and secured in an appropriate area to provide efficient and effective service, as one would not want to be "hunting" for the EBUS console and supplies while awaiting the procedure. Additionally, the proximity of other EBUS sites would also need to be considered so as to balance the efficacy of each site without competing or unnecessarily duplicating equipment. In the situation of multiple sites performing EBUS, one would aim to ensure each site would be able to be utilized appropriately and avoid any redundancy. If sites are too close in proximity or there are insufficient referrals and procedures, then one or multiple sites will be underutilized. If there is only one physician performing the procedures, then having more than one site may also be ineffectual and inefficient not only for that particular site but also for the physician's lost productivity due to the inefficiency of travel time.

BUSINESS PLAN

New or updated resources are essential to maintaining or starting an IP program, and these require capital funding.[1] To outline a method to achieve projected goals, a business plan details projections over 3–5 years and includes a market analysis, service line analysis, marketing, and financial overview.[4-6]

Market Analysis

A market analysis delineates the target of the service or product and is one of the most important components to the business plan. In the case of IP, the target is broad and includes the entire health care community as a whole including the physician groups, hospitals, and patients. One would need to consider the demand for the IP service, potential growth, and barriers to the service. Demand will very likely be low initially until there is increased awareness and the benefit and success of the service are demonstrated. As this improves, growth and increased revenue will follow. Barriers that should be considered include the support of and goals of the practice or administration, practice and referral patterns, as well as competition from other practices or services.

Service Line Analysis

A service line analysis incorporates the specifics of the intended IP service, the organizational structure, operation, equipment, and personnel. An obvious component to this would be defining the specific procedures to be provided by the IP service (Box 19.1). Identifying an organizational structure to the program as a part of the broader general pulmonary/critical care, thoracic surgery, or other department, is important to establish and develop the service. A thorough SWOT (strength, weakness, opportunity, and threat) analysis of the organization and service line should be performed. In addition, one needs to outline the location or locations in which procedures are performed and the clinical contexts that apply, such as inpatient or outpatient, procedure suite, operating room, and so on. Locations may be different depending on staff and resources with some centers choosing to have one dedicated procedural suite and others moving the procedures to an endoscopy suite, operating room, radiology suite, or other locations. This may be informed by available space, fixed locations of equipment, availability of supporting services (i.e., anesthesia, ultrasound, etc.), staffing, or other local factors.

BOX 19.1 Range of Interventional Pulmonology Procedures

Diagnostic Bronchoscopy
    Basic bronchoscopy
    Endobronchial ultrasound
    Navigational/robotic bronchoscopy
Therapeutic Bronchoscopy
    Electrocautery
    Argon plasma coagulation
    Laser
    Airway stenting
    Endobronchial valve placement
    Bronchial thermoplasty
Pleural Procedures
    Thoracentesis
    Chest tubes
    Tunneled pleural catheters
    Pleurodesis
    Medical thoracoscopy
Others
    Percutaneous tracheostomy
    Percutaneous gastrostomy tube placement

Scheduling protocols for clinical evaluations and procedures should also be established. The appropriate equipment, supplies, and technology should also be incorporated as part of this analysis. For instance, for bronchoscopy this would include a full range of bronchoscopes, EBUS, bronchoscope towers, associated supplies and disposables or any other intended equipment, cleaning equipment and space, and related supplies. Such an analysis revolves around the specifics of a procedure with different procedures such as thoracoscopy, tracheostomy, pleural procedures, and so on, each having unique needs. All this requires defining the range of the IP services (Box 19.1) and the role of the IP team in the process. One should consider where the IP service fits in the initial evaluation and management (E/M), perioperative, and longitudinal care for the patient. An active clinical presence in outpatient and inpatient setting would serve to aid in building rapport and broaden the referral base, hence further developing the IP practice. One must also consider the efficiency of care and to centralize the service line to avoid redundancies and duplication of equipment unnecessarily, as referenced earlier. The specific IP team members need to be identified, which may include medical assistants, nurses, respiratory therapists, and advanced practice providers such as an advanced practice nurse or physician's assistant. Each team member's roles should also be clearly defined in terms of the IP service and in the general practice.

Marketing

As conveyed earlier, building a referral base is fundamental to growing and sustaining a new service. A marketing strategy should be developed to raise awareness and understanding of the benefits of the burgeoning IP service. This may include "meet and greet" with departmental and interdepartmental colleagues and respective heads of departments, colleagues outside of the institution, and patients or their advocates. Other avenues include educational meetings or lectures such as grand rounds with associated departments including pulmonary, thoracic surgery, and oncology. An active presence in multidisciplinary conferences, such as a tumor board meeting, is also beneficial. Frequent interaction during multidisciplinary conferences or shared or closely related clinics allows frequent encounters and interactions with other providers to build a rapport and broaden a referral base. A shared multispecialty clinic works well, but in some settings this may not be feasible or logistically possible. In those situations, a virtual multidisciplinary clinic could be considered, which are meetings or clinics in which members may not communicate or meet face-to-face but rather review patients in a virtual context, electronically and/or separately. Another important aspect of marketing would be advertising. This could be done by simply posting flyers, informational packets, or other advertising materials throughout a practice or hospital community or even local or regional media. This could also include providing educational courses or seminars.[2,4,7] Further, more direct outreach to patients via conventional and social media along with medically relevant organizations or groups can be utilized. This could include interviews or advertisements on websites, blogs, radio, and television informing the community of the new IP service.

Financial Overview

Although a basic goal of a new service would be to generate revenue and remain financially solvent, it can be challenging in a new IP practice. It is important for the practitioners and administrators to avoid isolating IP into its own financial group. It should be analyzed as part of an overall program that contributes significantly to patient recruitment, downstream revenue, institutional

---

> **BOX 19.2 Components of Financial Analysis of an Interventional Pulmonology Program**
>
> 1. Projected volume
> 2. Expenses
>   (a) Fixed cost
>   - Facility cost
>   - Depreciation
>   (b) Variable cost
>   - Labor
>   - Supplies
>   - Repairs
> 3. Initial investment
> 4. Cash flows
> 5. Return on investment
> 6. Break-even analysis
> 7. Downstream revenue
>   Thoracic surgery
>   Radiation and medical oncology
>   Radiology services
> 8. Contribution margins

---

reputation, and patient satisfaction. Financial analysis of the IP program should include projected volume, revenue, expenses (fixed and variable), labor, and supplies (Box 19.2). Return on investment (ROI), break-even analysis, and pro forma projections are important to generate as part of the evaluation.[1] Current procedural reimbursement is neither time nor cost efficient, so other considerations to generate revenue and decrease costs should be entertained. Some facets to consider would be in the initial and longitudinal patient care allowing for capturing of revenue via E/M. Moreover, downstream revenue and contribution margins from procedures such as EBUS may be cited as this has been known to impact additional services and practices by radiology, thoracic surgery, pathology, and oncology.[2,4,8] Additionally, cost savings are afforded by IP given the high-quality and efficient care. This is especially important in financial "at-risk" models of care that cap the dollars available for patient care. Practice locations and staffing are other components to consider. Sharing office space or procedural areas with other specialists and/or departments may not only reduce associated costs but also increase referrals and revenue. An example is sharing office space with general pulmonologists or oncology groups, which leads to increased personal access, engagement, and discussions to drive further evaluations, procedures, and revenue. A shared procedural area and/or staff may reduce overhead, but may bring about other limitations, including lack of familiarity with advanced procedures, delays, or inefficiency in scheduling so monitoring efficiency and having the flexibility to adjust is important.

EQUIPMENT

As related to the goals outline earlier, the relevant equipment needs should be assessed and strategically planned. Initial costs to obtain and maintain equipment can be expensive. Direct costs would incorporate the equipment and related supplies (such as forceps, needles, etc.), whereas indirect costs would include costs associated with staff, space, storage, and administration. A rationale to assess equipment needs for medical necessity should be employed to avoid misusing funds for equipment that would be rarely used.[4,7,9] Understanding both the physician and especially the facility reimbursement per procedure can help plan for future costs and time to pay off the purchases and maintain supply needs.

INTERVENTIONAL PULMONOLOGY TEAM

A dedicated IP team enhances the efficiency of the IP service. An experienced team has familiarity with the nuances and specifics of each case and helps avoid delays and decreased productivity. The members and roles of the IP team should be clearly identified so as to avoid missing or duplicating steps. An IP team may include nurses, respiratory therapists, medical assistants, and advanced practice providers with notable caveats to each. Nurses may be involved throughout all phases of care, including initial evaluations, perioperatively, and in follow-up. Respiratory therapists are involved mainly in the perioperative phase, although limited by being unable to administer sedation. Advanced practice providers can be involved with all phases of care and further enhance the IP service by providing some procedural services, triage, and follow-up care in multiple contexts, both outpatient clinic and inpatient services. The team should be developed based on specific needs, member competencies, and local practice patterns.

MONITORING

After initiating a program, multiple elements should be assessed in follow-up to ensure the program is attaining the original goals and to guide any changes if needed. Routine assessments would include the types of and number of procedures, associated diagnoses, diagnostic yield, and complications, as well as other metrics such as procedural time and efficiency. The type and number of new inpatient and outpatient referrals and follow-up clinical visits may also be helpful in guiding the service. Fiscal measures to monitor would include service revenue, clinical and procedural reimbursements, as well as clinical and procedural costs. Those involved in the revenue cycle of billing and collection must have an intimate understanding of both general billing and reimbursement along with aspects that are unique to IP. Once collected, these data should be evaluated to assess for areas amenable for improvement. Why are some procedures more common and others less so? Is there a lack of need for some or is more education needed within the referral base? Are yields what are expected? Can the process support better yields, scheduling efficiency, and increase in satisfaction for patients and staff? Is billing being correctly done and in a timely manner? Are precertifications and appeals done correctly? Is there a pattern of denials that needs direct follow-up with an insurance carrier to avoid future issues? These are some of the questions a successful program repeatedly explores and uses to refine the process.

◼ SUMMARY

IP program development is challenging and exciting. Bringing needed services to an institution that may not yet understand the need can greatly improve patient care, quality, and experience. It can enhance the reputation of and referrals to an institution or practice. It is up to the IP service and their administrators to honestly assess the needs, plan for the proper introduction of new technologies and programs, and be open to change as needs evolve. Having new technology is not a goal in and of itself. Asking for equipment that will benefit patients and the institution and delivering on the promise of a new program is more important than offering a specific procedure. Growing an IP program takes focus and drive, often convincing people of a need that is real but that they do not realize it exists. Success in identifying and satisfying that need is a reward in and of itself.

REFERENCES

1. Desai NR, French KD, Diamond EJ, Kovitz KL. Value-based proposition for a dedicated interventional pulmonology suite: an adaptable business model. *Chest.* 2018;154(3):699–708.
2. French KD, Desai NR, Diamond E, Kovitz K. Developing an interventional pulmonary service in a community-based private practice: a case study. *Chest.* 2016;149(4):1094–1101.
3. Assessing the industry using Porter's five forces. *Vet Rec.* 2014;174(Suppl 1):3–4.
4. Kessler E, Wahidi MM. The business of bronchoscopy: how to set up an interventional pulmonology program. *Clin Chest Med.* 2018;39(1):239–243.
5. Beheshti MV, Meek ME, Kaufman JA. The interventional radiology business plan. *J Vasc Interv Radiol.* 2012;23(9):1181–1186.
6. US Small Business Administration. Write your business plan. <https://www.sba.gov/starting-business/write-your-business-plan>; Accessed 06.24.2017.
7. Colt H. Development and organization of an interventional pulmonology department. *Respirology.* 2010;15: 887–894.
8. Pastis NJ, Simkovich S, Silvestri GA. Understanding the economic impact of introducing a new procedure: calculating downstream revenue of endobronchial ultrasound with transbronchial needle aspiration as a model. *Chest.* 2012;141(2):506–512.
9. Kruklitis R, French K, Cangelosi MJ, Kovitz KL. Investing in new technology in Pulmonary Medicine – navigating the tortuous path to success. *Chest.* 2017;152(3):663–671.

INDEX

Page numbers followed by '*f*' indicate figures, '*t*' indicate tables, '*b*' indicate boxes.